Spirituality and Addiction

Spirituality and Addiction

Editors

Bernadette Flanagan
Noelia Molina

MDPI • Basel • Beijing • Wuhan • Barcelona • Belgrade • Manchester • Tokyo • Cluj • Tianjin

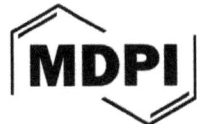

Editors
Bernadette Flanagan
Department of Applied Arts
Waterford Institute of Technology
Ireland

Noelia Molina
Spirituality Institute for Research and Education
Waterford Institute of Technology
Ireland

Editorial Office
MDPI
St. Alban-Anlage 66
4052 Basel, Switzerland

This is a reprint of articles from the Special Issue published online in the open access journal *Religions* (ISSN 2077-1444) (available at: https://www.mdpi.com/journal/religions/special_issues/Spirit_Addict).

For citation purposes, cite each article independently as indicated on the article page online and as indicated below:

LastName, A.A.; LastName, B.B.; LastName, C.C. Article Title. *Journal Name* **Year**, *Volume Number*, Page Range.

ISBN 978-3-0365-4705-3 (Hbk)
ISBN 978-3-0365-4706-0 (PDF)

Cover image courtesy of Damien Jackson.

© 2022 by the authors. Articles in this book are Open Access and distributed under the Creative Commons Attribution (CC BY) license, which allows users to download, copy and build upon published articles, as long as the author and publisher are properly credited, which ensures maximum dissemination and a wider impact of our publications.

The book as a whole is distributed by MDPI under the terms and conditions of the Creative Commons license CC BY-NC-ND.

Contents

About the Editors . . . . **vii**

Bernadette Flanagan and Noelia Molina
Introduction: Spirituality and Addiction
Reprinted from: *Religions* **2022**, *13*, 555, doi:10.3390/rel13060555 . . . . **1**

Amanda Dillon
Bible Journaling as a Spiritual Aid in Addiction Recovery
Reprinted from: *Religions* **2021**, *12*, 965, doi:10.3390/rel12110965 . . . . **5**

Lisete S. Mónico and Clara Margaça
The Workaholism Phenomenon in Portugal: Dimensions and Relations with Workplace Spirituality
Reprinted from: *Religions* **2021**, *12*, 852, doi:10.3390/rel12100852 . . . . **35**

Monique M. Verrier
A Psychospiritual Exploration of the Transpersonal Self as the Ground of Healing
Reprinted from: *Religions* **2021**, *12*, 725, doi:10.3390/rel12090725 . . . . **53**

Marcin Wnuk
Do Involvement in Alcoholics Anonymous and Religiousness Both Directly and Indirectly through Meaning in Life Lead to Spiritual Experiences?
Reprinted from: *Religions* **2021**, *12*, 794, doi:10.3390/rel12100794 . . . . **75**

Margaret Bullitt-Jonas
Climate Change, Addiction, and Spiritual Liberation
Reprinted from: *Religions* **2021**, *12*, 709, doi:10.3390/rel12090709 . . . . **87**

Lisete S. Mónico and Valentim R. Alferes
The Effect of Religious Beliefs and Attitudes in Intrinsic and Extrinsic Optimism and Pessimism in Players of Games of Chance
Reprinted from: *Religions* **2022**, *13*, 97, doi:10.3390/rel13020097 . . . . **103**

Paul Barrows and William Van Gordon
Ontological Addiction Theory and Mindfulness-Based Approaches in the Context of Addiction Theory and Treatment
Reprinted from: *Religions* **2021**, *12*, 586, doi:10.3390/rel12080586 . . . . **123**

Pádraic Mark Hurley
The Significance of 'the Person' in Addiction
Reprinted from: *Religions* **2021**, *12*, 893, doi:10.3390/rel12100893 . . . . **133**

Garret B. Wyner
Spiritual Addiction: Searching for Love in a Coldly Indifferent World
Reprinted from: *Religions* **2022**, *13*, 300, doi:10.3390/rel13040300 . . . . **147**

About the Editors

Bernadette Flanagan

Bernadette Flanagan completed her doctorate in Humanities (Spirituality) at the Milltown Institute, Dublin. Since that time, she has become an Associate Professor in Spirituality and led the development of MA and professional doctoral studies in Spirituality in Ireland. She has consulted to a wide range of organizations, both in Ireland and internationally, on dimensions of spiritual education, spiritual care and spiritual practice in such fields as healthcare, education, relational wellbeing, aging, addiction and leadership.

Noelia Molina

Noelia Molina holds a BSc in Biomedical Sciences and MSc in Molecular Pathology. She worked for 17 years as a Medical Scientist. She completed her Doctor in Philosophy (Spirituality) in 2016 at Dublin City University. Her doctoral dissertation investigated the transition to motherhood as a spiritual process. She has specialized in maternal mental health, helping women psychologically and spiritually through birth, infertility and miscarriage. In her psychotherapy practice, she has helped individuals through the journey of various addictions. Currently, she is the Programme Leader of the MA in Applied Spirituality in SETU (South East Technological University), Ireland.

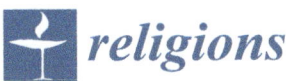

Editorial

Introduction: Spirituality and Addiction

Bernadette Flanagan and Noelia Molina *

Spirituality in Society and the Professions Research Group, Department of Arts, South East Technological University, X91 K0EK Waterford, Ireland; bernadette.flanagan@setu.ie
* Correspondence: noelia.molina@setu.ie

Citation: Flanagan, Bernadette, and Noelia Molina. 2022. Introduction: Spirituality and Addiction. *Religions* 13: 555. https://doi.org/10.3390/rel13060555

Received: 20 April 2022
Accepted: 2 May 2022
Published: 16 June 2022

Publisher's Note: MDPI stays neutral with regard to jurisdictional claims in published maps and institutional affiliations.

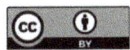

Copyright: © 2022 by the authors. Licensee MDPI, Basel, Switzerland. This article is an open access article distributed under the terms and conditions of the Creative Commons Attribution (CC BY) license (https://creativecommons.org/licenses/by/4.0/).

This collection of papers is inspired by years of collaboration in delivering academic programmes in Applied Spirituality. In particular, it has been observed in the annual intake of students for the MA in Applied Spirituality (South East Technological University), on which both editors teach, that there is a growing demand to interrogate what difference spirituality makes to diverse aspects of life—exercising leadership in a public service environment; teaching children to meditate; accompanying women in the transition to motherhood; or designing Instagram posts for spiritual seekers.

In this collection of essays, we turn the spirituality spotlight onto the inner drives in life which can shape our existence, consciously or unconsciously. The diversity of addictions discussed, and perspectives presented, aims to raise deeper questions regarding the nature of addiction. Rather than presenting addictions as diverse clinical challenges, the essays seek to reflect on addiction as a universal aspect of the human condition. The diversity of foci in the papers implicitly raises the question of what form of addiction is a force within any individual life. Engaging the phenomenon of addiction through the lens of spirituality seeks to highlight that the journey through addiction is more than undertaking a moral re-alignment in life; and is instead a re-focusing of the dynamic of the search for authenticity in a life.

In this Special Issue we hope that each contribution to the collection will, its own unique way, help to prepare the ground for some of those larger, more foundational conversations regarding addictions into the future. In reflecting on leveraging spirituality as a force for good in the face of addictions, the Special Issue seeks to engage an understandable wariness on the part of social workers (and other professionals) of 12-step programmes on grounds that their religious/spiritual dimension may not be appropriate in the 21st century.

While the academic study of spirituality in the society and the professions moves forward rapidly, the sheer variety of issues and challenges with which it is engaging often means that essays in a particular field such as spiritual awakening and disability; spiritual dimensions of aging; spiritual practices for ecological awakening may be distributed across intra-professional journals such as disability studies, gerontology or sustainability studies respectively. In this Special Issue one of the aims is to provide a collection of reflections from diverse professionals in one single volume on the subject of Addiction and Spirituality. This is a rare goal in publications and the exclusive focus on Spirituality and Addiction has only been achieved in a few select publications such as Christina Grof's, *Thirst for Wholeness: Attachment, Addiction, and the Spiritual Path* (1994) or more recently the special issue of the journal *Implicit Religion*, entitled 'Religion, Spirituality and Addiction Recovery' Vol 22/2(2019): guest edited by Wendy Dossett and Liam Metcalf-White. In the latter publication, Dossett and Metcalf-White similarly argued that the categories of religion, spirituality, and non-religion, as they relate to addiction recovery, need further analysis than they receive in the clinical literature.

The aim of the 21st century approach to addiction, religion and spirituality is to work towards an integrative mode of recovery. A recent statement from the Spirituality Interest Group of the International Society of Addiction Medicine (ISAM) (Marc Galanter and

Potenza 2021) recommended incorporating spirituality into research and clinical care in the treatment of addictions. Currently, most addiction treatments and clinical research are concentrated on pharmacological and behavioural approaches. This ISAM statement recognised that disciplines such as neuroscience, social science and psychology need to be engaged in clinical studies on the role of spirituality and religion. Thus, the spiritual construct can serve as a component of the 'recovery capital' for addiction.

This Special Issue highlights the nature of addiction as a multifactorial and complex experience within the human condition. Researching how spiritual resources which are unique to the individual (spiritual programmes, spiritual experiences, spiritual peer support groups) can be evaluated and incorporated in the recovery plan from any addiction is paramount to comprehend the profound inner world of any addiction. The evaluation and integration of spiritually oriented approaches will challenge the current three theoretical models from which the scientific and medical community operate: the medical/disease model, the moral/ethical model and the biopsychosocial model.

We hope that the rich and varied contributions to this issue can elucidate the crucial role of spirituality in the recovery of addiction. The contributions fall into two main types. The following four essays address foundational issues in the theory of addiction and spirituality:

Monique Verrier turns our attention to 'A Psycho-spiritual Exploration of the Transpersonal Self as the Ground of Healing'. She challenges psychotherapeutic models that are rooted in assumptions that the causes of addiction are some kind of lack of development, of confidence, of positive thoughts or impulse control. Instead, she locates the fulcrum of addiction recovery in the Transpersonal Self—the Soul, Heart, Presence, Higher Power, Authentic Self, etc. With the assistance of auto-ethnography she argues that the alchemy of healing occurs when that which can never be harmed makes contact with that which has been wounded. She testifies that non-dual awareness effects addiction recovery from the ground of being.

In their article, **Paul Barrows and William Van Gordon** evaluate the first generation and the new wave/second generation MBIs (mindfulness-based interventions) in the treatment of addictions. The authors investigate how some MBIs are spiritually de-rooted from the original Buddhist concept of *tisikkhā* (three trainings: higher virtue/higher mind/higher wisdom) principle, within which meditation is traditionally taught. They outline different types of MBIs which are openly spiritual in nature and can actively challenge the inner mechanism of addiction in the individual. Ontological Addiction Theory (OAT) is proposed as a new metaphysical model in which the deep belief of an inherently existing 'self' or 'I' could be seen to create an impaired functionality. The idea of a self that is empty of intrinsic existence provides, according to the authors, a clear strategy to stop the cycle of addiction at its source, by undermining self-attachment, by deconstructing the ego-self and by dismantling the maladaptive addictive beliefs that have accumulated.

A counter view on OAT (Ontological Addiction Theory) is taken up by **Pádraic Hurley**'s paper. The author does this by setting forth the implications of a 'Fourth Turning' in Buddhism, along with a 'post-metaphysical' turn in social science, philosophy and spirituality. These developments challenge the conventional separate, egoic-self framework in OAT by presenting an alternative view on the ontology of 'the person', which is proposed by developmental psychology as an 'integrative presence' developed through a healthy process of 'individuation'. The author agrees with the view of Van Gordon et al. (2016) that a lack of the egoic sense of self and consequent cravings for fulfilment fuel 'addictions'. However, this paper challenges the possible transcendental reductionism of OAT, in favour of the significance of 'the person' in addiction as a unifying/integrating/meditating quality to unite all parts into a meaningful pre-sense of 'wholeness' that can feel truly related and connected to the world.

Finally in this category is **Garret Wyner**'s paper which aims at deeply reflecting on spiritual addiction as a collective moral problem. By *spiritual addiction* Wynner means "a felt compulsion to seek surrogates in the absence of that spirit of unconditional love underlying core personality change". Hope is explored by Wynner as the core disposition for a spiritual religion of the heart. By presenting a case study, the author, elucidates such important attitudes in addiction therapy as holding the hope until the individual is ready to take the 'hope back' into his/her life and displaying empathetic attunement with the spirit of truth and love. This paper challenges the identification of the roots of spiritual addiction as only physical and psychological, and adds a social dimension, including morality and religion. The author argues that the end of the 'collective moral crisis' that is fuelling spiritual addiction, will be the conscious realisation of living with unconditional love and of experiencing a true intimacy of interpersonal connections.

The following five essays address special/applied issues in the theory of addiction and spirituality:

Amanda Dillon in 'Bible Journaling as a Spiritual Aid in Addiction Recovery' explores the newly emerging practice of Bible Journaling. In this spiritual practice Bible readers create visual reflections in their Bibles using diverse drawing materials. She has gathered drawing from a small sample of women who participate in online social media and she explores how the Bible journaling has played a role in their journey of recovery from drug addiction. The critical reflection on the bible visual reflections which are shared uses multimodal analysis, a methodological approach which provides a structured semiotic framework in which every feature of a visual creation is examined so as to explore how a journaler has made meaning of a biblical text for her recovery journey.

Lisete dos Santos Mendes Mónico and **Clara Margaça** investigated 'The Workaholism Phenomenon in Portugal: Dimensions and Relations with Workplace Spirituality'. The sample in this study i larger, and is comprised of a heterogeneous group of 306 Portuguese employees, who were surveyed using a 25-question Workaholism Battery test (2010) and the five dimensions of Workplace Spirituality test (2008: sense of community; individual and organizational values alignment; sense of contribution to the community; joy at work; opportunities for an inner life). In the analysis of the intersection between the experience of workplace spirituality and workaholism the authors explore whether workplace spirituality development has the potential to promote a balanced and healthy relationship with work.

Marcin Wnuk raises the question, 'Do Involvement in Alcoholics Anonymous and Religiousness both Directly and Indirectly through Meaning in Life Lead to Spiritual Experiences?' The sample for the study consisted of 70 Polish AA participants. Since addiction literature considered often lacked precise, well-established definitions for spirituality and for religiousness they have sometimes been used interchangeably in studies. The researcher is clear that the generalizability of findings will be limited to Roman Catholic AA participants from Poland. In such a population it was found that both religious commitment and AA involvement were together a support to transformation for alcohol-addicted individuals. The finding that non-religious or religiously sceptical AA participants still experienced similar benefits to the AA religiously-inclined members leads to a deeper reflection on the core spiritual experience that supports transformation. Both the theoretical and practical implications are discussed by the author.

Margaret Bullitt-Jonas' reflects on how an understanding of addictive behaviour can generate greater understanding of the reluctance to engage the climate crisis in 'Climate Change, Addiction, and Spiritual Liberation'. As in the life of an addict we today can seek to look away; to sees but not see; to change the subject. By reflecting on her own journey of recovery from food addiction, she identifies six transferable themes for awakening to the climate crisis: moving denial and truth-telling; stepping forth from isolation to community; grieving losses; taking moral responsibility; praying the Serenity Prayer; and nurturing love.

In her second essay in the collection **Lisete dos Santos Mendes Mónico** (with **Valentim Alferes** this time) attends to the way in which the effect of religious beliefs and attitudes of intrinsic and extrinsic optimism and pessimism in players of games of chance. The sample is composed of 271 recurring players of games of chance and gambling who answered a questionnaire on the measures of religious beliefs and attitudes, of optimism, and pessimism. Data analysis is performed by SPSS and AMOS. Results show that the influence of religious beliefs and attitudes is higher on optimism than on pessimism. These results show the importance of religious behaviours as self-regulatory mechanism for stability and promotion of optimism. This paper also opens research on the importance of distinguishing internal causes from external causes in the beliefs underlying optimism and pessimism.

It is our hope that these papers will help in understanding the importance of the incorporation of spirituality in research, and clinical treatments in the journey of addiction.

Author Contributions: Both authors contributed equally to the paper. All authors have read and agreed to the published version of the manuscript.

Funding: This research received no external funding.

Acknowledgments: The authors acknowledge the support provided by the Spirituality Institute for Research and Education, c/o Jesuit Provincialate, Milltown Park, Milltown Road, Dublin D06 W9Y7, Ireland whose excellent library provided consultation materials for the publication.

Conflicts of Interest: The authors declare no conflict of interest.

References

Marc Galanter, Helena Hansen, and Marc N. Potenza. 2021. The role of spirituality in addiction medicine: A position statement from the spirituality interest group of the international society of addiction medicine. *Substance Abuse* 42: 269–71. [CrossRef] [PubMed]

Van Gordon, William, Edo Shonin, Giulia Cavalli, and Mark D. Griffiths. 2016. Ontological addiction: Classification, aetiology and treatment. *Mindfulness* 7: 660–71.

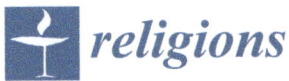

Article

Bible Journaling as a Spiritual Aid in Addiction Recovery

Amanda Dillon

School of Humanities, Waterford Institute of Technology, X91 K0EK Waterford City, Co. Waterford, Ireland; adillon@wit.ie

Abstract: Bible Journaling is a trend of the past decade whereby readers make creative, visual interventions in their Bibles, using coloured pens and pencils, watercolours, stickers and stencils, highlighting texts of particular resonance. Journaling, in its more conventional written forms, has long been recognised as a pathway to spiritual development. Significantly, Bible journaling is almost exclusively practiced by women and has a high level of interpersonal interaction attached to it, through open and mutual sharing of these creations, through various online social media fora. Gleaned from the sharing of women who journal for spiritual support, this article examines the role Bible journaling plays in aiding recovery from drug addiction. Multimodal analysis is a methodological approach that provides a structured semiotic framework in which to closely examine every feature of a creation such as a journaled page of a Bible, to examine how the journaler has made meaning of a text through their interventions on the page. Appreciating every mark, choice and placement of image, colour, typography as a motivated sign revealing the interest of the creator, the sign-maker, a detailed multimodal analysis is conducted of one page of a recovered drug-user's journaled Bible. As shall be demonstrated, profound insights into the appropriation of sacred texts for the spiritual life of a recovering addict can be gleaned in this process. Bible journaling reveals itself to be a highly valuable spiritual practice for those in addiction recovery. This interdisciplinary paper uniquely brings a methodological approach from the field of semiotics to the field of spirituality. Both the methodological approach and the subject of sacred text journaling may be of particular interest to spiritual directors, across many religions with a foundational sacred text, as a means whereby adherents can engage with a text in a deep, contemplative and creative practice that is personally, spiritually sustaining and motivating during a difficult phase of life.

Keywords: Bible journaling; biblical spirituality; drug addiction; journaling addiction; addiction recovery; multimodality; multimodal analysis

Citation: Dillon, Amanda. 2021. Bible Journaling as a Spiritual Aid in Addiction Recovery. *Religions* 12: 965. https://doi.org/10.3390/rel12110965

Academic Editors: Bernadette Flanagan, Noelia Molina and Greg Peters

Received: 9 August 2021
Accepted: 22 October 2021
Published: 3 November 2021

Publisher's Note: MDPI stays neutral with regard to jurisdictional claims in published maps and institutional affiliations.

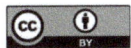

Copyright: © 2021 by the author. Licensee MDPI, Basel, Switzerland. This article is an open access article distributed under the terms and conditions of the Creative Commons Attribution (CC BY) license (https://creativecommons.org/licenses/by/4.0/).

1. Introduction

Within spirituality research, the practice of journaling has long been recognised as a particularly valuable and powerful means of self-reflection, discernment, discovery and healing (Progoff 1975, 1983; Budd 2002; Adams 2004; Pennebaker 2004; Moon 2004; Milner 1986; Lukinsky 1990). In recent times, a new phenomenon has emerged that adds an interesting dimension to the many, varied practices of journaling already carried out. Of course, it is recognised that many journalers have made recourse to the biblical text in the past (Peace 1995; Cepero 2008; Leonard 1995), but Bible journaling as researched in this article is a strikingly new development for two key reasons. Firstly, specially designed journaling Bibles are now printed with a wide, blank margin, alongside the text, on the page—leaving space for the reader's own reflections in this wide margin. It is a bespoke product where for the first time the journaler journals directly in their Bible. Secondly, this publishing innovation has sparked a new trend of journalers not only writing in these margins, as first envisaged by the publishers, but, significantly, also making other creative interventions in their Bibles. Included here are twelve photographs (Figures 1–12) of journaled pages created by the participants in this study. These pages shall not be commented on individually, apart from Figures 7 and 8. They are included to demonstrate to the reader the great richness and diversity of personal engagement that is evident on these pages: the chosen texts for reflection as well as a variety of meaning-making interventions made on the page, from naïve drawing with pencil crayons to the complex collation and overlaying of cut and paste images, symbols, stickers, tickets, textures, lettering, cards and other ephemera.

As can be seen in these images, there is a shift away from a predominantly written, verbal form towards a multimodal form, including the visual—drawing, painting, sketching and tracing—and pasting of images and patterns, in this journaling practice. More generally, a move towards creative and visual journaling practices is evidently popular (Hieb 2005) and specifically in relation to addiction recovery (Maisel and Raeburn 2008). Furthermore, the sense of touch is engaged with the inclusion of textures in the way of stickers, ribbons, felt, cords, tassels and bobbly, embossed papers. The results are highly innovative and creative, multimodal interventions being made in printed Bibles, reflective of the reader's own personal engagement with their sacred scriptures (Dillon 2020).

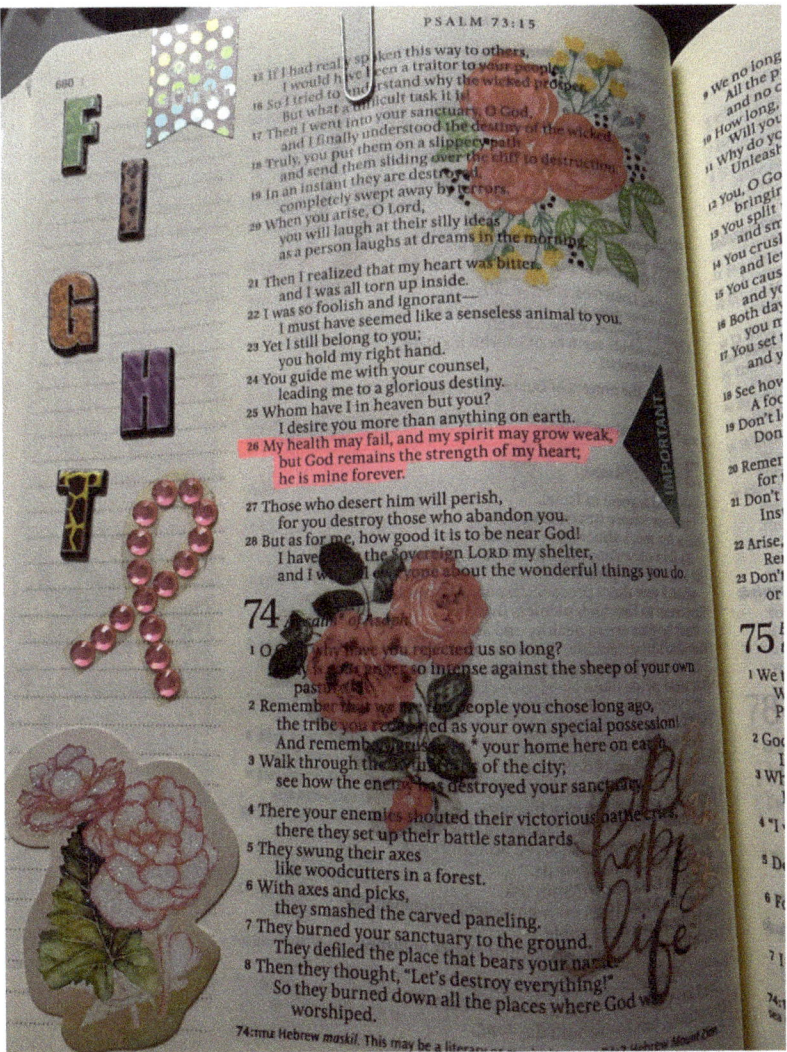

Figure 1. Psalm 73:26. With kind permission of the journaler.

Bible journaling of this type has emerged as a hugely popular spiritual practice among Christian women, in particular, as a means of engaging in a profound way with the biblical text. For many believers, the Bible is the primary resource for their personal faith in the Christian God.[1] Many churches in North America now have Bible journaling groups that gather weekly to do this together, often combined with Bible study and more experienced practitioners offering demonstrations of creative ideas (Fischer and Peiffer 2019; Nichols Hickman 2013). Beyond this, social media also provides a widely used platform for sharing ideas, skills, reviews of different journaling Bibles and materials and, most importantly, the journalers' own pages and artworks. Many Bible journaling groups have large numbers of followers on Facebook especially, one in the region of forty thousand members, and there is lively interest and activity on Instagram and Pinterest.

As shall be shown in this article, Bible journaling has proved highly beneficial for many women in recovery from various addictions. Addiction is at once a social issue and a spiritual issue (Alexander 2008; Plante 2018; Bedi and Pereira 2020). There is much written and produced about the opioid addiction crisis currently ravaging sectors of North American society (Stoicea et al. 2019; DeWeerdt 2019; Theroux 2017; Gibney 2021). This unprecedented rise in drug addiction sets up a formidable pastoral challenge for Christian churches, to which they have responded in different ways, some of which will be touched on here. The participants in this study have been on the receiving end of that outreach and care and concern. In the course of researching this article, I interviewed five women who kindly shared their process of Bible journaling, some of their pages and the spiritual and other benefits derived from engaging with the Bible in this way.

Firstly, I shall explain my methodological approach, followed by a brief and generalised overview of the participants in this study, before applying a multimodal analysis to one page of a journaled Bible (Figures 7 and 8). There are twelve photographs featured here of three of the women's journaled Bible pages, and as is immediately apparent, each one of these is worthy of a study all on its own. At the centre of this article is a detailed multimodal analysis of one journaled page of a Bible (Figures 7 and 8). My intention and hope is that this analysis reveals the depth of meaning that may be elicited from a close examination of the page, revealing the value of this spiritual practice for those in addiction recovery. See the end of the document for further details on references.

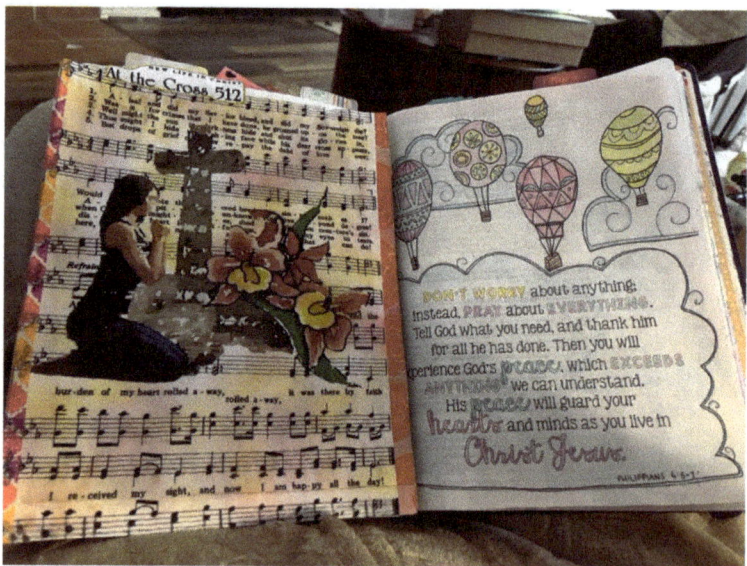

Figure 2. Philippians 4:6–7. With kind permission of the journaler.

2. Methodology: A Multimodal Analysis

This study initially arose out of a posting about addiction, in a very general sense, in a Facebook group, conducted with the permission of and through the administrators of the group. This is a large group with many thousands of members, dedicated to the members' common interest in and practice of Bible journaling. This quickly elicited a response from over thirty women sharing stories about many different journeys through almost every type of addiction and the role Bible journaling played in the various stages of their recovery. Many also shared images of their pages in this discussion. One of the characteristics of Bible journaling generally is the propensity of journalers to share their artworks and journaled pages by posting photos online in the multiplicity of social fora available. Special care is taken here to anonymise the women completely, bearing in mind that they may have shared one or more of these images in the public domain, beyond this particular Facebook group and this research process. The quotations from the women will not be linked to the featured artworks to further protect their identities and privacy.

Many women share their pages, some almost daily within the many groups like this Facebook group. I am constantly struck by the generous, supportive tone of the posts and comments, always encouraging and building up fellow journalers and readers. Any stigma that one might imagine would be associated with this topic in the context of conservative Christian Bible journaling and Bible study groups did not surface. Rather, those who identify as addicts, including addictions to food, drugs, alcohol or nicotine, receive responses of great compassion when discussing their situation, either current or historical. Five of those women then chose to engage in a semi-structured, private conversation. Three were kindly willing to share images of their journaled pages for the purposes of this publication. The reflections and testimonies of these women demonstrate that Bible journaling is a spiritual resource utilised by recovering and recovered women with addiction as a significant aid in their recovery.

There are people engaged in this practice all around the world, from South Africa to Singapore, but far and away the greatest number are located in North America. In parts this is related to:

1. Population size generally, the large population of Christians, and then the large number of Bible journaling Christians within that demographic.
2. Location of primary market for US journaling Bible publishers.
3. Energetic marketing of the Bible journaling products and peripherals (stationery, pens, highlighters, paints, paste-ins, etc.).
4. Importance of the Bible in Protestant and Evangelical churches especially.
5. Previous success of related creative, paper-based hobbies such as scrapbooking and colouring.
6. Social media platforms facilitating groups and the sharing of experience and expertise, products, etc. Of the initial over thirty women who responded to me in the social media groups, only a handful were not geographically located in North America. Those willing to participate in a research project, to discuss their experience of addiction and to share photographs of their pages were all from North America.

This article finds its theoretical foundation at the intersection of social semiotics and biblical reception history. The primary methodology employed in this article to engage with the journaled page is multimodal analysis. This is a social semiotic approach to cultural phenomena. Multimodal analysis is a theoretical semiotic framework applicable to all the semiotic modes at work simultaneously in any given artefact. In the instance of sacred text journaling these semiotic modes include densely-printed verbal text, highlighted text, handwritten words, drawings, paintings, stickers, patterned papers and tapes, colour and other additions such as ribbons. Contra Saussure—rather than finding a fixed meaning in the *sign* (word, image, sound, etc.)—those engaged with multimodal analysis understand *meaning-making* to be fluid and changeable, constantly evolving, much like language, and particular to social groups (Kress and van Leeuwen 2021; Van Leeuwen 2005; Jewitt 2014; Unsworth 2008).

This semiotic approach understands representation as a process in which the makers of signs, Bible journalers in this case, seek to make a representation of some concept, entity or object, in which their interest in the concept or object, at the point of making the representation, is a complex one. This interest arises out of the cultural, social and psychological history of the sign-maker and is framed and focused by the specific environment in which the sign-maker produces the sign. That "interest" is the source of the selection of what is seen as *the criterial aspect* of the object, and this criterial aspect is then regarded as adequately representative of the object in a given context. These criterial aspects are represented in what seems to the sign-maker, at the moment of sign-making, the most apt and plausible fashion, in the most apt and plausible representational mode (drawing, painting, cutting, pasting, highlighting). Sign-makers (journalers) thus have a meaning which they wish to express and express it through the semiotic mode(s) that make(s) available the subjectively felt, in the most plausible, most apt form (Kress and van Leeuwen 2021).

Multimodal analysis provides the means to describe the social-semiotic resource (journaling) of a particular group (sacred text journalers), the group's explicit and implicit knowledge about this resource and its uses in the practices of that group. The emphasis multimodal analysis places on *the criterial aspect* of the word, image, colour, etc., chosen by the sign-maker, makes this the richest and most appropriate approach to analysing the multimodal work of Bible journalers. Multimodal analysis values every choice of colour, texture, highlighted word, drawn image—every intervention—as a motivated *meaning-making* choice and sign on behalf of the journaler, informed by their particular social and religious context. In other words, while a drawing of a Disney mermaid character may seem incongruous or banal, when juxtaposed with and overlaid on an ancient sacred text, it must be understood as a conscious choice laden with meaning. In the context of sacred text journaling that meaning is also indicative of the hermeneutical process at play and may be revealing of personal transformation.

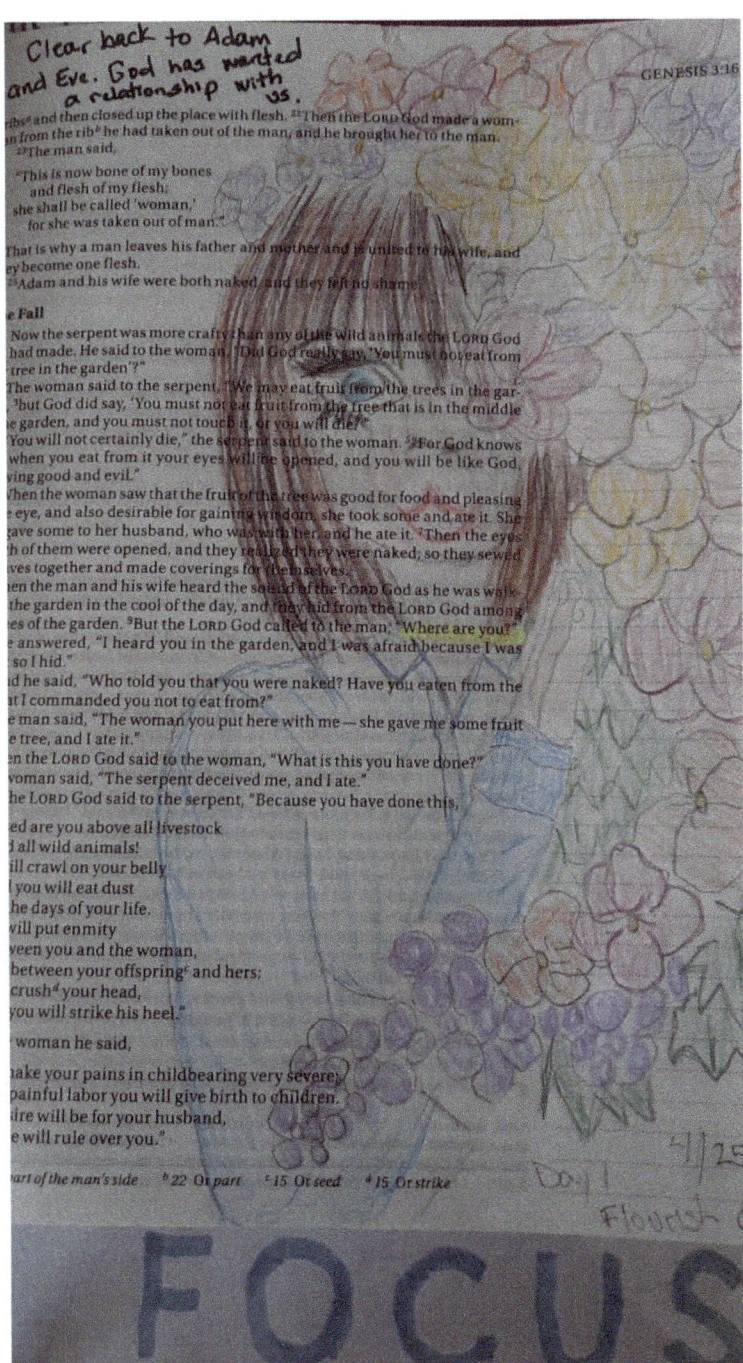

Figure 3. Genesis 3:9. With kind permission of the journaler.

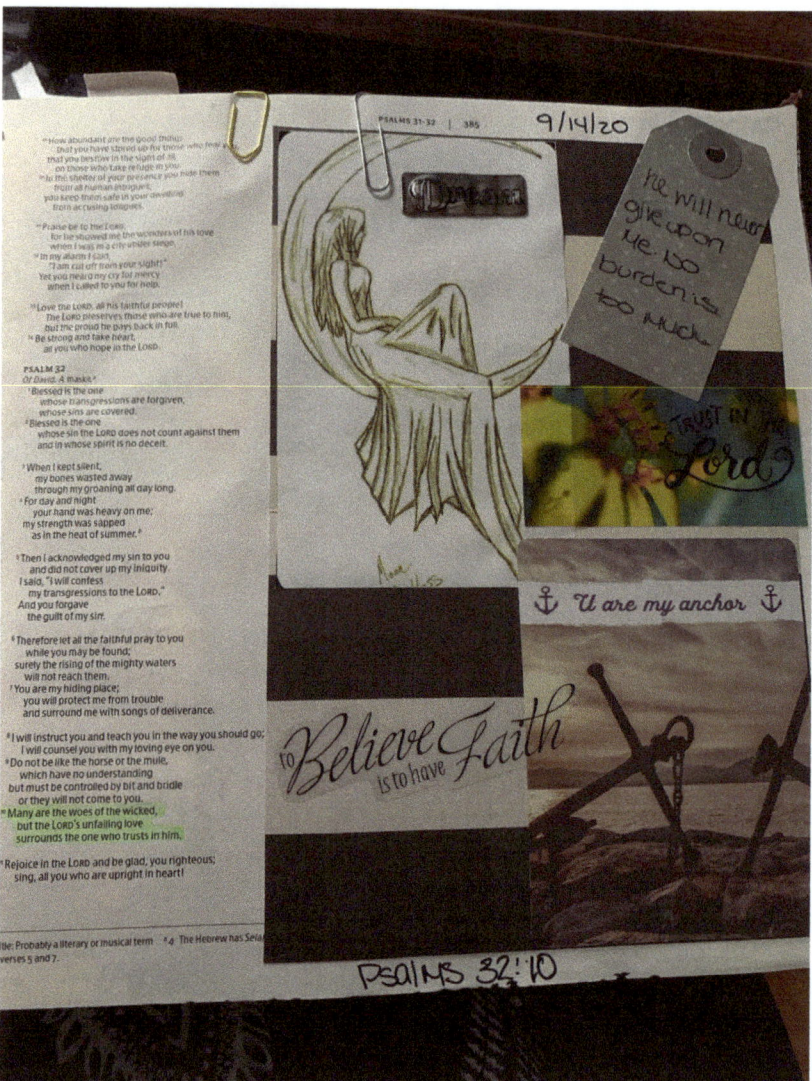

Figure 4. Psalm 32:10. With kind permission of the journaler.

3. An Overview of the Bible Journalers and Their Practice

The five participants were all women living in North America (Canada and the US), ranging in age from their late twenties to early fifties. The median age is mid-thirties. Four are caucasian, and one is of mixed indigenous ethnicity. They represent a broad socio-economic spectrum. In some instances, having fallen into poverty as a consequence of their drug addiction, they are still struggling to overcome that financial deprivation and establish lasting financial security in their lives. Four explicitly identify as cis-gender and heterosexual and are in marriages or long-term relationships. Three of the women have children. Two of the women had one or more of their children during the period of time that they were addicted to drugs and cite being a mother as their primary motivation for coming off drugs.

3.1. Pathways into Bible Journaling: Faith, Church and Addiction

The women interviewed here have different experiences of coming to Christian faith, and in turn Bible journaling. While most had some residual knowledge and encounters with churches as children, not all did. Some of their personal accounts bear out other recently advanced autobiographical theories about how and why people can suddenly stop their using (Grisel 2019; Szalavitz 2019). Different religious organisations feature in assisting them pastorally in their recovery.

> Growing up we never had Bibles or heard anything about King Jesus and my family was alcoholics and drug addicts, so of course I started using and drinking at a young age, fast forward to about maybe 7–8 years ago, I was at my lowest, my rock bottom so to speak. I was homeless and heavy into crystal meth. I journaled a lot of that noise and it helped me to keep my head. The one moment I remember clearly was standing on a street corner asking the Lord for something, anything, as I was just done (which was also an entry in a journal). I was led to a trailer called "Love Lives Here" and there met a servant of Christ Jesus who was ministering repentance and water baptism. I never heard such things before. I then started reading the Bible and really journaling my struggle. Now, here's where the journaling really came into action—I wrote everything: my fears about never getting clean, my fears about being homeless and sleeping on the street in the murder capital of this country. I also journaled all my moments of happiness, and things I was learning in the Bible stories, and about the people around me who inspired me. Journaling became my place where I could just sort things out where I could express things and be with the Father as no one else ever read my journals. My personal sort of documented walk [with the Lord].

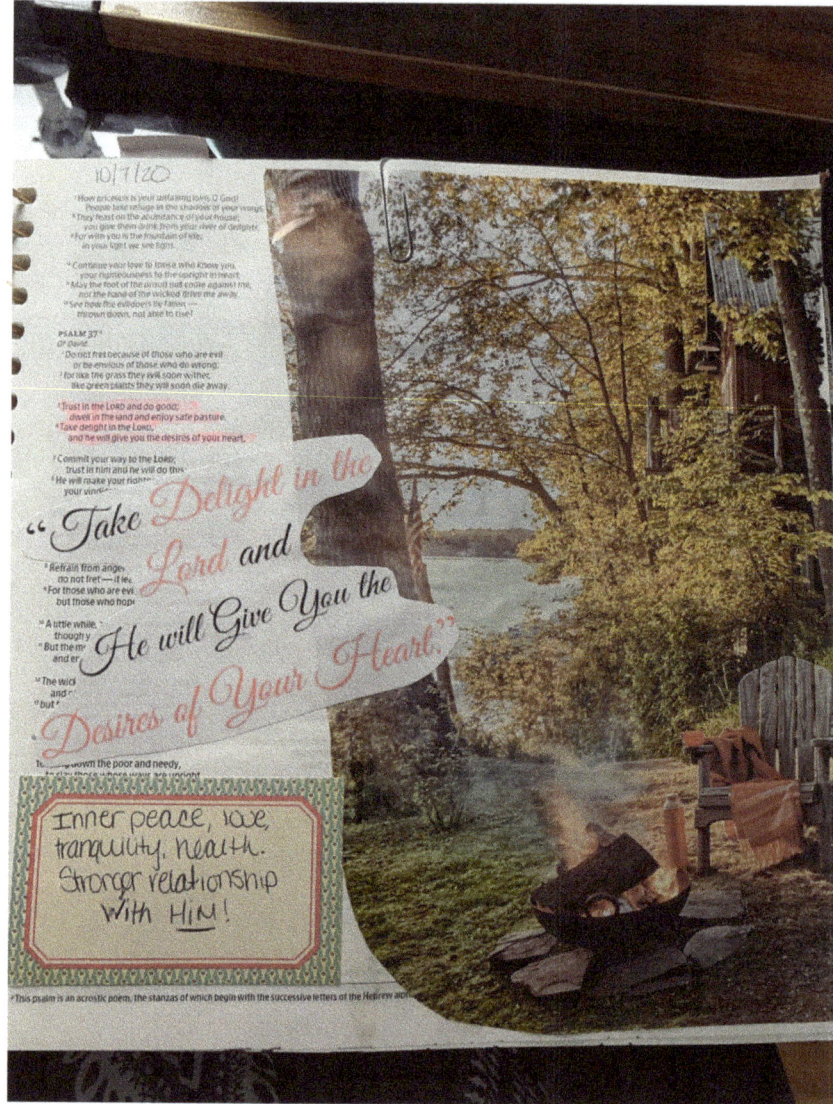

Figure 5. Psalm 37:3–4. With kind permission of the journaler.

Another women was addicted to the prescribed painkiller Percocet, ingesting 35 pills per day at the height of her addiction.

> I was baptised four years ago. Before I found God I had struggled in the area of addiction. I was also selling . . . I was in deep. Probably 35 Perc 30s a day.[2] I was awful. I threw all my relationships in the trash and didn't care . . . I grew up with an alcoholic and distant father who pushed me away constantly. My mother, the biggest source of strength had moved out of the state. My sister and brother both struggled with some addictions too and they lived in other states too. I felt like I had no one to turn to. Then one day I just stopped cold turkey. I had had enough. I was so tired of living my life that way! My children needed me more than I needed what I was doing. It wasn't until I quit that I literally felt God calling me.

I started out with Jehovah's Witnesses coming to my home teaching me the Bible. I was honest and told them point blank I didn't see myself attending their church but that I was more than happy to host them at my home (before Rona) in order to learn the Bible itself. She was such a sweet woman she came every week for over two years. My other half and I moved and we got a car and, finally, I was able to find my home at the Rock Church. This family here has been amazing.

Another woman describes her experience:

My addiction was to multiple substances. Pills, coke, heroine. I did a lot of things that I was not proud of. I lost my faith throughout all of that. I almost overdosed, and in that moment I snapped back to reality and said to myself I need God back in my life. I need him to help me, I need him to save me. I am now five years clean and my relationship with God is stronger than ever. Bible journaling was a new way for me to express myself and my love for God and all he has brought back into my life after losing it all to addiction.

Combinations of nicotine, alcohol and food also feature as an issue of concern. Some identify as completely addiction free now, whilst others continue to deal with nicotine and food addictions although now of lesser severity than at the height of their addiction. These ongoing conditions are a cause of anxiety for these women. "Having been a young addict I think cigarettes are more addictive than most drugs and alcohol. I wish when I had gone through treatment in 1985, they would have addressed it then, when I was 15. Back then they encouraged us to smoke cigarettes to replace drugs and alcohol," noted one woman.

All the women claim to be in a very different place spiritually, since beginning Bible journaling and joining groups that do so—even if this is online, as it has been for most over the last eighteen months of the Covid-19 pandemic. Four of the women cited anxiety as an ongoing issue. Two of the women are in therapy long-term. Journaling is part of the therapy for one. Two other women belong to Celebrate Recovery groups. These are groups that may be found across the US in Christian churches. Celebrate Recovery is a 12 step programme, not dissimilar to the AA and NA 12 step programme, but it is modified, including, significantly for some Christians, an explicit focus on Jesus Christ rather than the more ambiguous and personally adaptable "Higher Power" known of in the original 12 step programme.[3] The group sessions generally meet weekly around a broad range of issues that include anxiety as well as addiction. There are both large and small group sessions in these weekly meetings. The Celebrate Recovery (CR) programme includes resources such as a CR Bible, replete with added content such as testimonials, inventories and pointers to key inspirational texts, which three of the women use alongside the Bible they journal in. The motif "hurts, hang-ups and habits" is an inclusive phrase that recurs throughout the literature and language of the CR programme as it reaches beyond those who have clinical addiction issues to other emotional and psychological problems, large and small. It consciously moves the language away from the label of "alcoholic" or "addict" and recognises that addiction is complex and multifaceted in twenty-first century life.

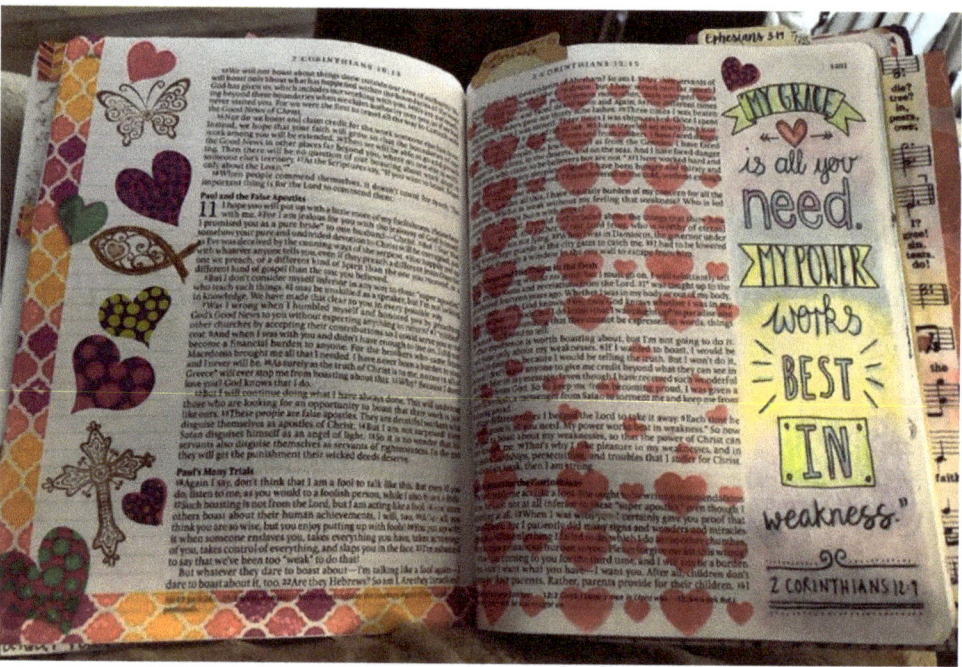

Figure 6. 2 Corinthians 12:9. With kind permission of the journaler.

Three of the women had no external intervention in their initial decision to stop their drug-taking. They spontaneously took a decision to do so having reached rock bottom, a place of desperation. Various factors played into this including the death of a dealing partner ("suicide-by-cop"), concern about their children and their role as a mother, homelessness and fear of danger. Some speak of having reached their lowest point of ultimate desperation and being afraid of dying by either accidental or deliberate overdose if they did not stop.

3.2. Practice

I have a few different Bible journals that I use.[4] I have the Inspire Prayer, the original Inspire, the Psalms/Proverbs Illustrating Bible, and the original Illustrating Bible, and various notebooks. I usually journal every day. When journaling, it just depends, I pray around it [Bible]. I have a devotional that I use, and sometimes I open the Bible to a random page and read and then select the verses that speak to me on that day. Sometimes, I select a text from my devotional, other times it's as simple as seeing a post on Facebook with a verse that jumps out at me.

Characteristic of Bible journaling in general, the women have more than one Bible and many supplementary resources including: 30-Day Daily Inventory, Devotionals or a Faith and Focus journal. The posts of others in the social media groups can also be a launching point into a particular text. Church retreat days, Bible study or Bible conferences with a journaling component can also direct someone to a particular text. One woman writes a "daily letter to God". Another says: "I usually do mine before bed as a reflection for the day. I have a whole devotional time process though. I have a few devotionals I go through, usually they have some sort of questions attached which helps me go a little deeper and not just surface level." One makes use of being on night shift at her job. "Since I work third shift usually, I work on it while I am at work a lot of the time. It's really nice. Keeps me grounded".

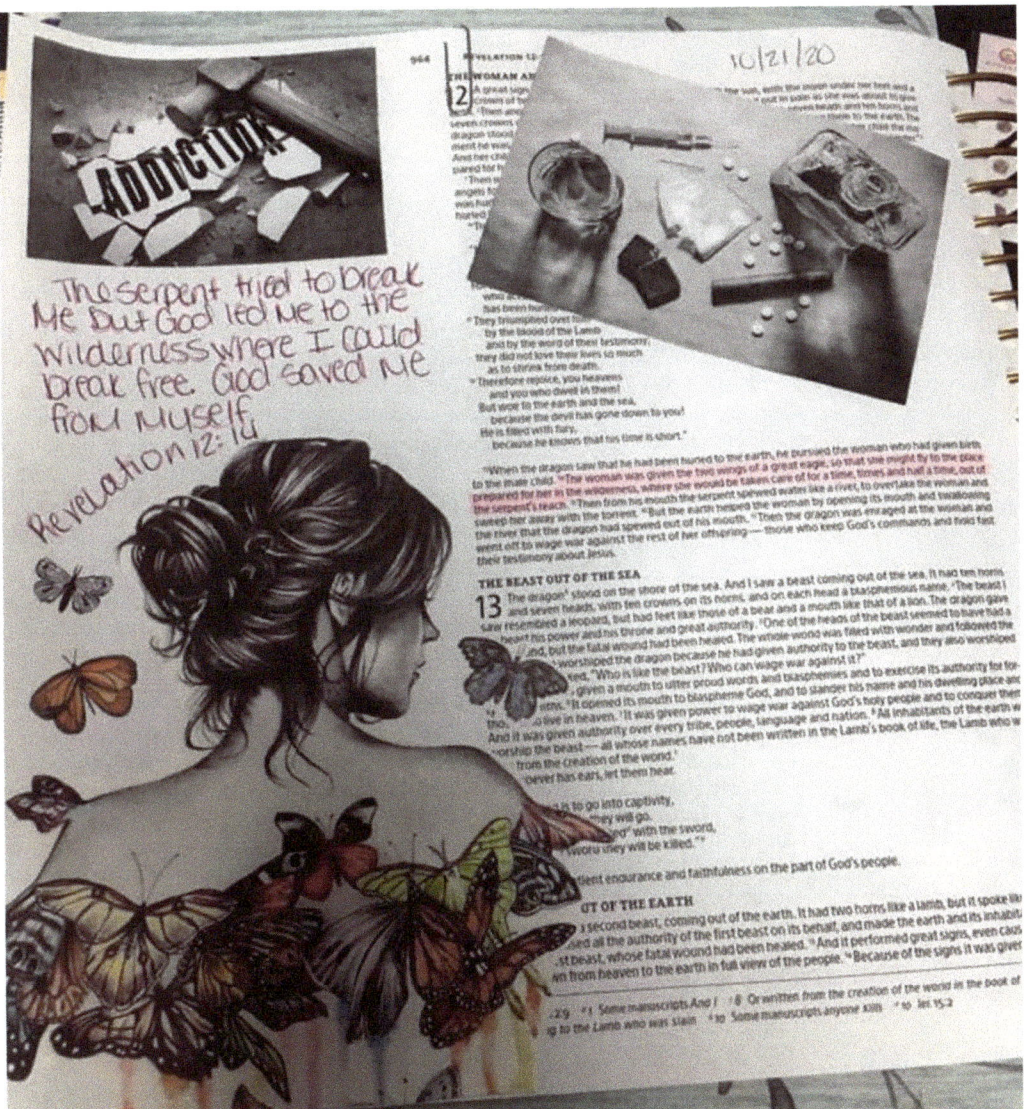

Figure 7. Revelation 12:14. With kind permission of the journaler.

4. A Multimodal Analysis of a Bible Journaled Page

Every one of the journaled pages that is featured in this article would make for a fascinating analysis such is the depth of reflection and quality of expression found on each respectively (Figures 1–6 and Figures 9–12). I elected to focus on the page seen in Figure 7 as it is immediately compelling on a visual level and the word-image relationship between the biblical text and the journaler's creative interventions on the page are striking for a multiplicity of reasons, as shall become apparent.

4.1. Thick Description

Before launching into a detailed multimodal analysis, I would like to begin with a short thick description of what we are looking at in Figure 7. This is a journaled left-hand (verso) page in a spiral-bound, journaling Bible (NIV) with a large blank, unlined, left-hand margin. There is a handwritten date in the top right corner: 10/21/20. The biblical text featured, on the right-hand half of the page, is from The Revelation to John 12–13:14, the last book of the New Testament. Almost exactly halfway down the right-hand column of printed text, in the middle of the page, the following verse (Rev 12:14) is highlighted in pink:

> The woman was given the two wings of a great eagle, so that she might fly to the place prepared for her in the wilderness, where she would be taken care of for a time, times, and half a time, out of the serpent's reach".

In the left-hand panel a black and white photographic image, one-fifth of the depth of the height of the page, has been pasted in the top left corner. It shows something resembling a rectangular white concrete block featuring the word "ADDICTION" in bold, compressed, black capitals (e.g., Helvetica Black Condensed). There is a heavy wooden hammer with a large metal head lying over the smashed lettering. Beneath this picture are six lines of text in the journaler's own handwriting clearly referring to the printed biblical text:

> The serpent tried to break me but God led me to the wilderness where I could break free. God saved me from myself. Revelation 12:14.

In the top half of the right-hand column is another black and white image, pasted in over the biblical text at about a thirty-degree angle, leaning over, down to the right. This photograph, taken from above, shows the paraphernalia of hard drug use, pills, an injecting needle and so on, cast with dramatic shadows. The images used here may be sourced from magazines or the internet.

Beneath the artist's handwritten verbal text is another pasted-in image of a young woman seen from behind. This is a focal point of the page. She faces to the right—towards the printed biblical text. We see her profile. She has long hair held up in a "messy" bun revealing bare shoulders. On her naked back are an array of fifteen or so multicoloured butterflies of many different shapes and patterns and sizes. Butterflies also fly around her, and one alights on her left shoulder. A blue butterfly, flying close to the right of her face, overlaps the biblical text, as does her right side, obscuring the text. Streaks of watercolour paint bleed off the edge of the page beneath the butterflies.

4.2. Composition

The pink-highlighted biblical text in the middle of the printed column provides the hermeneutical key to what is happening on this page: a multimodal journaling, mixing imagery with personal, verbal text, illustrating a liberation from addiction to freedom and personal transformation. This highlighted text, working in conjunction with the handwritten text slightly diagonally above it on the left, forms a visual divider separating the top half of the page, which deals with addiction, and the bottom half, which reveals liberation and transformation. In the vertical plane, there is a polarization, a sense of contrast between the top half and bottom half of the page. In both horizontal columns, left and right, verbal text forms a visual focus between the images of addiction and the image of the young woman. This central position in a vertical arrangement has a mediating quality. That is, the pink-highlighted biblical text (right) and the personal, handwritten appropriation of that text (left), as it applies directly to the life of this young woman, function here to mediate between her former life (above) and the "new creation", her new self-image (below).

Conventionally, and historically, in artworks dealing with Christian religious content, the upper third of the format signifies the realm of the divine and the lower third the earthly domain. If we apply this structure here, this arrangement is interesting for a number of reasons. It might seem ironic or even incongruous to place these images relating explicitly to addiction, the very thing that may be understood to have disrupted her relationship with God, in this "divine" area of the page. Reference, directly below, in her handwritten text to "the serpent", the symbol for the devil or evil in the Christian paradigm, implies she links the drug-taking with the influence of evil in some way.

Moreover, the opaque image on the right is placed directly over the biblical text. If we understand the scriptures as a foundational place of encounter with God for the reader, it follows that one potential meaning to this placement of the crooked, right-hand image is that the elements it features obscured and prevented her reading of the Bible, representing a disruption in her relationship with God. This drug habit formed a *barrier* between the artist and God.

The angle of the right-hand image is also significant. Considering first the elements within this photograph, it is worth noting that none of the items in the image are aligned with either the vertical or horizontal axis. Every element is at a slightly different diagonal angle and slightly differently angled from each other object. Only the injecting needle and the pipe show any consistency in their parallel arrangement. The placement is apparently random. By contrast, a highly ordered layout would conform to the grid of vertical and horizontal—one might expect this in a photograph of medical implements for a scientific journal, for example. Diagonals within a composition may enliven an image with dynamism, movement and energy but may also allude to disorder and dysfunction. That this image is then placed on the page at an angle reiterates the instability implied in the internal composition. Here,—at a downward-tilting 30-degree angle, unbalanced, not on an even keel, falling—even this slanting of the picture speaks to the disorder that the elements figured brought about in her life.

The placement of the addiction images in the upper third suggests that what they represent for the journaler is not in the down-to-earth realm of the journaler—where she has placed a representation of herself. Addiction has been placed in another realm, the divine realm. In other words, we might say, in the everyday discourse of Christian spirituality that this problem has been "handed over to God", that former drug-taking is now in the control of God and no-longer in her realm of reality. She is separated from it by the mediating biblical text, the Word of God that speaks of God's intervention in her life, which she has appropriated for herself. This is further confirmed in the past tense structure of the handwritten text.

The two addiction images are contained within rectangular boxes, with clearly defined, sharp edges. They are bounded. By contrast, the image of the young woman, larger than both, is not contained, but bleeds off the edges of the page to left and bottom and over the biblical text on the right. In keeping with the freedom it signifies, it is an expansive, organic, free shape reaching into the space around it, with further individual butterflies flying about, freely overlapping the text. It is a powerful, mystical and highly symbolic image. Moreover, great salience is added here in the bright colouring of the many butterflies, adding to the foregrounding of this image, as does its overlapping of the text. The bright colours not only illuminate the butterflies but also form a rainbow of sorts, running "down her back" off the page into space, flowing out into her life.

Human nakedness, in the context of the Bible, carries strong connotations of the creation narratives of Genesis (the opening book of the Bible). Her naked shoulders allude to new birth, emergence and freedom. There are many connotations one could assign to this illustrated figure in relation to the Bible. In her nakedness and surrounded by, arising even, from the vibrant, flowing, living beauty of nature, she may be seen as a type of Eve, in the positive sense of being an original creation of God, at home in the Edenic garden, before the Fall. In the New Testament, Paul makes reference to "a new creation": "So if anyone is in Christ, there is a new creation: everything old has passed away; see, everything has become new!" (2Cor. 5:17; and see Gal. 6:15). The sense of arising out of a kaleidoscope of butterflies links the women closely with the butterflies, she is a metamorphosed "butterfly" too. The flutter of butterfly wings picks up on the mention of wings in the highlighted text; the woman was given "wings" (of an eagle), and here is a woman with many wings.

The journaler herself says, "The butterflies symbolise the addiction leaving my body and becoming beauty in God's Grace".

The symbolic value of the butterfly in Christian art is closely linked to transformation. "A dual symbol whose short life and transcendent beauty signified vanity and futility, but whose three-stage cycle as a caterpillar, chrysalis, and butterfly denoted resurrection or new life. The chrysalis was interpreted as a symbol of sleep or death and the butterfly the new life that arises out of sleep or death. When either the Christ Child or his mother held the butterfly, it connoted the Resurrection" (Apostolos-Cappadona 2020). Within the Greek symbol system it represents the soul and its personification, Psyche (Hall 1994).

This pose of the woman is important here. Turning, both the bodily gesture and the mental disposition of shifting focus, is an enduring trope of the Hebrew and Christian scriptures. The verb "to turn" indicates a shift in understanding, behaviour, attitude and direction, sometimes simultaneously both psychological and physical. It may also include a radical transformation in material form brought about by God: Lot's wife turned to look back and was turned into a pillar of salt (Gen. 19:26); in Exodus, the plagues include the waters of the Nile River being turned into blood (Ex. 7:17, 20). Turning often signals a change in the narrative. Repeatedly, one hears of God "turning" attention and favour, or anger, towards or away from individuals or nations (Deut. 23:14; Num. 25:11; Judg. 4:2;). Prophets urge the people not to "turn" to idolatry (Lev 19.4, Deut. 11:16); travellers "turn" and set out on a journey (Gen. 18:22; Deut. 2:1); Moses "turns aside" to behold the spectacle of the burning bush (Ex. 3:3). The natural elements are subject to God's turning action: "and the Lord turned a very strong west wind" (Ex. 10:19). The New Testament continues the prophetic call to turn away from wrongdoing and turn towards the Lord (Matt. 18:3; Luke 1:16; Acts 14:15; Acts 26:18; Acts 26:18; Gal. 4:9). Again, as with the OT, turning is also linked with radical, material transformation brought about Jesus, such as the turning of water into wine at the wedding at Cana (John 2:9). In the journaler's choice of this illustration of the young woman, representing herself, she is indicating two different aspects of turning. Firstly, she has *turned* away from, *turned* her back on her previous life. Secondly, her head is *turned* towards the right and now looks towards the biblical text, the Word of God. There has been a fundamental change in her life, in her direction, away from a former way of life towards a new spiritual engagement with her God. This turning signifies radical psychological, spiritual and physical transformation.

In a semiotic analysis of the visual elements it is important to note the two different perspectives offered in the images used here—both of which further demonstrate the meaning-making at play. The two black and white photographs show their objects from directly above. This is referred to as the "bird's eye view" or interestingly, in this context, "god's eye view." This is an objective observation of the elements or situation, from a privileged position of power or authority. "It contemplates the world from a god-like point of view, putting it at your feet rather than within your reach of your hands" (Kress and van Leeuwen 2021). Again, this both reinforces the suggestion that the upper third is the realm of the divine on this creative construction. Mostly importantly, it also implies that the journaler herself shares this viewpoint and is able to "look down" upon these instruments of addiction from an objective standpoint, and from a position of both power over and detachment from her previous life.

When we turn to the illustration of the young woman, there is a marked change in perspective. The viewer is placed "on a par"—at the same "eye-level" as the woman illustrated here—in what is referred to as the close personal range, featuring the head and shoulders, indicating a high level of identification with the woman figured. Again, there is a high level of modality in terms of realism here, even though it is a conceptual, symbolic image. The black and white establishes a visual link with the images in the upper realm, but the addition of vibrant colours raises its salience and heightens the symbolic value of a coming to new life, a transition from the world of the black and white, the former life in addiction, blooming into the world of full colour, in this immediate and personal time and space.

Likewise, the modality of these two images is significant. Both are photographs suggesting a high-level of modality, in the sense of representing reality or "truth". They are not abstract, although the image on the left is conceptual rather than an image readily drawn from real life; it is contrived albeit looking very "realistic". The image on the right, may be said to have an almost analytical, scientific diagram feeling about it, systematically setting out the various items related to drug misuse; it could almost be labelled and featured in an educational resource explaining the function of each item. Again, I suggest that this high-level of modality demonstrates that the journaler has no illusions about this reality of this dimension of her past.

I suggest the mode of black and white photography here serves to add a temporal dimension. Black and white photography is indicative of a bygone era, BC—before colour. Potentially, it also hints that whatever colour, fun, bliss, vibrancy that she may have once experienced in this way of life has faded, has dissipated, and been replaced with the cold, hard facts. There is no romance about this static image. It is an image from another time demonstrating a further distancing of the self from this previous reality.

4.3. The Word-Image Relationship

4.3.1. "Break"

> The woman was given the two wings of a great eagle, so that she might fly to the place prepared for her in the wilderness, where she would be taken care of for a time, times, and half a time, out of the serpent's reach. (Rev 12:14)

As the pink-highlighted text is a particularly rich sentence of Scripture, it is worth spending some time opening up its meaning and the profundity it therefore lends to this page of journaling as personally appropriated by this journaler.

Above this picture of a woman is her own handwritten reflection: "The serpent tried to break me but God led me to the wilderness where I could break free. God saved me from myself. Revelation 12:14".

This is a striking sentence that mediates connections between the picture above it and that beneath it, as well as the focal sentence in the biblical text. It almost paraphrases the parallel printed text. It is also written more than once, in the same place, layered initially in pink, the same colour as the highlighted biblical text, making an explicit link visually between these two pieces of verbal text. It is then repeated, reinforced with a stronger, darker colour. The repetition highlights the importance of this reflection for the journaler. The word "break" is used twice here. Firstly, it refers to the action of "the serpent" upon her; secondly, it refers to her own action as being able to "break free". Again, in the first instance it appears directly beneath the image of the *broken* word "ADDICTION", the attempt of the serpent to *break* her through addiction, but she prevails and *breaks free* of the addiction. The placing of this handwritten text here directly correlates with the image above it, in a powerful multivalent way. This liberation is attributed to God who led her "to the wilderness" and who "saved" her from herself. The image is placed on the right up in the divine realm of the page, reiterating God's saving action.

4.3.2. "Wilderness"

The use of the deeply symbolic word "wilderness" occurs in the Rev 12:14 text too, described as "a place prepared for her, where she would be taken care of, out of the serpent's reach". This sentence is rich in the language of providence and loving, protective care. Virginia Burrus emphasizes in her exegesis that the woman is protected by the wilderness, which "cradles her body" (Burrus 1999). In the Bible, the wilderness is a complex trope—both a place of danger but also one of potential safety and provision. Leonard Thompson suggests that "wilderness" functions in Revelation "symbolically as a place similar to chaos with transformational potential for judgment, deliverance, nourishment, punishment, death, and rebirth" (Thompson 1997). "In Revelation place is bound up with destiny and contingency" writes Schüssler Fiorenza (1991), and Brian C. Jones points to the liminal aspect: "wilderness denotes both a place and an existential condition. It is a zone of liminality where individuals or groups encounter existential limits and where they are tested and transformed through numinous encounter (Oropeza). For humans, wilderness is a passageway, not a destination" (Jones 2009). Writing about this text, biblical scholar Yarbro Collins says the purpose of the story is "to interpret the present situation of his [the author's] first readers and to encourage them to take a particular stand. [...] The most illuminating way to read the story is as a paradigm or model of and for the experience of the first readers. They are expected to identify with the woman [...] The rescue of the woman evokes trust that these hardships are not in vain" (Yarbro Collins 1979). In other words, the journaler here has done exactly what the author intended and read herself into this text.

The manner of rescue involves themes from the exodus story. The two wings of the great eagle recalls a traditional metaphor for the deliverance from Egypt—"You have seen what I did to the Egyptians, and how I bore you on eagle's wings and brought you to myself" (Ex 19:4). The refuge taken in the desert calls to mind the wilderness wandering. In John's time, retreat to the desert symbolised readiness for the manifestation of God's rule. This figurative account of rescue does not necessarily imply literal protection from harm. In the context of the Apocalypse as a whole, it expresses a radiant trust in divine providence even in the midst of hardship and suffering. (Yarbro Collins 1979).

The eagle is a symbol of God's providence in Exod 19:4, Deut 32:10–12. "[God] enables her, like the children of Israel to reach the desert, which in both the OT and NT represents a place of provisional safety, of discipline, of waiting for the promises of God. It was thus in the Exodus period for the forty years before the Israelites entered the promised land; cf. Deut 8:2–10." Twice Elijah withdrew to the desert; 1 Kings 17: 2–3, 19:3–4. Yahweh lured his bride into the desert; Hosea 2:14. Isaiah commanded a highway to be made for the Lord there; Isa 40:3. The bride in the Song of Songs is said to come from the desert; Song 3:6–8, 8:5 (Massyngberde Ford 1975).

It is in the wilderness that John the Baptist prepared himself and the people for the Coming One (Luke 1:80, 3.2). In the synoptic gospels, following his own baptism, Jesus is led or driven out into the wilderness, by the Holy Spirit, as he prepares for his public ministry (Matt. 4:1; Mark 1:12; Luke 4:1).

4.3.3. "Nourish"

In other Bible translations (NRSV, ESV, KJV) the word "nourished" may appear in place of "taken care of". This also echoes previous occasions in which God nourished those in the wilderness: the Israelites are nourished with manna in the desert (Ex. 16:31–35; Num. 11:6–9; Deut. 8:3, 8:16; Josh. 5:12), as is Elijah (I Kings 17:4, 19:5, 7).

4.3.4. Conclusions

The belief of the journaling artist here is in this providential care and protection of a loving God who led her to "the wilderness" creating a "prepared place" in which she could break free from the hold addiction had on her life. As is seen in these previous instances of reference to the wilderness in the Bible, it is a liminal place of both provision and preparation. It would be safe, I suggest, to interpret this here as an acknowledgement, on the part of the journaler, of an experience of liminality in her recovery and of recognising this as having been a safe space of provisional care brought about providentially by God.

It is clear that this page illustrates profound personal transformation away from drug addiction and into a new, liberated life. The journaler has brought many different elements, both realistic and conceptual, to a page of biblical text, one sentence of which, laden with resonance, she has appropriated to her own life and woven into a beautiful, sophisticated, deeply personal, multimodal narrative describing God's liberating and salvific action in her own life.

4.3.5. And Then

In response to my request for the high-resolution image for the purpose of this publication, the journaler kindly sent the photo. However, it came with further additions to the page—something I had not expected—but, of course, within the context of this multimodal analysis proved fascinating and heartening. As you will observe on Figure 8, three further butterflies have been added to the page. They all appear on the right-hand side overlapping the printed biblical text. Several interesting factors may be observed here. Firstly, the butterflies are larger than those on and around the woman. Secondly, they overlap the biblical text but do not obscure it completely as they are semi-transparent. They do not, however, overlap or obscure the pink-highlighted text. It may be that the journaler has internalised this text, having appropriated it so intimately to her own journey, memorised it by heart and so can call to mind those words that may be obscured. It may also be indicative of emboldened spiritual autonomy taking flight and vigorously embossing her newfound inner strength and renewed sense of identity fully across the page, across her life.

I suggest the yellow central butterfly acts as a further pointer, drawing attention to this line of text. Thirdly, the highest of the butterflies on the page, has crossed over the former dividing line, as it were, of the pink-highlighted, printed text, into the upper realm. This butterfly almost touches or overlaps the bounded, rectangular black and black photograph, but does not. In other words, what is signified by this photograph remains firmly contained, sealed within that frame. This butterfly now sits prettily alongside her handwritten text, and as it is slightly pinkish in colour, makes a further visual link between the two pieces of verbal text, left and right. What is most significant about these additional butterflies, however, and closely tied to their increased size, is their texture. They are embossed butterflies made out of a type of plastic or silicone gel. These butterflies are not two-dimensional, but three-dimensional, they have form. This is a firmer, stronger, more durable material. One could trace the contours of the margins of the wings and the antennae. And we might trace this progression from the flat, flimsier, paper butterflies to the gel-embossed butterflies as marking an advance in the artist's strengthening confidence in her own recovery. As the butterflies fan out across the page, larger and more robust in material, in character, one intuits an ever-greater sense of blossoming, flourishing and freedom from the journaler. The energy of transformation is dynamic and expanding, taking up more space, with greater vigour, becoming the decidedly dominant feature on this page. The metamorphosis denoted by the butterfly symbol and its implications for her spiritual journey of recovery continues positively.

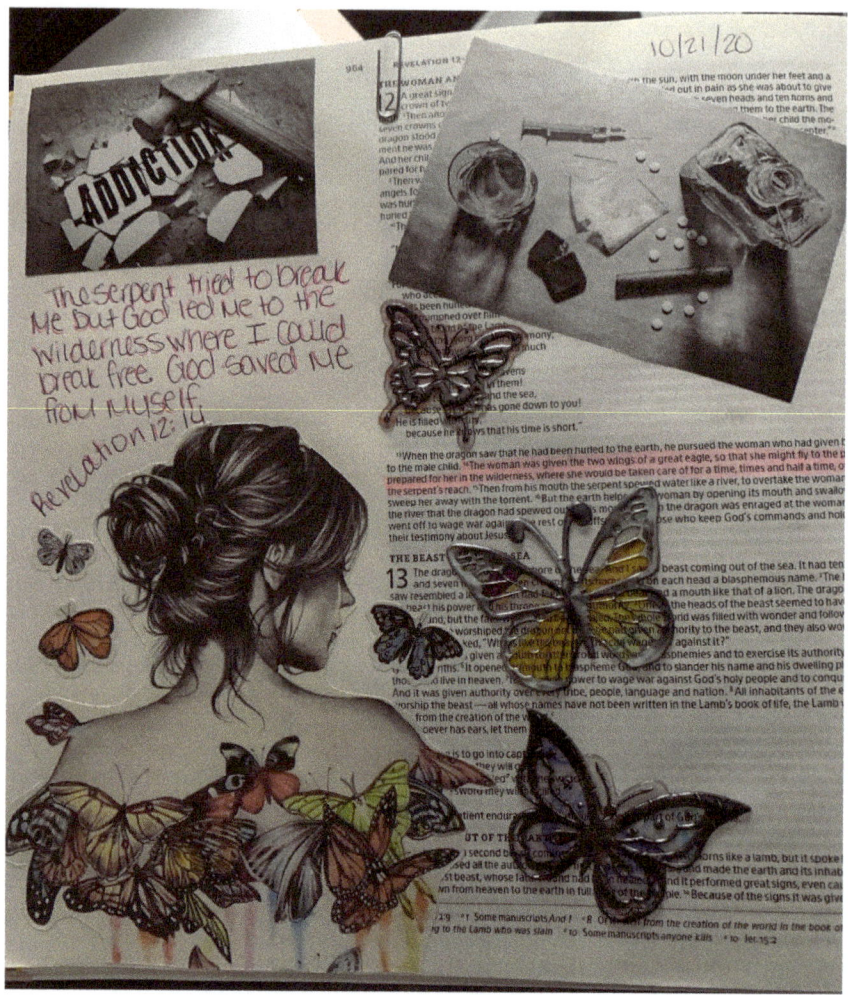

Figure 8. Revelation 12:14. With kind permission of the journaler.

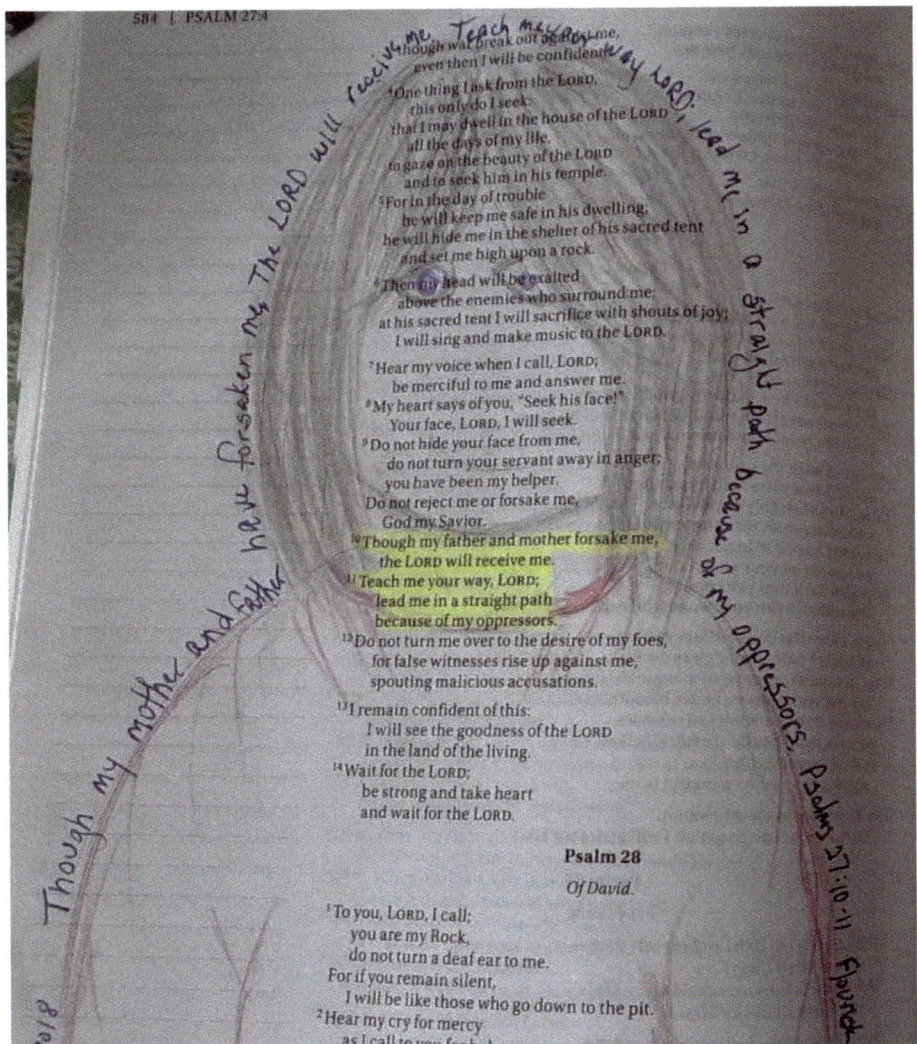

Figure 9. Psalm 27:10-11. With kind permission of the journaler.

5. A Necessary Note on Trauma and the Bible

It is important to acknowledge that trauma lies at the root of addiction for many people (Maté 2018; Etherington 2008; Alexander 2008). One may add to this that addiction itself may be experienced as a trauma and often brings further trauma into the life of an addict. Furthermore, scholars recognise the multiple catastrophes or impending catastrophes, be they natural disasters, war and migration or financial collapse, and add to that a global pandemic, political insurrection and further climate-change related environmental crises, as constituting our contemporary time as a "trauma paradigm" or "trauma culture" (Andermahr and Pellicer-Ortín 2013). Among those interviewed, a number referred to traumatic events: the death by suicide of a partner, overdose, homelessness, abusive parents or partners, to mention a few examples. Many also referred to experiencing high levels of anxiety on a day-to-day basis. What role might the Bible play in assisting the recovery from trauma?

Within Biblical studies, trauma studies has now become an area of interest and interdisciplinary research. According to Claassens, "Given the fact that ancient Israel found themselves repeatedly invaded and occupied by one empire after another, much of the biblical literature that emerged from Israel's traumatic past can thus be characterised as trauma literature" (Claassens 2020). The collective trauma experienced by the people spurred the prophets (such as Jeremiah) to write with the intention of making meaning out of their suffering for the traumatised people (Stulman 2014). "By means of poetry, throbbing with raw emotion and pain, as well as a number of narratives, reflecting multiple layers of trauma and suffering, the authors of the prophetic books sought to capture something of the violence the community had lived through" (Claassens 2020). This understanding of the biblical text as a type of "trauma literature" suggests it may offer the contemporary reader a narrative holding space in which to reflect upon their own trauma and contemplate God's response and care for individuals and nations in these situations. Already, we have seen how one apocalyptic passage (Rev 12:14) offered a meaning-making textual mirror for one recovered addict. There is, however, a flip side to this appreciation for the affirming dimension of biblical narratives, of which one has to remain vigilantly mindful. Equal to the recognition of this beneficial aspect, is an increasing critique of the abuse of the biblical text by undereducated and unloving pastors, church workers and believers. No doubt the Bible has always been manipulated to suit agendas, often antithetical to its driving message, in order to bully, stigmatise and, one may even go so far as to say, traumatise people. One only has to think of so-called gay-conversion therapies to know that there are victims of such abuse who would no doubt describe themselves as traumatised by certain interpretations and presentations of the Bible (Ó Tuama 2015). Gender is another area where misogynistic interpretations of women's value and role in family, church and society are recognised as causing profound emotional pain for many women in the church. In some denominations, these constructs purportedly drawn from the Bible, carry the monikers "Biblical Womanhood" and "Biblical Manhood" (Barr 2021; Byrd 2020; Kobes Du Mez 2020). One of the women in this study spoke of how journaling, including Bible journaling, is helping her work through her childhood experience:

> I believe journaling is God answering my prayers and showing me the answers he wants me to have. It is calming for me. My therapist has me journal everyday. Even if all I write is 'life sucks', 'I wanna smoke', 'Anxiety is high', 'Pain hurts', etc. It is me being real with where my thoughts are. My therapist and I have been able to uncover lies I believed ... such as because I was not a boy I was unlovable by God. Because I wrote my thoughts. Then she helps me change the lie with Scripture. It's a long process but one I'm willing to do ... must do in order for whole wellness.

> She has helped me heal a childhood where my Sunday School teachers told me regularly I was "Satan's child" ... where my twin brother was the perfect child. Boys were the chosen ones in what I grew up with. It contributed to my addictions to numb the feelings.

Valuing the Bible as a spiritual resource for healing from addiction or emotional pain carries with it the parallel necessity of knowing that it is also used to cause emotional pain and trauma.

6. Limitations to This Study and Future Directions

There are a few notable limitations to this study. Firstly, the size of the cohort is restricted to five participants. Clearly, the potential for a larger sized cohort is available but would require greater resources and capacity. The highly personal nature of an inquiry into the intimate life stories of people who have suffered from addiction, and all the negativity that invariably brings into one's life, requires a great deal of awareness, planning and care for the protection of people's privacy and respect and concern for their vulnerability throughout the process. Secondly, only one journaled page is given a thorough multimodal analysis. An analysis of a page of each of the three journalers' submissions, to this study, would profoundly enrich the investigation. It would allow for more concrete assertions about the value of Bible journaling as a spiritual resource in this very particular context of addiction. Finally, this article has focused on an in-depth multimodal analysis and has demonstrated the value of this methodological approach in drawing out the meaning-making processes at work, in this fascinating reception of a text by a Bible reader and her interventions on the page in response to that. This approach foregrounds the criterial choices made by the creator of the multimodal artefact, allowing them to "speak" for themselves. An interesting further step might have been the inclusion of one or more art therapists in a discussion around their perceptions of the featured page or pages. Would they, approaching the pages with a different disciplinary (psychology) framework, arrive at similar or different analyses of the expressive content displayed?

Noting these limitations immediately opens up potential directions for further research. Multimodal analysis places the creator's productive meaning-making choices at the centre of its enquiry. It provides the scientific discourse for a thorough semiotic analysis of a semiotic event or artefact. It allows for both an in-depth analysis of one item, such as the page analysed here, or a broad analysis of multiple items of similar significance. A large scale meta-analysis into multiple pages of Bible journaling in this context of addiction would allow for the cross referencing of the choices of biblical text, the visual treatment of the biblical text (highlighting, accentuating, obscuring, etc.), the choices of key symbolic tropes (i.e., butterfly), the treatment of human figures, the representation of the "self" in some way, the addition of further text (by hand or pasted in), free drawing and use of imported images (drawn by other artists and sourced online, in magazines, etc.), the representation of the divine, the representation of addiction, the modality of colour, composition, scale, texture and point of view. It is my firm contention that multimodal analysis has much to offer those working in the spiritual and psychological care of people with addiction issues as a resource for understanding the self-expressive, multimodal communication of people who journal.

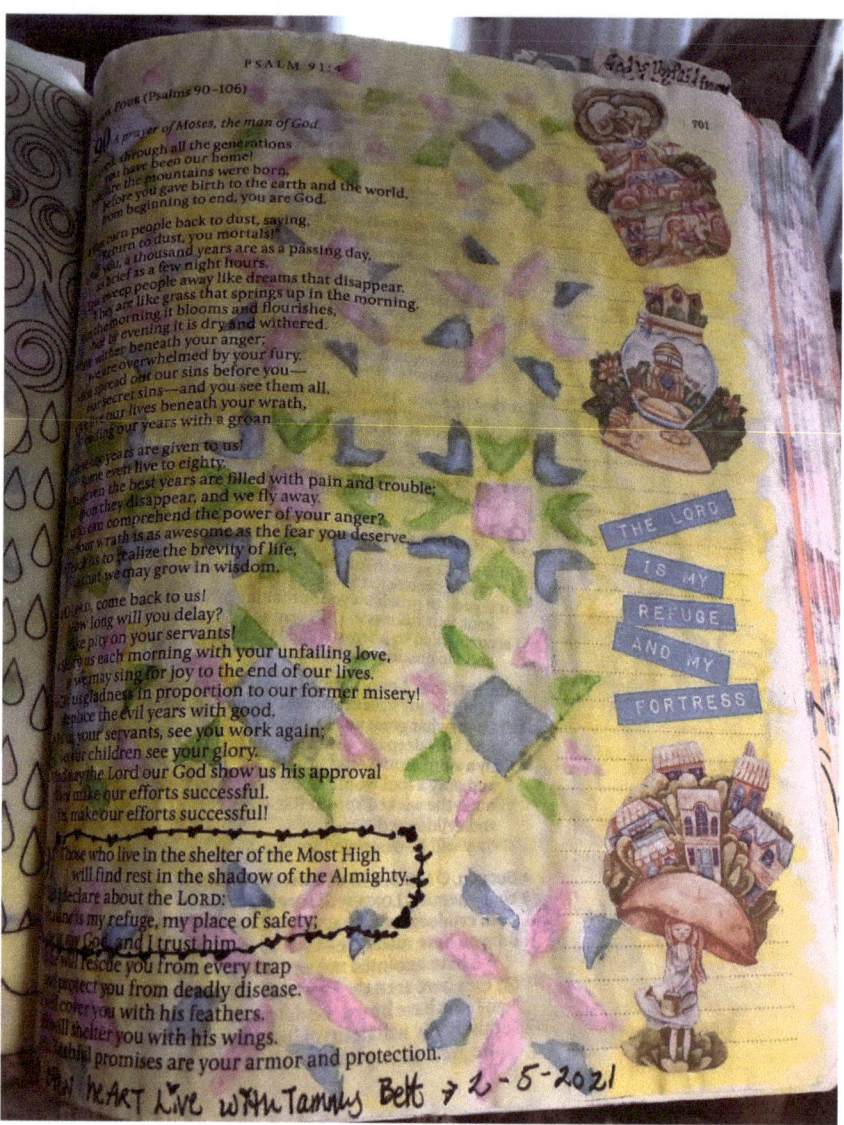

Figure 10. Psalm 91:1-2. With kind permission of the journaler.

7. Conclusions

> Our images reveal that we are holographic creatures, living multiple stories.
> (Allen 1995)

In one respect, the Bible journaling phenomenon is a consequence of the expansive US Bible publishing business that is constantly looking for new ways to market the Bible. Whilst initially intended for written journaling, it has developed in unexpected ways due to the ingenuity of readers. Many of the techniques journalers use may be recognised as having possibly originated in the multimillion-dollar scrapbooking and colouring hobbies that have preceded it. The mass marketing of Bibles in the US has also meant the individual ownership of multiple copies of the Bible and therefore a different approach to the material book (Beal 2012). Nonetheless, it may be argued that the journaling readers have set the course for these Bibles and new iterations are a response to consumer demands (wider margins, thicker paper, spiral binding, etc.). Such is the interest and momentum in Bible journaling, it is difficult to see it waning anytime soon as a significant spiritual practice for a large number of Bible readers.

Observing the importance of this practice for those who engage in it, one wonders how this might be relevant to other religious groups in relation to their sacred Scriptures and holy books. Dillon (2020) has shown that Jewish and Muslim journalers are slowly yet increasingly involved in journaling with their sacred texts but in a markedly different way, in that they journal alongside their holy book in a separate journal and not directly into and on the pages of their holy books. Interventions directly in the material book of Scripture would not be acceptable in these faiths. Nonetheless, very beautiful pages featuring, for example, calligraphic treatment of an individual ayah embellished with arabesque or floral designs may be seen in the work of Muslim journalers of the Quran (Hassan 2016). Jewish and Muslim journalers are also more circumspect in the public sharing of their journaling. Within online Christian-dominated Bible journaling groups there are a very small number of journalers who identify themselves as Jewish and share their work. However, it is difficult to discern, as yet, groups with a distinctly Jewish leadership, membership and Hebrew Bible focus. With regard to Muslim journalers, these social media groups are generally not publicly open and are more controlled in terms of membership.

The plain journal market is one that continues to develop and expand. Plain journals with well-designed covers featuring the Om symbol, Sanskrit texts and graphic designs and artwork from the Dharmic religions are available. I suggest it should be possible to develop dedicated journals with selected texts from the Scriptures of other faiths, as features within the journal and focus points for contemplation and reflection in written or visually creative form. Indeed, journals of this type may already be available in regions where these religions are practiced and be used in similarly creative ways.

As the journaling of biblical texts has proven to be of great support to those in recovery from addiction, and other mental health issues such as anxiety, I suggest that adherents of other religions struggling with or in recovery from an addiction would likewise find spiritual support, inspiration, courage, strength and benefit from a similar journaling practice with their own venerated texts.

As one woman mentions, her therapist uses Bible journaling as one means to work with her client in reframing negative childhood messaging she received from her church. In some contexts, this approach might be deemed to belong to the realm of spiritual direction rather than professional therapy. Spiritual directors may well decide this practice would beneficially suit certain directees. Those who use art therapy would be well served by some knowledge of multimodal analysis and the social semiotics of visual expression.

In Bible journaling, many women find a spiritual practice that supports them in their recovery from addiction and the establishment of a new self-image. Through Bible journaling, these women contend with their pasts and acquire a new status understanding themselves as forgiven and loved by their God and supported through God's promises in Scripture. Their pain is assuaged, losses faced and a new future heralded. The foundational text of their faith is engaged with in a very tactile and immersive way: keywords reiterated in stickers, letters cut from magazines, naive drawings and pencil-crayoned self-portraits alongside highlighted verses, weaving images and words together in a newly wrought interpretation that speaks directly to their particular situation. Through this practice, many women take what was and what never was and create what is "me", "a new creation" (2 Cor 5:17) able to carve out a new life and cope with the challenges of living.

Bible journaling emerges, in the last five or six years, as a new contemplative and reflective practice, performed almost exclusively by women. Through this creative engagement with their holy Scriptures, women become first-hand receivers and interpreters of these texts, in the private domain of this personal devotional reading and creative intervention. They become the first interpreters of a divine word spoken to them and internalised through this lengthy and elaborate, creative engagement. This practice generally happens either individually, or in small groups of women, and is shared in online groups that are likewise almost exclusively female. In other words, this is biblical interpretation and appropriation happening beyond and outside of the often highly controlled, patriarchal and male-clerical space of the organised religion of Sunday morning. These women are becoming authoritative readers and interpreters of their own Scriptures. This is profoundly significant and, I contend, must have enduring consequences for their mental health, their lives, their families and their churches as they develop spiritual autonomy in relation to, and with, their holy texts.

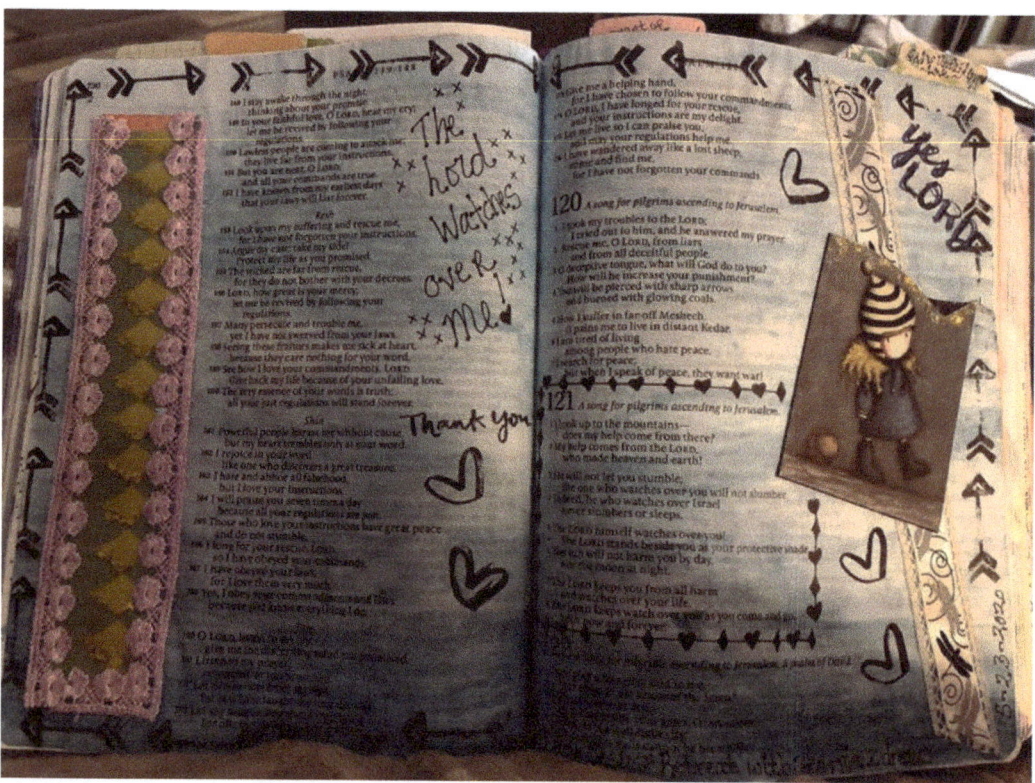

Figure 11. Psalm 121. With kind permission of the journaler.

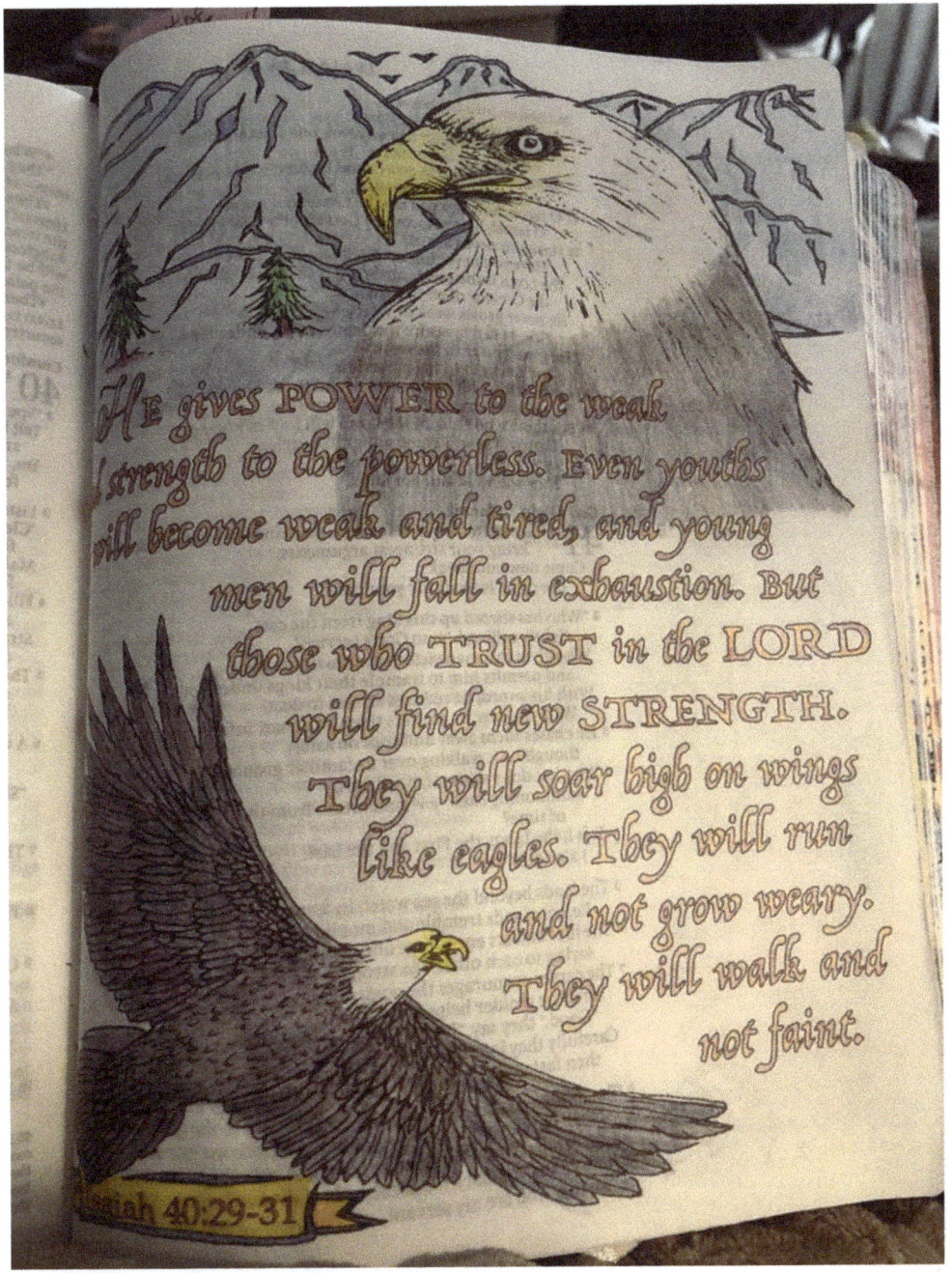

Figure 12. Isaiah 40:29–31. With kind permission of the journaler.

Funding: This research received no external funding.

Institutional Review Board Statement: Ethical review and approval were waived for this study, due to the methods being applied complying with professional reflective practice analysing images. No new interventions or artworks were created in the course of the research conducted.

Informed Consent Statement: Informed consent was obtained from all subjects involved in the study.

Conflicts of Interest: The author declares no conflict of interest.

Notes

[1] The Bible, as it exists today and is named and discussed in this article, consists of three parts: the Hebrew Bible, the Apocrypha, and the New Testament. The Hebrew Bible or Tanakh contains the canonical collection of Hebrew Scriptures, including the Torah ("Teaching"), Nevi'im ("Prophets") and Ketuvim ("Writings"), composed between roughly 900 BCE (possibly later) and 160 BCE in Hebrew or Aramaic. The Hebrew Bible shares much of its content with its ancient Greek translation, known of as the Septuagint. It is important to note that these texts predate the emergence of Christianity and the Christian writings of the first and second centuries CE. The Hebrew Bible is also venerated by Christians. It came to form the first and larger part of the Christian Bible and is referred to as the Old Testament, in the Christian Bible. Within Christianity, the Roman Catholic church, Eastern/Greek/Ethiopian Orthodox churches and some Protestant churches recognise and include varying numbers of additional books as belonging to a second division, within the OT, named the Apocrypha. There are many differing traditions across denominations and religious groupings concerning which books belong in the canons of Scripture. The New Testament consists of 27 books. It was composed and redacted over a period of about a century, by diverse authors, in Greek, between about 40 CE and 140 CE. It was recognised as a canon of Scripture formally in the Christian church in the fourth century. The Bible contains texts recognised as divinely inspired by adherents of Judaism, Christianity, Islam and other faiths.

[2] Percocet 30 mg. Percocet is a medication used to help relieve moderate to severe pain. It contains an opioid pain reliever (oxycodone) and a non-opioid pain reliever (acetaminophen).

[3] The 12 step programme has many strong advocates within the addiction recovery literature, including from those who vouch for it enabling spirituality to be factored into a holistic approach to and for the person in recovery (see Plante 2018; Rohr 2011; Ringwald 2002). Others, however, are critical of this method and how the spiritual dimension is dealt with (see Szalavitz 2019).

[4] Bible journaling has proven extremely lucrative for the publishing industry. Almost every US Bible publisher now offers many versions of a journaling Bible. Many popular translations are available as a journaling Bible, including but not limited to CSB, ESV, GNT, NAB, NIV, NKJB, NLT and NRSV, and where relevant, include Catholic editions. Some publishers have a multiplicity of versions, packaged in a variety of formats, targeted at different demographics. Some publish selected books of the Bible, such as the Psalms and Proverbs, separately. Journalers' choices are made based on both preferred translation as well as the attractiveness and functionality of the book design. Comparing and contrasting these many different translations and editions are frequent topics of discussion in the many dedicated social media groups. Many journalers have more than one Bible journal 'on the go' at any one time, sometimes preferring one translation of a particular text over another. Some journal a Bible as a gift. One woman, not included in this study, was journaling her journey through drug addiction recovery as a legacy she would be handing on to her children in time, in order that they might understand what she been through and how these texts had shaped her recovery.

References

Adams, Kathleen. 2004. *Scribing the Soul: Essays in Journal Therapy*. Denver: Center for Journal Therapy.
Alexander, Bruce K. 2008. *The Globalisation of Addiction: A Study in Poverty of the Spirit*. Oxford: OUP.
Allen, Pat B. 1995. *Art is a Way of Knowing*. Boston: Shambala.
Andermahr, Sonya, and Silvia Pellicer-Ortín. 2013. *Trauma Narratives and Herstory*. Basingstoke: Palgrave Macmillan. [CrossRef]
Apostolos-Cappadona, Diane. 2020. *A Guide to Christian Art*. London: T&T Clark Bloomsbury.
Barr, Beth Allison. 2021. *The Making of Biblical Womanhood: How the Subjugation of Women Became Gospel Truth*. Ada: Baker Publishing.
Beal, Timothy. 2012. *The Rise and Fall of the Bible: The Unexpected History of an Accidental Book*. New York: Houghton Mifflin Harcourt.
Bedi, Ashok, and Joseph H. Pereira. 2020. *The Spiritual Paradox of Addiction, The Call for the Transcendent*. Lake Worth: Nicholas Hays, Inc.
Budd, Luann. 2002. *Journal Keeping, Writing for Spiritual Growth*. Downers Grove: IVP.
Burrus, Virginia. 1999. An Immoderate Feast: Augustine Reads John's Apocalypse. In *History, Apocalypse, and the Secular Imagination: New Essay's on Augustine's City of God*. Edited by Mark Vessey, Karla Pollmann and Allan D. Fitzgerald. Bowling Green: Philosophy Documentation Centre, pp. 183–94.
Byrd, Aimee. 2020. *Recovering from Biblical Manhood and Womanhood: How the Church Needs to Rediscover Her Purpose*. Grand Rapids: Zondervan.
Cepero, Helen. 2008. *Journaling as a Spiritual Practice: Encountering God Through Attentive Writing*. Downers Grove: IVP.
Claassens, L. Juliana M. 2020. *Writing and Reading to Survive: Biblical and Contemporary Trauma Narratives in Conversation*. Sheffield: Sheffield Phoenix Press.
DeWeerdt, Sarah. 2019. Tracing the US opioid crisis to its roots. *Nature* 573: S10–S12. [CrossRef]

Dillon, Amanda. 2020. Be Your Own Scribe: Bible Journaling and the New Illuminators of the Densely Printed Page. In *From Scrolls to Scrolling: Sacred Texts, Materiality, and Dynamic Media Cultures*. Edited by Bradford A. Anderson. Berlin and Boston: De Gruyter, pp. 157–78. [CrossRef]
Etherington, Kim. 2008. *Trauma, Drug Misuse and Transforming Identities. A Life Story Approach*. London: Jessica Kingsley Publishers.
Fischer, Melissa, and Kate Peiffer. 2019. *Bible Journaling for the Fine Artist*. Mission Viejo: Quatro.
Gibney, Alex. 2021. The Crime of the Century. HBO Documentary. Available online: https://www.hbo.com/documentaries/the-crime-of-the-century (accessed on 27 July 2021).
Grisel, Judith. 2019. *Never Enough: The Neuroscience and Experience of Addiction*. London: Scribe.
Hall, James. 1994. *Illustrated Dictionary of Symbols in Eastern and Western Art*. London: John Murray.
Hassan, Sumayah. 2016. What is Quran Journaling? How do you set up your Quran Journal? November 27. Available online: https://www.recitereflect.com/what-is-quran-journaling/ (accessed on 27 July 2021).
Hieb, Marianne. 2005. *Inner Journeying Through Art-Journaling: Learning to See and Record your Life as a Work of Art*. London: Jessica Kingsley Publishers.
Jewitt, Carey. 2014. An Introduction to Multimodality. In *The Routledge Handbook of Multimodal Analysis*, 2nd ed. Edited by Carey Jewitt. London: Routledge, pp. 14–27.
Jones, Brian C. 2009. Wilderness. In *NIDB*. Nashville: Abingdon, vol. 5, pp. 848–52.
Kobes Du Mez, Kristin. 2020. *Jesus and John Wayne: How White Evangelicals Corrupted a Faith and Fractured a Nation*. New York: Liveright.
Kress, Gunther, and Theo van Leeuwen. 2021. *Reading Images, The Grammar of Visual Design*, 3rd ed. London: Routledge.
Leonard, Alison. 1995. *Telling Our Stories: Wrestling with a Fresh Language for the Spiritual Journey*. London: Darton, Longman and Todd.
Lukinsky, Joseph. 1990. Reflective Withdrawal Through Journal Writing. In *Fostering Critical Reflection in Adulthood: A Guide to Transformative and Emancipatory Learning*. Edited by Jack Mezirow and Assoc. San Francisco: Jossey-Bass.
Maisel, Eric, and Susan Raeburn. 2008. *Creative Recovery, A Complete Addiction Treatment Program That Uses Your Natural Creativity*. Boulder: Trumpeter.
Massyngberde Ford, J. 1975. *Revelation*. AYB. New Haven: Yale University Press.
Maté, Gabor. 2018. *In the Realm of Hungry Ghosts: Close Encounters with Addiction*. London: Vermillion.
Milner, Marion. 1986. *A Life of One's Own*. London: Virago.
Moon, Jennifer A. 2004. *A Handbook of Reflective and Experiential Learning: Theory and Practice*. London: RoutledgeFalmer.
Nichols Hickman, Lisa. 2013. *Writing in the Margins: Connecting with God on the Pages of Your Bible*. Nashville: Abingdon Press.
Ó Tuama, Pádraig. 2015. *In the Shelter: Finding a Home in the World*. London: Hodder and Stoughton.
Peace, Richard. 1995. *Spiritual Journaling: Recording Your Journey Toward God*. Colorado Springs: NavPress.
Pennebaker, James W. 2004. *Writing to Heal: A Guided Journal for Recovering from Trauma & Emotional Upheaval*. Denver: Center for Journal Therapy.
Plante, Thomas G. 2018. *Healing with Spiritual Practices: Proven Techniques for Disorders from Addictions and Anxiety to Cancer and Chronic Pain*. Santa Barbara: Praeger.
Progoff, Ira. 1975. *At a Journal Workshop: Writing to Access the Power of the Unconscious and Evoke Creative Ability*. New York: Penguin.
Progoff, Ira. 1983. *Life-Study, Experiencing Creative Lives by the Intensive Journal Method*. New York: Dialogue House.
Ringwald, Christopher D. 2002. *The Soul of Recovery: Uncovering the Spiritual Dimension in the Treatment of Addictions*. Oxford: OUP.
Rohr, Richard. 2011. *Breathing Under Water: Spirituality and the Twelve Steps*. Cincinnati: St Anthony Messenger Press.
Schüssler Fiorenza, Elizabeth. 1991. *Revelation: Vision of a Just World*. Edinburgh: T&T Clark.
Stoicea, Nicoleta, Andrew Costa, Luis Periel, Alberto Uribe, Tristan Weaver, and Sergio D. Bergese. 2019. Current perspectives on the opioid crisis in the US healthcare system. A comprehensive literature review. *Medicine* 98: 20. [CrossRef] [PubMed]
Stulman, Louis. 2014. Reading the Bible through the Lens of Trauma and Art. In *Trauma and Traumatisation in Individual and Collective Dimensions: Insights from Biblical Studies and Beyond*. Edited by Eve-Marie Becker, Jan Dochhorn and Else K. Holt. Göttingen: Vandenhoeck and Ruprecht, pp. 177–92.
Szalavitz, Maia. 2019. *Unbroken Brain: A Revolutionary New Way of Understanding Addiction*. New York: Picador.
Theroux, Louis. 2017. Dark States—Heroin Town. BBC Documentary. Available online: https://www.bbcstudios.com/case-studies/louis-theroux-dark-states-heroin-town/ (accessed on 27 July 2021).
Thompson, Leonard L. 1997. *The Book of Revelation: Apocalypse and Empire*. Oxford: OUP.
Unsworth, Len. 2008. *Multimodal Semiotics: Functional Analysis in Contexts of Education*. London: Routledge.
Van Leeuwen, Theo. 2005. *Introducing Social Semiotics*. London: Routledge.
Yarbro Collins, Adele. 1979. *The Apocalypse*. Dublin: Veritas.

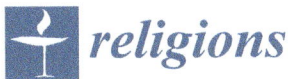

Article

The Workaholism Phenomenon in Portugal: Dimensions and Relations with Workplace Spirituality

Lisete S. Mónico [1],* and Clara Margaça [2]

[1] Faculty of Psychology and Educational Sciences, University of Coimbra, 3000-115 Coimbra, Portugal
[2] Faculty of Psychology, University of Salamanca, 37005 Salamanca, Spain; claramargaca@usal.es
* Correspondence: lisete.monico@fpce.uc.pt

Abstract: Workaholism phenomenon affects a quarter of the employed world population. The concept has been used to describe hardworking employees, which is not resulting from external requirements. Considering that organizations with well-developed workplace spirituality have employees more committed to achieving self-development, but also to serve the company, the relationship between workaholism and workplace spirituality is not straightforward, remaining unclear. The principal aim of this research is to analyze the workaholism phenomenon, considering patterns of workaholic and non-workaholic workers and their relationships with dimensions of workplace spirituality. The sample is comprised of a heterogeneous group of 306 Portuguese employees, who were surveyed by the Workaholism Battery, five dimensions of Workplace Spirituality, and a sociodemographic questionnaire. Cluster analysis defined three workaholic profiles (24% of the sample), and five non-workaholic profiles. Workplace spirituality dimensions differed according to worker profile and associations with work involvement, work enjoyment, and compulsive work addiction. Enthusiastic addicts and work enthusiasts showed the highest workplace spirituality, contrasting mainly with Reluctant hard worker, Disenchanted workers, and Unengaged workers, but also with work addicts. Workaholism is a complex and multidimensional phenomenon, whose dimensions are distinctly related to workplace spirituality. Workplace spirituality development can promote a more balanced and healthy relationship with work.

Keywords: workaholism; workplace spirituality; worker profiles; Portuguese employees

Citation: Mónico, Lisete S., and Clara Margaça. 2021. The Workaholism Phenomenon in Portugal: Dimensions and Relations with Workplace Spirituality. *Religions* 12: 852. https://doi.org/10.3390/rel12100852

Academic Editors: Bernadette Flanagan and Noelia Molina

Received: 27 July 2021
Accepted: 20 September 2021
Published: 11 October 2021

Publisher's Note: MDPI stays neutral with regard to jurisdictional claims in published maps and institutional affiliations.

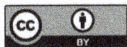

Copyright: © 2021 by the authors. Licensee MDPI, Basel, Switzerland. This article is an open access article distributed under the terms and conditions of the Creative Commons Attribution (CC BY) license (https://creativecommons.org/licenses/by/4.0/).

1. Introduction

The workaholism phenomenon affects a quarter of the employed population and it is described as a tendency to be obsessed with work duties and to work excessively hard. Furthermore, an all-consuming devotion to work is related to a set of undesirable consequences. This concept has been used to describe hardworking employees, which is not resulting from external requirements. Workaholics have persistent thoughts about work, experience negative emotions when not working (Clark et al. 2020), feel compelled to work as addicted, being deprived of activities in other areas of life, including family and relationships. Several researches provide robust evidence that workaholism is an addiction to work that leads to many negative individual, interpersonal, and organizational outcomes (Clark et al. 2016), and is characterized by working excessively (Schaufeli et al. 2008). According to Balducci et al. (2020a), there is a certain consensus regarding the definition of workaholism: being obsessed with work, a significant psychological dysfunction characterized by an excessive concern with work, and an uncontrollable internal desire to invest too much in work activities.

In Portugal, in 2010, it was estimated that 10% of workers would be workaholics (Cristão 2010), a behavior that causes negative emotions (e.g., guilt, anxiety, disappointment) and unpleasant activated emotions (e.g., irritability, hostility). In addition, the compulsion to work hinders the psychological disconnection from work and can influence the individual's ability to recover negatively, which also has an impact on physical health (Ornek and Kolac 2020). In 2019, Forbes pointed out that 66% of millennials suffered from workaholism, a trend that has worsened with the pandemic that has plagued all corners of the world since the end of that year (Stahl 2019).

In the workplace, the experience of being connected to others and the community environmental work, as well as the recognition that employees have an inner life that nourishes and is nourished by significant work, where they endow their energy, is associated with workplace spirituality (Foster and Foster 2019). According to Bella et al. (2018), workplace spirituality facilitates the promotion of opportunities for personal growth and fulfillment, as well as opportunities for significant contribution to society. Thus, it allows meeting individuals' needs for inner life, purpose, and community, which translates into a more sustainable way of working and living. Considering that organizations with well-developed workplace spirituality have employees more committed to achieving self-development, but also to serve the company, the relationship between workaholism and workplace spirituality is not straightforward, remaining unclear.

As a result of Covid-19 pandemic, the limits between work and personal life have become a very tenuous line. This happens because working from home is ingrained into family life, which affects relationships, as well as physical and mental health. Globalized competition, characteristic of modern societies, contributes to perpetuating workaholic behavior, which is reflected in a long workday, reinforced by tangible (e.g., promotion) and intangible (e.g., compliment) rewards (Balducci et al. 2020a). Thus, workplace spirituality can be a key factor; it is a multidimensional construct and a positive means to improve the success and competitiveness of organizations, as well as employees' well-being. The promotion of the workplace spirituality dimension is related to more responsible and pro-social behaviors (Dhiman and Marques 2016). Bearing in mind that the workplace is considered an inseparable part of human life and a source of values in communities, organizations can be seen as spiritual entities (Fairholm 1996). In this way, and in line with the 2030 Agenda, it is possible to affirm that workplace spirituality contributes to sustainability, insofar as the inherent values (i.e., a sense of community, care for others and for nature) will influence the future generations (Afsar and Badir 2017; Rezapouraghdam et al. 2019). Hence, workplace spirituality can be a path to sustainable development.

The principal aim of this study is to analyze the workaholism phenomenon, considering patterns of workaholic and non-workaholic workers, and their relationships with dimensions of workplace spirituality.

2. Background

2.1. Workaholism: Work Addicts or Work Engaged?

Especially in Western countries, the world of work has undergone profound changes in the past forty years. Today's workers have no time to leave the office, work longer days, and still take work home (Aziz and Tronzo 2011). Oates (1971) refers that a workaholic is a person "whose need for work has become so excessive that it creates noticeable disturbance or interference with his bodily health, personal happiness, and interpersonal relations, and with his smooth social functioning" (p. 4). Spence and Robbins (1992) define this concept as a set of attitudes, classified into three components: work involvement (limits between work and personal life), drive (internal motivation), and enjoyment of work (satisfaction obtained with work). It is described as an internal motivation to become overly involved in work, ignoring other areas of daily life (Porter 1996); vicious behavior (Atroszko et al. 2019) that leads to mood swings, withdrawal symptoms, conflict (Griffiths 2005); behaviors that include: working on breaks and during meals, not being able to delegate work; or yet, according to Ng et al. (2007), it encompasses three dimensions—affective (enjoying the act of working), cognitive (obsessed with work), and behavioral (working more hours than is due).

Several studies pointed out that workaholism as being associated with worse general well-being indices (e.g., Balducci et al. 2018; Schaufeli et al. 2008), as well as worse physical and mental health, and is related to many negative outcomes, such as burnout, job stress, work-life conflict (e.g., Clark et al. 2016). Therefore, workaholism cannot be seen as a positive characteristic indicating a healthy passion and enthusiasm for one's work not even to be associated with higher job performance (Balducci et al. 2020b). But, rather, as an unhealthy characteristic of a vicious behavior that can have destructive consequences for the individual's emotional, social and physical well-being (Stoeber and Damian 2016). It is important to note that the concepts of workaholism and engagement at work are often confused. The main difference between both is related to motivation, the trigger of behaviors. Briefly, workaholics feel an internal compulsion to work, whereas engaged workers see the act of working as intrinsically pleasurable (Subramanian 2018).

It is important to highlight that, with the mandatory confinement caused by the Covid-19 pandemic, the forced work-at-home scenario may have caused an increase in the workaholism situation (Molino et al. 2020; Spagnoli and Molinaro 2020). If there are benefits (such as reduced travel time), the consequences include a blurred line between work and family, social isolation, employees bearing the costs (e.g., pay for the internet), and work more than the due time (Vyas and Butakhieo 2020).

2.2. Spirituality: A Linkage between Workplace and Wellbeing

Workplace Spirituality (WS) has been the subject of several studies in recent years as a prominent reality (Mónico et al. 2016). In a plural society, where tolerance and spiritual and cultural freedom are sought, is crucial a true understanding of the place of different religions and spiritualities in the organizational environment (Wall and Knights 2013). Several studies were reported WS as a necessary determinant of employee commitment, job satisfaction and work-life balance satisfaction (e.g., Garg 2017). Research conducted by Pawar (2016) highlights that WS has a positive relationship with emotional, psychological, social, and spiritual well-being. However, a study by Foster and Foster (2019) revealed that most employees considered that spirituality was not something they felt comfortable discussing or appropriate to practice in the workplace.

Spirituality is independent of any religion or belief system, considered as a complex, multi-cultural and multi-dimensional concept (Mónico et al. 2016; Zsolnai and Illes 2017), and possesses a social basis and a social dimension (Oman 2015). It refers to an inner experience of an individual and can also be understood as the capacity to find and construct meaning about life and existence and to move toward personal growth, responsibility, and relationship with others (Myers and Williard 2003).

Samah et al. (2012) highlight the role of the organization as fundamental in the development of the spiritual needs of its employees. A study conducted by Kolodinsky et al. (2008) highlighted that WS is positively related to involvement and job satisfaction, organizational identification, and negatively related to organizational frustration. Another study demonstrated that there is a positive correlation between psychological capital and workaholism, and both have positive and direct repercussion on WS (Pedreira and Mónico 2013). Spirituality, when integrated into the professional environment, can lead to a greater seek for fulfillment (Fry 2003), as well as the development of a sense of community, through a connection with something greater (Marques et al. 2005). In other words, spiritual individuals tend to consider their role in employment to be significant (Tepper 2003), as spirituality is related to the commitment to the organization, which triggers an increase in engagement (Pawar 2016), personal and positive values (Murray and Evers 2011), as loyalty to the organization (Rego and Cunha 2008). According to Roof (2015), spirituality can significantly affect engagement, which translates into a direct relationship between spirituality-engagement. Hence, the significant effort of an engaged employee reflects pleasure at work, unlike the workaholic who does it out of compulsion (Clark et al. 2020). Several studies (e.g., Rahman et al. 2019; van der Walt and Klerk 2014) highlighted that spirituality in the workplace triggers positive results for organizations because it is strongly associated with engagement at work. According to Duchon and Plowma (2005), these concepts are associated with the sense of fulfillment and completeness, allowing employees to express themselves as a whole and to feel safe psychologically in the workplace, synonymous of a significant motivational effect (Bickerton et al. 2015).

3. Method

3.1. Participants

The sample is comprised of a heterogeneous group of 306 Portuguese employees from a wide variety of jobs and Portuguese's enterprises. A diverse sample of respondents was intended, including both genders, different ages, professions and positions, experiences and work systems. Of these respondents, 55.9% were female and 44.1% were male, with an average age of 40.34 years, (SD = 10.93). Regarding education, 30.1% of participants completed basic education, 34.6% completed secondary education and 35.3% completed higher education. With regard to the professional situation of the respondents, the majority are employed (56.9%), followed by State workers (20.6%) and businesspersons (14.4). The rest fall into the categories of self-employed professionals (3.6%) and student workers (4.6%). It is important to highlight that 31.4% of the sample occupies some leadership position. With regard to the number of employees of the organization where the participants work, the majority (35.0%) work in a company with a maximum of 10 employees or in companies with 11 to 50 employees (29.7%). Participants have an average of 12 years of working time in the current organization. When analyzing the monthly net salary, almost half of the sample (45%) earns between 501 and 1000 euros monthly; another half receives up to 500 euros (20.9%) or between 1001 and 1500 euros (20.3%). The remaining participants receive between 1501 and 2000 (8.5%) and a salary above 2000 euros (4.9%). Table 1 presents the sociodemographic characteristics of participants.

Table 1. Sociodemographic characterization of the sample [N = 306].

		Sample			
		n	%	M	SD
Gender	Female	171	55.9		
	Male	135	44.1		
Age	(min 18, max 69 years-old)			40.34	10.93
Education	Basic Education	92	30.1		
	Secondary Education	106	34.6		
	Higher Education	108	35.3		
Professional Situation	Employed	174	56.9		
	State workers	63	20.6		
	Businesspersons	44	14.4		
	Self-employed	11	3.6		
	Student-workers	14	4.6		
Leadership Position	Yes	96	31.4		
	No	210	68.6		
	Stay in the organization (min 0, max 56 years)			12.09	10.50
N° employees per organization	Up to 10	107	35.0		
	Between 11 and 50	91	29.7		
	Between 51 and 200	42	13.7		
	More than 200	66	21.6		
Net Salary	Up to 500 euros	64	20.9		
	Between 501 and 1000 euros	138	45.1		
	Between 1001 and 1500 euros	62	20.3		
	Between 1501 and 2000 euros	26	8.8		
	More than 2000 euros	16	4.9		

3.2. Research Tools

3.2.1. The Workaholism Battery

This battery (WorkBat), performed by Spence and Robbins (1992), is the widest instrument used in the investigation of workaholism, which is composed of different aspects of the relationship of employees with work and with the use of free time. The version adopted in this research was based on a standardized translation-back-translation procedure of the original by Andreassen et al. (2010). The whole questionnaire, composed of 25 items measured through a 5-point Likert scale (1-strongly disagree to 5-strongly agree), showed good reliability (α = 0.80). Confirmatory factor analysis supports the tri-factor model (CMIN/DF = 2.53, NFI = 0.68, RMSEA = 0.071; one error term correlated between items belonging to the same factor, based on the highest modification indices): (F1) Work Involvement—the use of time and energy in or out of work (8 items; ex: "I feel guilty when I miss work"); (F2) Drive—the internal motivation of people to work, level of drive to work (7 items; ex: "I often feel that there is something inside me that makes me work"); and (F3) Enjoyment of Work—the level of pleasure from work obtained through responses (10 items; ex: "I work more than is waited for me closely for its fun").

3.2.2. Workplace Spirituality Scale

For the assessment of spirituality in workplace, it was adopted a 6-point Likert scale (1-This sentence is completely false to 6-This sentence is completely true) from Rego and Pina e Rego and Cunha (2008), composed of 17 items with excellent reliability (α = 0.93). The second-order factor model showed an acceptable fit (CMIN/DF = 2.873, NFI = 0.91, RMSEA = 0.078), composed of five dimensions: (F1) Team's sense of community—the sense of community and common purpose, team spirit and mutual care among members (5 items, α = 0.93; e.g., "People in my group/team feel part of a family"); (F2) Alignment between organizational and individual values—the compatibility of the individual's values and inner life with the organization's values, mission and purposes (5 items, α = 0.88; e.g., "I feel good about the values that prevail in my organization"); (F3) Sense of contribution to the community—the relationship between work and personal values (3 items, α = 0.80; e.g., "I see that there is a connection between my work and the benefits for society as a whole"); (F4) Sense of enjoyment at work—the sense of pleasure and enjoyment at work (2 items, α = 0.78; e.g., "I feel joy in my work"); and (F5) Opportunities for the inner life—the organization's respect to the individual's spiritual values and the spirituality of the workers (2 items, α = 0.75; e.g., (reversed item): "My spiritual values are not valued in my workplace").

3.3. Procedure

Data collection was carried out in person by a research team, in Portugal, including the Autonomous Regions of Madeira and Azores, before the pandemic period. This team was composed by students of the subject Methodology of Research in Psychology of the integrated master in Psychology of the University of Coimbra. All the formal and ethical procedures of data collection were respected. Information was given about the purpose of the study and how participants should respond, explaining to them that the participation was anonymous and data will be used exclusively for academic purposes, despite can be suspended at any time. Participants agreed to informed consent, with the guarantee of the protection of their data, which includes anonymity and confidentiality. The inclusion criteria to be in the sample was that the employees have at least six months of professional experience and are currently working. Therefore, the type of enterprise or business structure was not defined.

3.4. Data Analysis

The tabulating and data analysis were performed through the statistical programs SPSS and AMOS (IBM Corp 2013). Missing values (1.6%) were replaced through series mean method Skewness and kurtosis values indicate a normal distribution, |Sk| < 1.30 and |Ku| < 1.73.

Reliability was calculated by Cronbach's alpha (Nunnally and Bernstein 1994). The score of 0.80 was taken as a good reliability indicator (Urbina 2014), and 0.70 as acceptable (Hair et al. 2018). Confirmatory factor analysis (CFA) was carried out with the maximum likelihood estimation method. Goodness of fit was analyzed using CMIN/DF (normed chi-square), NFI (normed fit index), and RMSEA (Root Mean Square Error of Approximation) (Kline 2011; Schumacker and Lomax 2016). Modification indices (MI) were used to determine how the fit of the model could be improved (Bollen 1989), and we considered freeing the parameters with higher MI inside each factor.

The predictive power of the dimensions was tested using hierarchical regression analysis. This method allows the researcher to enter independent variables cumulatively according to some specified hierarchy that is dictated in advance by the theory and logic of the research (Tabachnick and Fidell 2007). The assumptions of the hierarquical multiple regression were analyzed. Normal distribution and homogeneity were validated graphically. Independence of errors was obtained through the Durbin-Watson statistic, with scores between 0.92 and 1.28. The Variance Inflation Factor was used to diagnose multicollinearity, none of the variables being collinear (VIFs < 2.95).

After the descriptive statistics and intercorrelation matrix, two-step cluster analysis were performed with the WorkBat dimensions, leading to a classification of the participants into groups (low/high) in each dimension, and subsequently in the workaholic profiles. This is a hybrid approach that first uses a measure of distance to separate groups and after a probabilistic approach to choose the ideal subgroup (Kent et al. 2014). Using this technique allow to determine the number of clusters based on a statistical measure of fit, through the use of categorical and continuous variables simultaneously, analyzing the outliers (Kent et al. 2014). Several studies have proved this analysis to be one of the most reliable in terms of the number of subgroups detected, probability of classification of individuals into subgroups, and reproducibility of findings in clinical and other types of data (Gelbard et al. 2007; Kent et al. 2014). The distance measure was calculated by the Log-Likelihood method. The classification of clusters was done by using the Schwarz's Bayesian Criterion, which indicated for each dimension of WorkBat the number of clusters with good quality of discrimination (silhouette measure of cohesion and separation >0.50).

A Multivariate Analysis of Variance (MANOVA) was subsequently conducted to test whether the workaholic profiles differ from each other regarding workplace spirituality. The assumptions for the reliable use of this test (Hair et al. 2018) were analyzed. Pillai's Trace was used because it is a powerful statistic procedure and very robust to modest violations of normality and equality of the covariance and variance matrix, Box's M = 189.26 $F(105, 12261.67) = 1.50$, $p = 0.001$. Post-hoc Bonferroni tests for multiple comparisons were performed.

4. Results

Table 2 presents the descriptive and intercorrelations of workaholism and workplace spirituality. On average, participants scored 4.24 (SD = 0.87) on the global workplace spirituality scale, slightly exceeding the midpoint of each scale, the same occurring for the three dimensions of the WorkBat. A correlation matrix was created to assess the levels of association among the variables. As displayed in Table 2, it is notable that the majority of the correlations were statistically significant, except for the correlations between Drive and TsenseCommunity ($r = 0.071$), the Involvement and oppInnerLife ($r = 0.039$), and between Drive and oppInnerLife ($r = -0.029$). According to Cohen's classification (Cohen 1988), high correlations are greater than 0.50, moderate correlations are between 0.30 and 0.50, and low correlations of 0.10 and 0.30 and 0.10 a zero. It should be noted that the correlation between the global scales was positive and moderate ($r = 0.40$, $p < 0.01$).

Table 2. Descriptive statistics (min, max, M, SD) and correlation matrix.

	Min.	Max.	Mean	SD	2	3	4	5	6	7	8	9
1. WorkBat-Work Involvement	2.25	5.00	3.42	0.54	0.342 **	0.277 **	0.165 **	0.115 *	0.175 **	0.173 **	0.128 *	0.039
2. WorkBat-Drive	1.14	5.00	3.15	0.66	1	0.274 **	0.131 *	0.071	0.180 **	0.148 **	0.115 *	−0.029
3. WorkBat-Enjoyment of work	1.10	5.00	3.02	0.64		1	0.496 **	0.376 **	0.402 **	0.441 **	0.594 **	0.230 **
4. WS_globalscale [i]	1.00	6.00	4.24	0.87			1	0.875 **	0.908 **	0.712 **	0.784 **	0.570 **
5. WS_TsenseCommunity [ii]	1.00	6.00	4.11	1.09				1	0.730 **	0.440 **	0.595 **	0.419 **
6. WS_Aligment [iii]	1.00	6.00	4.12	1.02					1	0.592 **	0.652 **	0.416 **
7. WS_senContribComun [iv]	1.00	6.00	4.51	1.05						1	0.646 **	0.228 **
8. WS_senseJoyment [v]	1.00	6.00	4.5	1.02							1	0.344 **
9. WS_OppInnerLife [vi]	1.00	6.00	4.23	1.27								1

[i] WS: Workplace Spirituality; [ii] WS_TsenseCommunity: Team's sense of community; [iii] WS_Aligment: Alignment between organizational and individual values; [iv] WS_senContribComun: Sense of contribution to the community; [v] WS_senseJoyment: Sense of enjoyment at work; [vi] WS_OppInnerLife: Opportunities for the inner life. ** $p < 0.01$; * $p < 0.05$.

To understand whether the workaholism dimensions can be predicted from the dimensions of workplace spirituality, it was conducted a hierarchical multiple regression (Table 3), controlling variables such as gender, age, education, stay in the organization, and a leadership role in the organization. This analysis allowed testing which dimensions of workplace spirituality had an effect on workaholism.

Table 3. Hierarchical Multiple Regression of dimensions of workaholism predicted by workplace spirituality.

*DV: Work Involvement	R	R^2	R^2_{adj}	ΔR^2	b	SE	ß	t
	0.272	0.074	0.043	0.035				
Gender (1 = male; 2 = female)					−0.08	0.06	−0.07	−1.22
Age (years)					0.00	0.00	−0.08	−0.98
Education (years)					0.00	0.01	−0.01	−0.09
Leadership role (1 = yes; 0 = no)					0.18	0.07	0.16	2.54 *
Stay in the organization (years)					0.00	0.00	−0.02	−0.31
WS_senseCommunity					−0.02	0.04	−0.03	−0.39
WS_Aligment					0.06	0.05	0.12	1.24
WS_senContribComun					0.07	0.04	0.14	1.71
WS_senseJoyment					0.00	0.05	−0.01	−0.08
WS_OppInnerLife					−0.02	0.03	−0.05	−0.74
*DV: Drive	0.286	0.082	0.050	0.044				
Gender (1 = male; 2 = female)					0.05	0.08	0.04	0.67
Age (years)					−0.01	0.00	−0.11	−1.36
Education (years)					−0.01	0.02	−0.04	−0.67
Leadership role (1 = yes; 0 = no)					0.23	0.09	0.17	2.69 **
Stay in the organization (years)					0.00	0.00	0.08	0.97
WS_TsenseCommunity					−0.09	0.05	−0.14	−1.66
WS_Aligment					0.15	0.06	0.24	2.49 *
WS_senContribComun					0.04	0.05	0.06	0.73
WS_senseJoyment					0.02	0.05	0.03	0.38
WS_OppInnerLife					−0.06	0.03	−0.11	−1.70
*DV: Enjoyment of work	0.634	0.402	0.382	0.349				
Gender (1 = male; 2 = female)					−0.01	0.06	−0.01	−0.14
Age (years)					−0.01	0.00	−0.16	−2.36 *
Education (years)					0.03	0.01	0.11	2.30 *
Leadership role (1 = yes; 0 = no)					0.15	0.07	0.11	2.27 *
Stay in the organization (years)					0.00	0.00	0.06	1.00
WS_TsenseCommunity					0.01	0.04	0.02	0.23
WS_Aligment					−0.02	0.05	−0.03	−0.34
WS_senContribComun					0.08	0.04	0.12	1.94
WS_senseJoyment					0.33	0.04	0.52	7.61 ***
WS_OppInnerLife					−0.01	0.03	−0.01	−0.25

*DV: Dependent Variable; *** $p < 0.001$; ** $p < 0.01$; * $p < 0.05$.

After statistical control of sociodemographic variables, it was possible to observe that not all the workplace spirituality' dimensions had the same importance in increasing workaholism' components. Regarding the shared variance of the dependent variable (R2), the predictors of this model explain 7.4% of Involvement, 8.2% of Drive, and 40.2% of Pleasure.

Considering control variables, only leadership role was a significant positive predictor of Involvement, Drive, and Enjoyment of work, with higher scores in these WorkBat dimensions estimated for individuals occupying a leadership position (e.g., director, CEO, manager, department responsible, etc.). For the dimension Drive, only leadership role and Alignment factor had a significant and positive prediction. Finally, for the third dimension of the workaholism (Enjoyment of work), it was possible to found age as a negative predictor, but also three positive and significant predictors: education, leadership role, and Sense of enjoyment at work.

Definition of Profiles of Workers

Each dimension of the Workaholism Battery was individually submitted to cluster analysis. Two clusters were obtained for Involvement, Drive, and Enjoyment of work, with good quality of discrimination (see Table 4).

Table 4. Number of clusters, quality of discrimination, number of participants in each cluster (n, %) and means (M) for the dimensions of the Workaholism Battery.

WorkBat Dimensions:	Number of Clusters (C)	Quality of Discrimination	C1—Low % (n)	M	C2—High % (n)	M
Work Involvement	2	0.7	63.7% (n = 195)	3.09	36.3% (n = 111)	4.00
Drive	2	0.7	65.4% (n = 200)	2.78	34.6% (n = 106)	3.86
Enjoyment of work	2	0.7	68.0% (n = 208)	2.68	32.0% (n = 281)	3.73

The joining of the participants' belonging to each of the clusters in the three dimensions of WorkBat led to the emergence of eight different profiles of workers, three representing workaholic profiles and five non-workaholic profiles:

Enthusiastic Addicts—They report high scores in the three dimensions of the workaholism scale (Spence and Robbins 1992). These "positively involved workers" (Aziz et al. 2010, p. 628), prototype of the ideal worker, spend a lot of time at work and think about it, but because working is a passion, by virtue of the enormous energy and positive affectivity that characterizes them. However, according to Aziz et al. (2010), both personal relationships and health can be harmed by excessive dedication to work. Additionally, they are "intrinsically and strongly motivated by loyalty, self-development and responsibility, and also, but to a lesser extent, by the level of their salaries" (Buelens and Poelmans 2004, p. 449). They are satisfied with the salary, the social relations, and did not intend to leave the organization. Although they do not report health complaints, they reported many conflicts between work and family.

Work Addicts—They have high scores on the dimensions of the scale of involvement with work and drive for work, and low scores on the dimension of pleasure from work (Spence and Robbins 1992). These workers spend too much time at work and thinking about it, maintaining a very unbalanced relationship between work and private life, despite work not being something they truly appreciate, they are perfectionists and have great difficulty in delegating tasks (Aziz et al. 2010). These workers report few sleeping hours and reduced free time. They have many conflicts at work and also family-work conflicts. Furthermore, they reveal dissatisfaction with salary, family, relationships.

Work Enthusiasts—those who achieve high scores on the scales of involvement and pleasure from work, and low scores on the drive to work (Spence and Robbins 1992). They are characterized as very hard-working, they like what they do, are always present and animated, and work long hours, even though the quality of their work is poor (Aziz et al. 2010). Enthusiastic workers are balanced people and have the ability to compensate in their physical and mental health for the effects of excess time spent at work—they also demonstrate a certain immunity to stress. Their high motivation seems to be stimulated "by all the factors that make people work harder, including money, responsibility, loyalty, and self-development" (Buelens and Poelmans 2004, p. 454).

Reluctant Hard Workers—This profile presents high scores in involvement dimension and low scores in drive and enjoyment dimensions of the workaholism scale (Spence and Robbins 1992). These workers reported relatively long working hours with a strong perception of pressure and a low perception of growth organizational culture. They intend to leave the organization, and are dissatisfied with the salary, the superior and even with their colleagues.

Alienated Professional—These workers score below the mean on the scales of involvement, and above the mean on drive to work and enjoyment (Spence and Robbins 1992). They are internally driven and happy but not really committed with the work. This might be a group of professionals devoted to their professional skills, but not to their job or organization.

Disenchanted Workers—These workers score below the mean on the scales of involvement and pleasure with work, and above the mean on drive to work (Spence and Robbins 1992). Aziz et al. (2010) consider it to be the most problematic profile, due to they are extremely poor in satisfaction and in a sense of purpose, their psychological results are very poor, they experience high levels of stress and they are the ones who spend the least time at work. According to Buelens and Poelmans (2004), these workers are tremendously alienated, unmotivated and dissatisfied with their work in all aspects.

Relaxed Workers—They have low scores on the work engagement and work drive scales, and high on work pleasure (Spence and Robbins 1992). Unmotivated by salaries, they do not experience great pressure at work and manage to maintain a good relationship between work and family life. They are workers with high emotional well-being, they present only some complaints at the psychosomatic level (Aziz et al. 2010). Although they appreciate the challenges at work, they just don't get involved with it (Buelens and Poelmans 2004).

Unengaged Workers—This profile presents low scores in all dimensions of the workaholism scale (Spence and Robbins 1992). These workers do not have great motivation to work, being at the service strictly contracted hours. Their lives are not guided by great satisfaction or a sense of purpose, are accommodated to professional careers and are not subjected to great pressure at work (Aziz et al. 2010).

In Table 5 it is possible to analyze each typology profile of worker in our sample, attending to the cluster (low/high) in each WorkBat dimension. The largest number comprised the unengaged workers (27.1%), followed in turn by disenchanted workers (17.6%), alienated professionals (16.7%), enthusiastic addicts (12.4%), relaxed workers (10.5%), work addicts (8.5%), and, finally, by reluctant hard workers and work enthusiast (3.9% and 3.3%, respectively). Represent workaholic profiles 24.2% of the sample, composed of Enthusiastic addicts (12.4%), Work addicts (8.5%), and Work enthusiasts (3.3%).

Table 5. Complete Spence and Robbins' typology (Spence and Robbins 1992) of worker profiles: samples' n and %.

WorkBat Dimensions:	Work Involvement	Drive	Enjoyment of Work	Worker Profile	n (%)
Cluster:	High	High	High	1—Enthusiastic addicts	38 (12.4)
	High	High	Low	2—Work addicts	26 (8.5)
	High	Low	High	3—Work enthusiasts	10 (3.3)
	High	Low	Low	4—Reluctant hard worker	12 (3.9)
	Low	High	High	5—Alienated professional	51 (16.7)
	Low	High	Low	6—Disenchanted workers	54 (17.6)
	Low	Low	High	7—Relaxed Workers	32 (10.5)
	Low	Low	Low	8—Unengaged workers	83 (27.1)

Note: adapted from Buelens and Poelmans (2004), p. 444.

A MANOVA was conducted to test whether the profiles differ from each other regarding Workplace Spirituality dimensions. A significant multivariate effect was obtained, Pillai's Trace = 0.308, $F(35, 1490) = 2.79$, $p < 0.001$, observed power = 1.00, $\eta^2_p = 0.065$ (multivariate effect size of 6.5%). Univariate tests are displayed in Table 6. Workplace spirituality dimensions differed according to the worker profile (univariate effect sizes between 11% and 22%), excluding Opportunities for the inner life ($p = 0.211$). Enthusiastic addicts and work enthusiasts presented the highest workplace spirituality. Work enthusiastic scored the highest value in the Sense of enjoyment at work, and Reluctant hard workers score the lowest value in the Alignment between organizational and individual values.

Table 6. Descriptive statistics (M; SD), Univariate tests (F), effect size (η^2_p) and observed power (1-β) of worker profiles.

Worker Profile:	Enthusiastic Addicts (n = 38)		Work Addicts (n = 26)		Work Enthusiast (n = 10)		Reluctant Hard Worker (n = 12)		Alienated Professional (n = 51)		Disenchanted Worker (n = 54)		Relaxed Worker (n = 32)		Unengaged (n = 83)		F	η^2_p	Observed Power
	M	SD	M	SD	M	SD	M	SD	M	SD	M	SD	M	SD	M	SD			
WS_TsenseCommunity	4.73	0.92	4.16	1.55	4.5	1.2	3.63	1.32	4.34	0.86	3.68	0.93	4.42	0.85	3.85	1.08	5.30 ***	0.11	0.998
WS_Aligment	4.80	0.86	4.21	1.27	4.42	1.18	3.58	1.31	4.46	0.7	3.82	0.94	4.25	0.76	3.74	1.02	7.12 ***	0.14	1.000
WS_senContribComun	5.15	1.03	4.36	1.05	5.1	0.52	4.23	1.61	4.71	0.86	4.21	0.95	4.86	0.82	4.15	1.05	6.08 ***	0.12	1.000
WS_senseJoy	5.22	0.65	4.06	1.42	5.4	0.7	4.29	1.42	4.89	0.7	4.11	0.79	4.89	0.66	4.09	1.01	11.7 ***	0.22	1.000
WS_OpptnerLife	4.55	1.33	4.12	1.5	4.3	1.32	3.88	1.54	4.38	1.1	4.11	1.1	4.58	1.22	4.01	1.33	1.38	0.03	0.586

*** $p < 0.001$.

Post-hoc Bonferroni tests were performed to examine the profiles' mean differences regarding the Workplace Spirituality (see Table 7 for significant mean differences). Regarding the Sense of community dimension, the biggest difference concerns the Enthusiastic addicts and Reluctant hard Worker profiles and the smallest difference concerns the Alienated professional and Disenchanted workers profiles, with a value of mean difference of 0.663. Regarding the Alignment dimension, the biggest difference concerns the Enthusiastic addicts and Reluctant hard Worker profiles and the Enthusiastic addicts and Unengaged workers. The smallest difference concerns the Alienated professional and Disenchanted workers profiles. Regarding the Sense of Contribution to Community dimension, the biggest difference concerns the Enthusiastic addicts and Unengaged workers profiles. The smallest difference concerns the Alienated professional and Unengaged workers profiles, with a value of mean difference of 0.558. Finally, regarding the Sense of enjoyment at work dimension, the biggest differences concern the Work Enthusiast and Work Addicts, and the Work Enthusiast and Disenchanted workers. The smallest difference concerns the Relaxed Workers and Disenchanted workers profiles.

Table 7. Workplace Spirituality means difference of each profile and multiple comparison tests between profiles.

Dependent Variable (WS Dimension)	Profiles	Mean Difference	SE	p
Alignment between organizational and individual values (WS_senseCommunity)	Enthusiastic addicts—Reluctant hard Worker	1.096	0.346	0.047
	Enthusiastic addicts—Disenchanted workers	1.050	0.221	0.000
	Enthusiastic addicts—Unengaged workers	0.878	0.204	0.001
	Alienated professional—Disenchanted workers	0.663	0.204	0.036
	Relaxed Workers—Disenchanted workers	0.746	0.233	0.042
Alignment between organizational and individual values (WS_Aligment)	Enthusiastic addicts—Reluctant hard Worker	1.218	0.317	0.004
	Enthusiastic addicts—Disenchanted workers	0.986	0.203	0.000
	Enthusiastic addicts—Unengaged workers	1.060	0.187	0.000
	Alienated professional—Disenchanted workers	0.647	0.187	0.017
	Alienated professional—Unengaged workers	0.721	0.17	0.001
Sense of contribution to the community (WS_senContribComun)	Enthusiastic addicts—Disenchanted workers	0.939	0.21	0.000
	Enthusiastic addicts—Unengaged workers	0.995	0.195	0.000
	Alienated professional—Unengaged workers	0.558	0.177	0.049
	Relaxed Workers—Unengaged workers	0.71	0.207	0.019
Sense of enjoyment at work (WS_senseJoy)	Enthusiastic addicts—Work Addicts	1.166	0.232	0.000
	Enthusiastic addicts—Disenchanted workers	1.113	0.139	0.000
	Enthusiastic addicts—Unengaged workers	1.133	0.179	0.000
	Work Enthusiast—Work Addicts	1.342	0.340	0.003
	Work Enthusiast—Disenchanted workers	1.289	0.314	0.001
	Work Enthusiast—Unengaged workers	1.310	0.305	0.001
	Alienated professional—Work Addicts	0.834	0.220	0.005
	Alienated professional—Disenchanted workers	0.781	0.178	0.000
	Alienated professional—Unengaged workers	0.802	0.162	0.000
	Relaxed workers—Work Addicts	0.833	0.241	0.017
	Relaxed Workers—Disenchanted workers	0.780	0.204	0.004

Figure 1 represents how the individuals perceive Workplace Spirituality in each worker profile, regarding the six workplace spirituality dimensions. In order to make it easier to perceive the differences among the profiles, standardized scores were used, based on the means of each workplace spirituality dimension. As we can see, Enthusiastic addicts and Work enthusiasts present the highest scores, contrasting mainly with Reluctant hard worker, Disenchanted workers, and Unengaged workers.

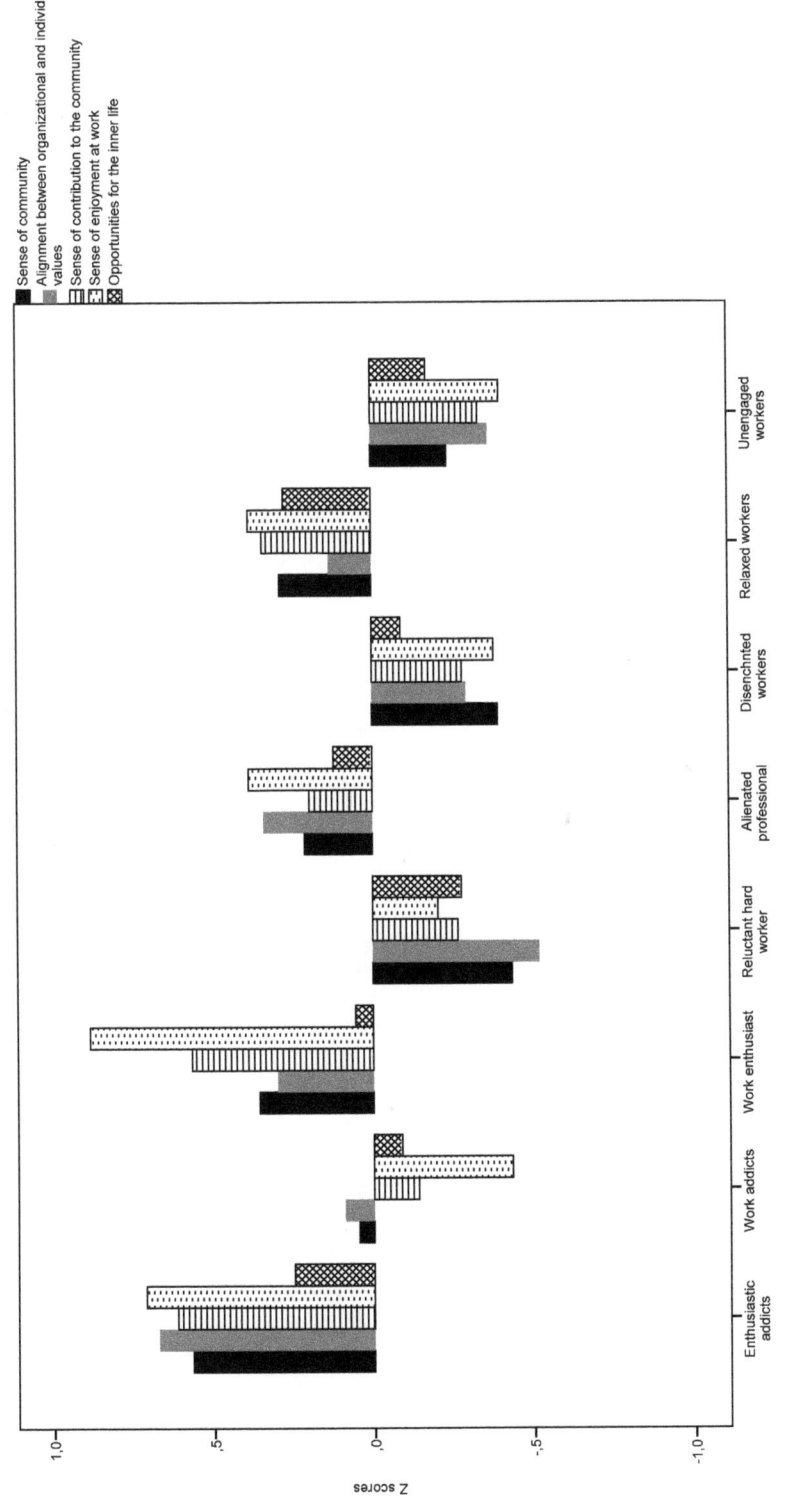

Figure 1. Workplace Spirituality dimensions in each worker profile: standardized scores.

5. Dicussion

The main objective of the article was to provide a better understanding of the study of workaholism, namely on the different profiles of workers and their respective relationships with the dimensions of the workplace spirituality. It was possible to observe that there is a low and positive relationship between the global scale of workplace spirituality and the workaholism dimensions Work Involvement and Drive, although a moderate relationship with Enjoyment of work. Assuming that spirituality is an internal resource that individuals can turn to, it is possible to assume that the higher the levels of workplace spirituality, the greater the probability of developing some worker profile involving a high Enjoyment of work (Enthusiastic addicts, Work enthusiasts, Alienated professional, or Relaxed Workers, according to Spence and Robbins' typology).

The results are in line with other studies carried out in Portugal (e.g., Pedreira and Mónico 2013). However, is pertinent to highlight the two other dimensions of WorkBat, and also other measures of workaholism. Indeed, some literature reveals a distinct approach. Spirituality can be understood as a resource to combat negative habits, reduce stress, contribute to general well-being (Goltz 2011), increase organizational commitment (Vandenberghe 2011), inspire greater performance (Smith and Futrell 2014), and allay the negative consequences of workaholism (Saxton 2016). Organizational climate, productivity/performance, commitment, trust, emotional intelligence, psychological capital, among other variables, have also been positively associated with workplace spirituality (e.g., Krishnakumar and Neck 2002; Mónico et al. 2016; Pedreira and Mónico 2013; Rego et al. 2007).

Considered as ideal and positively involved workers, addicted enthusiasts and enthusiastic workers, characterized by their balance between physical and mental health and work, are the groups that present the highest levels of workplace spirituality. The results are corroborated by the work of Rust and Gabriels (2011), when they state that when there is harmony between the company and the integration of employees' personal values (e.g., spirituality), everyone can aspire to greater things. Accordingly, as pointed out by Preziosi and Marschke (2011), the world of work in the 21st century wants to prosper more and more and, therefore, there is a need for both organizational leaders and their employees to use the spiritual resources, due to it will also make a significant contribution to society at large.

The cluster analysis allowed us to verify that it is the work enthusiast group who score the highest in the sense of pleasure and enjoyment at work. This result is consistent with the literature (e.g., Buelens and Poelmans 2004), which states that work enthusiasts are happy workers, love their jobs and avoid conflict both at workplace and at home. These behaviors can be related to the fact that they have a positive mindset, high levels of social intelligence (Buelens and Poelmans 2004) and the possibility of living their spirituality in the workplace. In addition to improving employee performance, as well as well-being and quality of life, through reducing stress, burnout and workaholism (Karakas 2010), spirituality catapults organizational effectiveness by providing employees with a sense of interconnectedness and community.

In contrast, it is the reluctant hard worker (those whose perception of organizational growth is low), the disenchanted worker (characterized by the alienation, lack of motivation and dissatisfaction with work at various levels) and the unengaged worker (lack of a sense of purpose, accommodated to their careers), who have lower levels of spirituality. It is worth emphasizing the finding of Killinger (2006), who states that the stress caused by workaholism can lead to loss of spirituality, chronic diseases, pain, and guilt.

6. Conclusions

This research contributed to the literature on workaholism by creating a analyze model of a workaholic and non-workaholic worker profiles, and studying the relationships with workplace spirituality. The literature points out that workplace spirituality has gained increasing attention in the organizational research field, considering this dimension a multidimensional construct and an alternative to improve employees' general well-being (e.g., Kinjerski 2013; McKee et al. 2011). Workaholism is a complex and multidimensional phenomenon, whose dimensions are distinctly related to workplace spirituality. Hence, workplace spirituality development can promote a more balanced and healthy relationship with work. This study also made it possible to understand how a soft skill, such as spirituality, can be a core value influence the development of a particular worker profile.

Workplace spirituality is associated with the inner life of employees, the connection with others, and the search for meaningful work in the community. In this way, when find a purpose in the professional activities, they act in an engaged way, applying the potential for the benefit of the organization. In addition to making them more productive over time, the incorporation of this value in organizations can influence the reduction of workaholic profiles and, consequently, the phenomenon of sustainability (Rezapouraghdam et al. 2019). On the one hand the Covid-19 pandemic led to job losses, influencing the increase in symptoms such as stress, depression and substance abuse, on the other hand it masked the boundaries between professional and family life, with the introduction of the concept 'working from home'. Therefore, the role of workplace spirituality is relevant, because it can play a vital role in improving mental well-being when it is properly accepted and practiced in organizations (Hisam and Sanyal 2021). Twenty-first century employees, despite following the various changes in the world of work (e.g., technology), seek and need a professional context that allows them to find a sense of purpose in harmony with the internal and personal values (Abdul Latiff 2021). In an organization that excels and respects the value of spirituality (of each one) it allows shaping behavior and professional performance, improving productivity and reducing addictive behaviors.

From a practical and professional point of view, our results can be particularly useful in the design of workshop on this topic. Spiritual workplaces encourage employees' sense of community, foster feelings of engaging in meaningful work, and support integrity, respect, responsibility, and personal/individual growth (e.g., Giacalone and Jurkiewicz 2003; Dhiman and Marques 2010; Kinjerski 2013). This type of initiative can allow organizations that adhere to the spiritual mindset to be more successful, ensure the happiness of the employees and are even more aware of their environmental and sustainable responsibilities. The findings reinforce the importance of the role of universities in improving the offer of programs that foster not only the economic aspect of entering the labor market, but also the importance of the idiosyncrasies of workers. Thus, policy makers and institutions responsible for creating labor-market orientations programs, should pay more attention and bring personal values to traditional training and education.

The present article has some limitations that should be addressed in future studies. The variables used in this study allowed us analyze the workaholism profiles and the relationships with the workplace spirituality dimensions of Portuguese workers. Although we strongly believe that these outputs are positive and promising, it is important to introduce new variables, measures, and theories that allow drawing a more consistent model. Regarding the sample, we consider that in the future it may be extended to other countries to evaluate cultural differences, which would permit to observe a broader range of results. For a better evaluation of the worker profiles it would be important to consider a longitudinal research to better understand the constructs' dynamic.

Author Contributions: Conceptualization, L.S.M. and C.M.; methodology: L.S.M.; software, C.M. and L.S.M.; formal analysis, L.S.M.; writing–original draft preparation and editing, C.M. All authors have read and agreed to the published version of the manuscript.

Funding: This research received no external funding.

Institutional Review Board Statement: Not applicable.

Informed Consent Statement: Informed consent was obtained from all subjects involved in the study.

Data Availability Statement: The data presented in this study are available on request from the first author, e-mail: lisete.monico@fpce.uc.pt.

Conflicts of Interest: The authors declare no conflict of interest.

References

Abdul Latiff, Noraidah. 2021. The Effect of Workplace Spirituality on Employee Performance. *Issues and Perspectives in Business and Social Sciences* 1: 22–27. [CrossRef]

Afsar, Bilal, and Yuosre Badir. 2017. Workplace spirituality, perceived organizational support and innovative work behavior: The mediating effects of person-organization fit. *Journal of Workplace Learning* 29: 95–109. [CrossRef]

Andreassen, Cecile, Jørn Hetland, and Ståle Pallesen. 2010. The Relationship between workaholism: Basic needs satisfaction at work and personality. *European Journal of Personality* 24: 3–17. [CrossRef]

Atroszko, Pawel, Zsolt Demetrovics, and Mark Griffiths. 2019. Beyond the myths about work addiction: Toward a consensus on definition and trajectories for future studies on problematic overworking. *Journal of Behavioral Addiction* 8: 7–15. [CrossRef]

Aziz, Shahnaz, and Casie Tronzo. 2011. Exploring the relationship between workaholism facets and personality traits: A replication in American workers. *The Psychological Record* 61: 269–86. [CrossRef]

Aziz, Shahnaz, Karl Wuensch, and Howard Brandon. 2010. A Comparison among worker types using a composites approach and median splits. *The Psychological Record* 60: 627–42. [CrossRef]

Balducci, Cristian, Lorenzo Avanzi, and Franco Fraccaroli. 2018. The Individual "Costs" of Workaholism: An Analysis Based on Multisource and Prospective Data. *Journal of Management* 44: 2961–86. [CrossRef]

Balducci, Cristian, Paola Spagnoli, and Melisa Clark. 2020a. Advancing Workaholism Research. *International Journal of Environmental Research and Public Health* 17: 9435. [CrossRef]

Balducci, Cristian, Guido Alessandri, Sara Zaniboni, Lorenzo Avanzi, Aura Borgogni, and Franco Fraccaroli. 2020b. The impact of workaholism on day-level workload and emotional exhaustion, and on longer-term job performance. *Work & Stress* 35: 6–26. [CrossRef]

Bella, Rircardo, Osvaldo Quelhas, Fernando Ferraz, and Marlene Bezerra. 2018. Workplace Spirituality: Sustainable Work Experience from a Human Factors Perspective. *Sustainability* 10: 1887. [CrossRef]

Bickerton, Grant, Maureen Miner, Martin Dowson, and Barbara Griffin. 2015. Incremental validity of spiritual resources in the job demands-resources model. *Psychology of Religion and Spirituality* 7: 162–72. [CrossRef]

Bollen, Kenneth. 1989. *Structural Equations with Latent Variables*. New York: John Wiley & Sons.

Buelens, Mark, and Steven Poelmans. 2004. Enriching the Spence and Robbins' typology of workaholism: Demographic, motivational and organizational correlates. *Journal of Organizational Change Management* 17: 440–58. [CrossRef]

Clark, Melissa, Jesse Michel, Ludmila Zhdanova, Shuang Pui, and Boris Balts. 2016. All work and no play? A meta-analytic examination of the correlates and outcomes of workaholism. *Journal of Management* 42: 1836–73. [CrossRef]

Clark, Melissa, Rachel Smith, and Nicholas Haynes. 2020. The Multidimensional Workaholism Scale: Linking the conceptualization and measurement of workaholism. *Journal of Applied Psychology* 105: 1281–307. [CrossRef] [PubMed]

Cohen, Jacob. 1988. *Statistical Power Analysis for the Behavioral Sciences*. New York: Routledge Academic.

Cristão, Catarina. 2010. Cerca de 10% dos portugueses são viciados no trabalho. Diário de Notícias, (Online). Available online: http://www.dn.pt/inicio/ciencia/interior.aspx?content_id=1547056&seccao=Sa%FAde (accessed on 21 April 2021).

Dhiman, Satinder, and Joan Marques. 2010. The role and need of offering workshops and courses on workplace spirituality. *Journal of Management Development* 30: 816–35. [CrossRef]

Dhiman, Satinder, and Joan Marques. 2016. *Spirituality and Sustainability*. Cham: Springer.

Duchon, Dennis, and Donde Plowma. 2005. Nurturing the spirit at work: Impact on work unit performance. *The Leadership Quarterly* 16: 807–33. [CrossRef]

Fairholm, Gilbert. 1996. Spiritual leadership: Fulfilling whole-self needs at work. *Leadership & Organization Development Journal* 17: 11–17.

Foster, Scott, and Anna Foster. 2019. The impact of workplace spirituality on work-based learners: Individual and organizational level perspectives. *Journal of Work-Applied Management* 11: 63–75. [CrossRef]

Fry, Louis. 2003. Toward a theory of spiritual leadership. *The Leadership Quarterly* 14: 693–727. [CrossRef]

Garg, Naval. 2017. Workplace Spirituality and Employee well-being: An empirical exploration. *Journal of Human Values* 23: 129–47. [CrossRef]

Gelbard, Roy, Orit Goldman, and Israel Spiegler. 2007. Investigating diversity of clustering methods: An empirical comparison. *Data and Knowledge Engineering* 63: 155–66. [CrossRef]

Giacalone, Robert, and Carole Jurkiewicz. 2003. Right from wrong: the influence of spirituality on perceptions of unethical business activities. *Journal of Business Ethics* 46: 85–97. [CrossRef]

Goltz, Sonia. 2011. Spiritual power: The internal, renewable social power source. *Journal of Management, Spirituality & Religion* 8: 341–63. [CrossRef]

Griffiths, Mark. 2005. Workaholism is still a useful construct. *Addiction Research and Theory* 13: 97–100. [CrossRef]

Hair, Joseph, William Black, Barry Babin, and Rolph Anderson. 2018. *Multivariate Data Analysis*, 7th ed. Hoboken: Pearson Prentice-Hall.

Hisam, Mohammed, and Shouvik Sanyal. 2021. Impact of workplace spirituality on organizational commitment–a study in an emerging economy. *Turkish Journal of Computer and Mathematic Education* 12: 984–1000. [CrossRef]
IBM Corp. 2013. *IBM SPSS Statistics for Windows, Version 22.0*. Armonk: IBM Corp.
Karakas, Fahri. 2010. Spirituality and Performance in Organizations: A literature review. *Journal of Business Ethics* 94: 89–106. [CrossRef]
Kent, Peter, Rikkle Jensen, and Alice Kongsted. 2014. A comparison of three clustering methods for finding subgroups in MRI, SMS or clinical data: SPSS twostep cluster analysis, latent Gold and SNOB. *BMC Medical Research Methodology* 14: 113. [CrossRef]
Killinger, Barbara. 2006. The Workaholic Breakdown Syndrome. In *Research Companion to Working Time and Work Addiction*. Edited by Ronald Burke. Cornwall: Elward Elgar, pp. 61–88.
Kinjerski, Val. 2013. The spirit at work scale: Developing and validating a measure of individual spirituality at work. In *Handbook of Faith and Spirituality in the Workplace*. Edited by Judy Neal. New York: Springer, pp. 340–83.
Kline, Rex. 2011. *Principles and Practice of Structural Equation Modeling*, 3rd ed. New York: The Guilford Press.
Kolodinsky, Robert, Robert Giacalone, and Carole Jurkiewicz. 2008. Workplace values and outcomes: Exploring personal, organizational and interactive workplace spirituality. *Journal of Business Ethics* 81: 465–80. [CrossRef]
Krishnakumar, Sukumarakurup, and Christopher Neck. 2002. The "what". "why" and "how" of spirituality in the workplace. *Journal of Managerial Psychology* 17: 153–64. [CrossRef]
Marques, Joan, Satinder Dhiman, and Richard King. 2005. Spirituality in the workplace: Developing an integral model and a comprehensive definition. *Journal of the American Academy of Business* 7: 81–91.
McKee, Margaret, Cathy Driscoll, E. Kevin Kelloway, and Elizabeth Kelle. 2011. Exploring linkages among transformational leadership, workplace spirituality and well-being in health care workers. *Journal of Management, Spirituality & Religion* 8: 233–55. [CrossRef]
Molino, Monica, Emanuela Ingusci, Fulvio Signore, Amelia Manuti, Maria Luisa Giancaspro, Vincenzo Russo, Margherita Zito, and Claudio Cortese. 2020. Wellbeing costs of technology use during covid-19 remote working: An investigation using the italian translation of the Technostress Creators Scale. *Sustainability* 12: 5911. [CrossRef]
Mónico, Lisete, Nathalia Mellão, Luiza Nobre-Lima, Pedro Parreira, and Carla Carvalho. 2016. Emotional intelligence and psychological capital: What is the role of workplace spirituality? *Revista Portuguesa de Enfermagem e Saúde Mental* 3: 45–50. [CrossRef]
Murray, Margaret, and Frederick Evers. 2011. Reweaving the fabric: Leadership and spirituality in the 21st Century. *Interbeing* 5: 5–15.
Myers, Jane, and Kirk Williard. 2003. Integrating spirituality into counselor preparation: A developmental, wellness approach. *Counseling and Values* 47: 142. [CrossRef]
Ng, Thomas, Kelly Sorensen, and Daniel Feldman. 2007. Dimensions, antecedents, and consequences of workaholism: A conceptual integration and extension. *Journal of Organizational Behavior* 28: 111–36. [CrossRef]
Nunnally, Jum, and Ira Bernstein. 1994. *Psychometric theory*. New York: McGraw-Hill.
Oates, Wayne. 1971. *Confessions of a Workaholic: The Facts about Work Addiction*. New York: World Publishing.
Oman, Doug. 2015. Defining Religion and Spirituality. In *Handbook of the Psychology of Religion and Spirituality*. Edited by Raymond Paloutzian and Crystal Park. New York: The Guilford Press, pp. 23–47.
Ornek, Ozlem, and Nurcan Kolac. 2020. Quality of Life in Employee with Workaholism. In *Occupational Health*. Edited by Orhan Korhan. London: IntechOpen, Available online: https://www.intechopen.com/online-first/quality-of-life-in-employee-with-workaholism (accessed on 21 April 2021). [CrossRef]
Pawar, Badrinarayan. 2016. Workplace spirituality and employee well-being: An empirical examination. *Employee Relations* 38: 975–94. [CrossRef]
Pedreira, Luanda, and Lisete Mónico. 2013. Workaholism and Psychological Capital: Repercussions on workplace spirituality. *International Journal of Developmental end Educational Psychology* 2: 535–44.
Porter, Gayle. 1996. Organizational impact of workaholism: Suggestions for researching the negative outcomes of excessive work. *Journal of Occupational Health Psychology* 1: 70–84. [CrossRef]
Preziosi, Robert, and Eleanor Marschke. 2011. How sales personnel view the relationship between satisfaction and spirituality in the workplace. *Journal of Organizational Culture, Communications and Conflict* 15: 71–110.
Rahman, Muhammad, Mahmud Zaman, Md Afan Hossain, Mahafuz Mannan, and Hasliza Hassan. 2019. Mediating effect of employee's commitment on workplace spirituality and executive's sales performance: An empirical investigation. *Journal of Islamic Marketing* 10: 1057–73. [CrossRef]
Rego, Arménio, and Miguel Pina e Cunha. 2008. Workplace spirituality and organizational commitment: An empirical study. *Journal of Organizational Change Management* 21: 53–75. [CrossRef]
Rego, Arménio, S. Souto, and Miguel Pina Cunha. 2007. Espiritualidade nas organizações positividade e desempenho. *Comportamento Organizacional e Gestão* 13: 7–36.
Rezapouraghdam, Hamed, Habib Alipour, and Huseyin Arasli. 2019. Workplace spirituality and organization sustainability: A theoretical perspective on hospitality employees' sustainable behavior. *Environment, Development and Sustainability* 21: 1583–601. [CrossRef]
Roof, Richard. 2015. The association of individual spirituality on employee engagement: The spirit at work. *Journal of Business Ethics* 130: 585–99. [CrossRef]
Rust, Braam, and Cecilia Gabriels. 2011. Spirituality in the workplace: Awareness of the human resource function. *African Journal of Business Management* 5: 1353–64.

Samah, Siti, Abu Silong, Kamaruzaman Jusoff, and Ismi Ismail. 2012. Relationship between spirituality and academic leader effectiveness. *International Conference on Human and Social Sciences* 2: 33.

Saxton, Michael. 2016. Workplace Spirituality, Workaholism, and Gender: A Quantitative Study of Higher Education Employees at a Small, Private College in the Northeastern United States. Ph.D. thesis, Capella University, Minneapolis, MN, USA.

Schaufeli, Wilmar, Toon Taris, and Willem van Rhenen. 2008. Workaholism, burnout, and work engage-ment: Three of a kind or three different kinds of employee well-being? *Applied Psychology* 57: 173–203. [CrossRef]

Schumacker, Randall, and Richard Lomax. 2016. *A Beginner's Guide to Structural Equation Modeling*, 4th ed. New York: Routledge.

Smith, Garry, and Charles Futrell. 2014. The inspired salesperson: Linking spirituality to performance. *Marketing Management Journal* 24: 172–85. [CrossRef]

Spagnoli, Paola, and Danila Molinaro. 2020. Negative (Workaholic) Emotions and Emotional Exhaustion: Might job autonomy have played a strategic role in workers with responsibility during the Covid-19 crisis lockdown? *Behavioral Sciences* 10: 192. [CrossRef]

Spence, Janet, and Ann Robbins. 1992. Workaholism: Definition. Measurement. And Preliminary Results. *Journal of Personality Assessment* 58: 160–78. [CrossRef] [PubMed]

Stahl, Ashley. 2019. Millenials: The Most Unhealthy Generation at Work. Forbes (Online). Available online: https://www.forbes.com/sites/ashleystahl/2020/12/30/millennials-the-most-unhealthy-generation-at-work/?sh=70be717d7b12 (accessed on 21 April 2021).

Stoeber, Jachim, and Lavinia Damian. 2016. Perfectionism in Employees: Work engagement, workaholism, and burnout. In *Perfectionism, Health, and Well-Being*. Edited by Fuschia Sirois and Danielle Molnar. New York: Springer, pp. 265–83.

Subramanian, Kalpathy. 2018. Workaholism—Does working more impact productivity? *International Journal of Innovative Trends in Engineering* 40: 69–75.

Tabachnick, Barbara, and Linda Fidell. 2007. *Using Multivariate Statistics*. Boston: Pearson Education, Inc.

Tepper, Bennet. 2003. Organizational citizenship behavior and the spiritual employee. In *Handbook of Workplace Spirituality and Organizational Performance*. Edited by Robert Giacalone and Carole Jurkiewicz. New York: M.E. Sharpe, pp. 181–90.

Urbina, Susana. 2014. *Essentials of Psychological Testing*. Hoboken: Wiley.

van der Walt, Freda, and Jeremias de Klerk. 2014. Workplace spirituality and job satisfaction. *International Review of Psychiatry* 26: 379–89. [CrossRef] [PubMed]

Vandenberghe, Christian. 2011. Workplace spirituality and organizational commitment: An integrative model. *Journal of Management, Spirituality & Religion* 8: 211–32. [CrossRef]

Vyas, Lina, and Nantapong Butakhieo. 2020. The impact of working from home during the COVID-19 on work and life domains: An exploratory study on Hong Kong. *Policy, Design and Practice* 4: 59–76. [CrossRef]

Wall, Tony, and John Knights. 2013. *Leadership Assessment for Talent Development*. London: Kogan.

Zsolnai, Laszlo, and Katalin Illes. 2017. Spiritually-inspired creativity in business. *International Journal of Social Economics* 44: 195–205. [CrossRef]

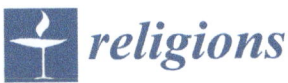

Essay

A Psychospiritual Exploration of the Transpersonal Self as the Ground of Healing

Monique M. Verrier

Holistic Counseling in Psychology, John F. Kennedy School of Psychology, National University, Pleasant Hill, CA 94523, USA; moniqueverriertherapy@gmail.com or mverrier@email.jfku.edu

Abstract: This paper focuses on the transpersonal Self as the psychological and spiritual healing factor in psychotherapy and addiction recovery, and illustrates the importance of bringing awareness of the Self and the energy of wholeness into focus with clients in the therapeutic process. The concept and experience of Self is explored through the psychospiritual therapeutic model of Internal Family Systems and through a spiritual lens of the nondual wisdom traditions derived from Advaita Vedanta and aspects of Kashmir Shaivism. Obstacles to the recognition of Self, approaches to facilitating this recognition, and the therapeutic benefits of knowing the essential Self are examined through the author's personal experience with these models and their use in overcoming depression, anxiety, eating disorders and addiction. Psychotherapeutic interventions that support making contact with the Self are examined as well as the implications of Self-knowing on personal relationships, behavior and inner experiences, as well as how one relates to others and the world.

Keywords: addictions; eating disorders; existential psychology; healing; Internal Family Systems; nonduality; psychotherapy; transpersonal psychotherapy

---

Citation: Verrier, Monique M. 2021. A Psychospiritual Exploration of the Transpersonal Self as the Ground of Healing. *Religions* 12: 725. https://doi.org/10.3390/rel12090725

Academic Editors: Bernadette Flanagan and Noelia Molina

Received: 10 August 2021
Accepted: 31 August 2021
Published: 5 September 2021

Publisher's Note: MDPI stays neutral with regard to jurisdictional claims in published maps and institutional affiliations.

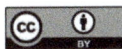

Copyright: © 2021 by the author. Licensee MDPI, Basel, Switzerland. This article is an open access article distributed under the terms and conditions of the Creative Commons Attribution (CC BY) license (https://creativecommons.org/licenses/by/4.0/).

1. Introduction

Many psychotherapeutic models, such as the psychoanalytic, psychodynamic, behavioral and cognitive approaches, are either explicitly or implicitly rooted in an assumption that the cause of psychological pathology and dysfunction is some kind of lack: of development, growth, self-esteem, confidence, trust, self-love, emotional regulation, positive thoughts, impulse control, etc. I offer here an alternative perspective that people innately possess all the qualities and inner resources they need for total mental and spiritual health no matter what their psychological background or experience. We do not become whole, we are whole. We are wholeness veiled by the addition of psychological constructs and beliefs that seem to obscure this truth, including the very belief that we are lacking or not whole. A therapist's or counselor's understanding from this perspective may minimize the possibility of unintentional reinforcement of beliefs and self-constructs around the sense of lack that further contributes to the obscuring of Self as wholeness for clients. This orientation supports clients' recognition of the transpersonal, essential Self right now, and deepens that knowledge of Self into firm inner grounding, supporting what might otherwise be a challenging healing process by promoting innate safety and relaxing psychological ego defenses.

The path to knowing the Self is varied but often starts with a divesting of what is not essential to our Being. It is a path of subtraction, unburdening, and uncovering. A curious phenomenon occurs in this process of divesting, which is that we fall deeper into an ever-widening circle of Self that is paradoxically *more* inclusive of experience. In this lessening, we become more expansive and the freedom to be our unique person occurs gently and effortlessly. It is the impersonal path of Self to the deepest and most intimate personal expression of who we are.

Through direct and skilled guidance, we can come to know the nature of ourselves as wholeness, having both immediate and gradual effects. The touching into our Being is direct and yet gradually deepens and transforms from the inside out. Knowing our Self is ordinary, ever present, and yet often overlooked. For this reason, client Self-led counseling might also be an overlooked therapeutic approach that could help soften defenses and increase security from a grounded base. There is a common misunderstanding that it takes years of ego building or exploring personality traits before we can really know ourselves. However, everyone knows themselves. Our Self is what we all refer to when we say 'I', but we rarely explore the nature of that 'I' (Spira 2017a). This paper will explore the nature of Self through a psychotherapeutic model with a spiritual lens, *Internal Family Systems* (Schwartz and Sweezy 2020), and through the spiritual model of the nondual wisdom, explored through a psychological lens. In both these models, the awareness of Self is established as the primary ground upon which further self-exploration and healing grows. I acknowledge that there are myriad theories on the nature of Self, Jungian theory being chief among them, and thus my analysis here is necessarily selective as it is beyond the scope of this paper to address them all (for an overview of different approaches to Self the reader is referred to Daniels 2002a, 2002b). I share my own experience in psychotherapy and spiritual exploration as a way of showing the power of conscious awareness of our essential Self to liberate oneself from the maze of the mind and psychological suffering that often underpins addiction and compulsive behaviors.

The following account of my personal experience is what I found to be valuable in my healing and may not be the appropriate path for others. It requires a certain amount of willingness and capacity to explore the self in a transpersonal way. Medical support and addressing environmental deficiencies may also be required. In the exploration of my experience, my hope is to bring to light the unintentional ways that counselors might reinforce and perpetuate their clients' identification with core beliefs of brokenness, defectiveness, unacceptableness, and separation. Uncovering the ever-present, never broken, whole aspect of Being and bringing it to the light of awareness and into the therapy or recovery process can facilitate the healing of those aspects of ourselves that are lost, hurt, confused and in need of connection. The alchemy of healing occurs when that which can never be harmed makes contact with that which can, revealing that what appears to be shadow is really those apparent aspects of ourselves that seem to block the light of our being. Certain terms and words will be used in specific ways. For a list of definitions, the reader may refer to Appendix A.

2. The Whole Story: A Psychotherapy Journey

I started psychotherapy at age 11 at my own request due to a deep depression. My initiating therapy at that age points starkly to the unresolved inner conflict that continued for more than 30 years: the subtle core belief that there is something wrong with me or something fundamentally missing and the equally hidden yet unrelenting conviction that this, in fact, cannot be true. Somewhere deep inside me I knew that there was something wrong, and I also knew as well that the idea of 'something wrong' was wrong and that I needed help connecting to what I knew was true. I was not able to articulate or explain these feelings at the time and this is only something that I can reflect on half a lifetime later. All I knew then was that something was not right and that I had a desperate longing for something I could not pinpoint or define. It was only many years later that I understood this feeling as a longing for myself, the nature of which is life itself.

The beginning of my work with the Jungian Analyst who was to be my therapist for over 30 years started with minutes-long silences whereby I had the undivided attention of a caring and attentive person. The silences were punctuated with 'what are you feeling?'—something I perceived as a trick question and one that I loathed and for which 'fine' was always the answer. This was my first experience with the Jungian style of leaving wide open spaces for 'something' to emerge. When I discovered the sand tray, I was relieved, as that was my way out of the 'what are you feeling?' situation. My sand tray pictures spoke for me.

Fast forward a few years...I was definitely in touch with my feelings and I had a much better understanding of what happened to me in my family. However, my mind had become a mouse in a maze of circular thoughts scurrying around confusing tight spaces and dead ends. I had become very depressed and anxious, something that would only get worse throughout my teenage years and early adulthood. An eating disorder that started as a child grew in severity, and by the time I was 15, I was exhibiting alcohol abuse. By my early twenties, I was on the path toward alcoholism. My self-esteem was very low, I had painful ruminating thoughts, and I completely seized on these negative ideas running rampant in my mind. The only solution to these painful experiences was food, and later, alcohol. Each time I delved into the reasons for my behavior, I came up with the same answer: I must be damaged or weak, simply incapable of handling life. My mind became a murky pond. When I finally found my way through it, I felt like my head had finally popped above the dark water and I could see and breathe again. That would not be until 31 years after the start of my therapy.

2.1. A Maze of the Mind or a Labyrinth of the Soul

In *Awakening the Heart: East/West Approaches to Psychotherapy and the Healing Relationship* (Welwood 1983), Thomas Hora tells the story of a man who had been in analysis for several years due to his problem of nail biting. When asked by a friend how the analysis was going, he proclaimed it was 'wonderful.' When asked if he had stopped biting his nails, he answered, "No, but now I know why I do it" (Hora, in Welwood 1983, p. 132). This was exactly my experience. I could have written volumes on why I did what I did, but I was still doing it, which added to my suffering. Now I 'knew better' but I was not 'doing better.' I could see all the psychological threads but was hopelessly entangled in them. I saw how my psychological self was put together, but as I still identified with this self, I felt destined to live out this painful conditioned patterning, since it seemed like 'me.' Ram Dass points out,

> Psychotherapy, as defined and practiced by people like Erikson, Maslow, Perls, Rogers, the neo-Freudians, or the neo-Jungians does not in the ultimate sense transcend the nature of ego structure. They really seem to be focused on developing a functional ego structure with which you can cope effectively and adequately with the existing structure. They have very little to say about how deeply identified you are with the ego structure.
>
> (Ram Dass in Welwood 1983, p. 34)

After years of therapy, I was functional within my culture; had a grasp on reality; knew myself as a distinct person; performed well enough at my job despite the constant anxiety; and could tolerate basic emotions. I had done a good job of figuring out the maze and had worked out how to manage some of the trickier parts and dead ends. However, internally, I was deeply confused and suffering. Conceptual pathways to healing that I discovered along the way, such as redemption, self-empowerment/self-esteem building, self-actualization, and transformation sometimes added to my burden. I utterly failed at these 'tasks' and that added more to my conviction that I was just simply broken beyond hope. By age 33, my eating disorder had taken to riding in the sidecar of alcoholism and despite the antidepressants I had been taking for 10 years, I still suffered from depression and had anxiety around even the smallest life pressure. I lived my life as safely as possible to mitigate my fear. I had done a lot of work in therapy—uncovering repressed emotions, understanding my role in my family and examined extensively the deficiencies in my early environment. I had mourned the mother I needed but never had, felt compassion for the lost, vague little girl I once was, and pieced together the story of me. Yet, I suffered to the point of despair.

I figured there must be more to know, more to discover, some secret repressed in my subconscious that once brought to consciousness would hold the answer to my healing. I did not realize through all those years that my assumption of and identification with a psychological conditioned self, a self-image or ego, was setting me on a path of identifying with an image of brokenness, of not being adequate. In the search for the fix, I was inadvertently reinforcing the idea that my very self was broken or damaged. It had not yet occurred to me that, although thoughts can be disturbing, feelings can be painful and hurtful, there was no hurt or disturbed self to be found. When I finally turned inward to look for this broken person, all I found were mutable thoughts, images, memories, and feelings—all contributing to a sense of self, but no broken, damaged person could be found.

In *The Paths of Ego* (Welwood 1983), Hora quotes a French psychiatrist who says, (translated to English), "We don't get well because we remember, but we remember as we get well" (p. 133). Getting well, for me, meant exploring the truth of my own existence, my own Being, before I could go any further in uncovering my past. In order to begin healing beyond general emotional stability, I did not necessarily need a big understanding of the meaning of life, I just needed to peek around the edges of who I understood myself to be, and in order to do that, I needed to ask the right questions. In discussing existential psychotherapy, Hora (Welwood 1983) explains that we do not probe the past, " ... we allow it to reveal itself in the course of gaining a better understanding of what is" (p. 134). I felt the pain of probing the past without the proper understanding of 'what is' in broader terms and this was causing more harm than good after a while. Hora goes on to say that (in existential psychology) we do not ask 'Why?' and we do not ask 'Who is to blame?' or 'What should I do?' I came to see that these types of questions are asked from the perspective of the self who feels broken and needs to be fixed. The answers led me deep into stories of resentment, self-pity and failed therapy strategies to fix a deficient self, leading to more despair for which the only remedy was more alcohol. The failure of the broken self to heal the broken self reaffirmed the belief in a broken self. What I was truly craving was a deep understanding of what Hora calls 'what is' as it relates to the nature of being and truth that aligned with my actual experience in the background of the depression.

In my persistence to not fall into a black hole and to overcome my addictions, I analyzed every dream and symbol, probed for memories, tried countless types of therapeutic interventions and recovery methods, all giving me a temporary sense of direction and control that provided a double-edged sword: a sense of hope—the carrot that I would chase for more than 30 years—and then despair. Even my anti-strategy strategies of 'letting go,' 'giving over' or 'surrender' were approached with an effortful doing. There was always a 'me' that needed to 'do' the surrendering, the letting go. I had not yet understood that what needed to be surrendered *was me,* or who I thought myself to be, and that *letting go was my true nature.* I came to see that a mental contraction into an idea of 'me' was tasked with 'letting go' and this mental activity, in turn, *created a sense of self* that was then further identified with. Later, it became clear that my default is letting go and all efforts to let go only add to that which seems to need to be let go of. A clever little trap.

Hora (Welwood 1983) goes on to say that in existential therapy, mainly, we ask two questions: 'What is the meaning of what seems to be?' and 'What is what really is?' What really started healing on a deep level was posing the implicit questions 'what *seems* to be?' and 'what really *is*?' What does the world and self appear to be and what is the reality of the world and who I am? In analysis, I had ferreted out all the psychological patterns. I had identified the letters and recognized the patterns of words and had seen the sentence that was my story and truly felt its emotional impact. However, the sentence was utterly out of any broader context. It meant nothing on its own—a dangling incomplete sentence of 'me' that I stared at and tried to make sense of for decades. It did not occur to me that the person who was trying to make sense of it was actually one of the words in the sentence—a word not seeing itself as a word and not realizing that the missing word that rendered the sentence nonsensical was simply the fact of not seeing who I *thought of* as myself as one of the words—in other words, a *part of the story.* From that word's *point of view*, there was always going to be something missing from that sentence because the word (the identified self) was embedded in the story.

Many years later, I realized that what I was longing and searching for was that which is essential to me within a larger context and that nothing I tried to see from the vantage point of that which was generated from within the story, stemming from a misunderstanding about who I was, would ever be capable of seeing *what is*. The confusion I felt exemplified the issue that the contemporary nondual teacher Rupert Spira (2017b) raises: "The mind cannot know the nature of reality until it knows its own nature" (p. 27) and from this standpoint, the sentence of 'me' was never going to make sense from the perspective of one of the words in the sentence. Spira (2017b) further explains that knowing the nature of mind does not mean to study *the content* of the mind, but rather to discover the essential nature of the mind. What I had not yet seen was that the *words* in the sentence change, and what is constant is the space in between the words, that which is *essentially* me. What I had yet to discover was that with a broader perspective, the maze of my mind could become a labyrinth of liberation—a single windy path to the center of my Being. One path in and the same path out.

A Mental Maze Becomes a Labyrinth of Liberation

I finally realized that the maze of my mind was entirely thought-created, consisting of memories, judgements, worries, interpretations, predictions and expectations, all circling around a felt concept of 'me', which was then tasked with various means to solve itself. Mazes are multicursive and branchlike, causing the follower to choose between different paths in order to reach some destiny or goal. Some of these paths lead to dead ends and turnarounds, causing the follower to go in circles (Kingsley 2010). There are several ways in and out. In order to 'solve' a maze, more thought is created—more 'figuring out,' learning, memory, and finding patterns. As an analogy of mental and emotional processes, it is easy to see how the maze can seem never ending. It seemed that the more I tried to understand the maze, the deeper and more complicated it became. Trying to solve it seemed to somehow create more of it.

I now see this process that I associate with the maze as an occurrence within a larger and more profound journey: that of the labyrinth. The objectives of a maze are very different from that of a labyrinth. Solving a maze involves making sense of experiences, learning details particular to that part of the maze, and makes use of memory and future projection. I see the labyrinth as related to *what is*, and is not so much something we do but is simply what is happening. The experience of the maze for me now seems like an abundance of activity undertaken while, in actuality, I was slowly moving forward in the labyrinth toward a deeper understanding of the Self. The labyrinth path may seemingly lead further away from the center (in this case, the knowing of Self) and then fold towards it again in twists and turns, but the path is unicursive, so the only choice is forward toward the center or away, back toward the single entrance/exit. In explaining the history of mazes and labyrinths in art, and the interpretive difference between a maze and a labyrinth, Kingsley explains, "The labyrinth is regarded as a more solemn undertaking [than the maze] associated with ritual and spiritual and religious journeys" (Kingsley 2010, p. 90). For me, what initiated the change from a mental maze to a spiritual path was turning toward my thoughts with curiosity and openness. As the nondual teacher and psychologist, Dr. Gail Brenner (2018), suggests, "Instead of swirling in the content of the thoughts, you open up to seeing them with wisdom and clarity" by relaxing attention "away from involvement into the safe haven of being aware" (p. 92). It was this small shift in focus toward the Self beyond the ego that fundamentally changed my course.

The beginning of my discovery of the transpersonal Self and the primacy, constancy, and eternal quality of the essential nature of myself started with a feeling and an image that came to me during a meditation in which I sensed the ever-changing nature of everything and all experiences: pets, friends and partners who had come and gone; various homes, the changing cells in my body, ideas, feelings—all of it was sensed as flowing through and around a golden thread that was strong, constant and seemed to have no beginning or end. This golden thread started before the story of 'me' and I simply knew it would still be present after my body and mind ceased to be, yet I knew also that this thread *was me*—an immutable Self. That was the first time ever in my life that I knew that I could handle all change, that the death of my loved ones, or any loss, while painful and difficult, could not take anything essential from me or damage or diminish me in any way. I had never felt this way before but the certainty has grown ever since.

It was years later, upon hearing the myth of Ariadne (GreekMythology.com 2021) and the golden thread that she gives to Theseus in order to find his way out of the labyrinth and back to her (his true love) as he journeyed to the center to slay the minotaur, that both the images of the golden thread and the labyrinth made sense to me. I have come to see the thread as the constant and ever-present essence of Being on the one path that can only ever lead back to our Self—our true heart. What changed my experience of the maze of my mind into a labyrinth of liberation was a loosening of focus on the mutable inner and outer objects of experience and a curiosity in and growing awareness of the golden thread that weaves through all of it. At the time I was in Jungian therapy, this wider scope of life, this labyrinth that I had not yet come to see as my own Self, I had known only esoterically as a spiritual path, a religion, a philosophy, a self in which I might be a fragment of the collective unconscious that I may have access to (again, from beyond myself). From my own perception, Jung's ([1954] 1970) concept of individuation, which he believed usually started around mid-life, perhaps is what I contributed to this Self, but it was something that I had known as a child, and is perhaps more in line with what some other cultures have described as the essence of life, Buddhahood, or other known applications of such a term. Once I was able to name it, I knew it for what it had always been in my life and the concepts of mythology that I had learned in Jungian therapy helped me see this path through this labyrinth path.

The path of the labyrinth to the center of Self brought me from a life of depression, fear, and addiction to a life of joy and love of life. I no longer take the antidepressants that I was told by the medical community that I would probably need for life. Anxiety is an old friend that visits from time to time, but I feel a security that is not dependent on circumstances and a groundedness that is not created but rather simply present. I no longer suffer from alcoholism or eating disorders. Intimate relationships and close friendships feel safe. I have a broad range of emotions and an acute sensitivity, but I feel in the flow of life and have an intimacy with all of my experience.

2.2. Longing for Self: Finding the Center of the Labyrinth

As someone deeply interested in human experience, during this journey, I spent a lot of time reflecting on what helped me and what might help others who are stuck in the maze of the psychological self. What I came to see was that my seemingly fragmented psyche consisted of splits or aspects of a self that together formed a psychological system (Schwartz and Sweezy 2020; Fisher 2017); I completely identified this system as 'me' and therefore was unavailable to be present with the psychological system *as an experience* (Fisher 2017); I suffered from a belief that I was separate from the world and others that formed an existential wound—the sense that I was bound to the limitations and destiny of temporary body and finite mind. All of these together created and maintained the sense of a separate inside self that was apart from and fearful of the outside world. This insecurity required some kind of anchoring in a world of apparent objects (Spira 2016a), which took root in addictions, and at other times, relationships. It became apparent that persistent *thought* (mental processes), reinforced by a felt sense in the body, created this overall sense of separation and the fragmented psyche resulted from this same body-mind process that gave rise to the assumption of an inner 'separate self.' I was unaware of and completely unidentified with any aspect of myself beyond this sense of a separate self and the psychological system that developed to maintain it.

In essence, I was unaware of what I have come to see as my transpersonal Self or what I call True Nature—the self beyond the contents of mind or experience. I had become lost and identified with these psychological parts of myself consisting of emotional memory, images, and thoughts, and therefore had no ground upon which to stand in order to do any meaningful therapeutic work. The present Self became veiled by the superimposition of 'past' self-stories, sensed through thought, memory and sensations. Janina Fisher (2017) describes this as "having no vantage point in the here and now from which to look back and view what happened 'then'" (p. 40). My experience is that the transpersonal Self is only here and now and therefore presence is what was required for healing.

2.2.1. The Path of Unbecoming

By the time I arrived at my second therapist's office, I was emotionally exhausted by my self-inflicted wanderings in the maze, which had itself become addiction like, as the compulsion to 'heal' or resolve my psychological conflicts overwhelmed me. The presence of and relationship with my childhood therapist had an immeasurable impact on my healing, but the many years of ego building 'failures' had left me worn. The relationship with my second therapist began the journey of "being" instead of "searching" or "doing". This was a process not of becoming someone but one of unbecoming. Rather than searching for myself and shining a laser beam on unconscious material, all that was required was playful curiosity and a soft relaxed mental focus. This soft focus is what I have likened to an inner version of the yogic gaze or drishti (Life 2007)—a soft but prolonged, continuous, single-pointed focus on an inner point that is stable and unmoving—what I later recognized as my essential Self. Gently focusing on this immutable part of me allowed me to find an internal anchor independent of experiences that come and go.

2.2.2. The Healing Factors

From this vantage point, I see that a process unfolded that facilitated healing psyche and spirit. The stages of this process prepared the ground for further healing by touching into what is essentially me and discerning what aspects are not essential to my Being. While sensing into the essential Self, I turned toward what I had previously identified as me to *welcome it* into a new relationship and integrate it by taking it into my Being. Eventually, I allowed this new way of being to *realign* my thoughts, feelings, relationships and activities. I continue to *cultivate mindfulness* of the habitual thinking, beliefs, and mental processes that create an apparent veiling of my Self, and which reinforces the identification with a separate insecure self.

This therapeutic approach embraces a clear and direct path to knowing the Self, and from that perspective, progressively realigns, reorients, restructures, and facilitates the processing of old conditioning and feelings, especially the ones rooted deep in the body, by attending to those painful beliefs and feelings. This essentially flips the usual psychotherapy process around whereby we explore what is *essentially true* first and then from that grounding, sorting through and seeking to make sense of that which *appears to be true*. I found that what impeded so much of my previous efforts to heal was that I simply could not fully process or integrate 'what appears to be true' from the vantage point of 'what appears to be true.' In other words, most psychotherapy will focus on the client's associations, meaning making, interpretations, and beliefs around the psychologically constructed self—all of which appears true to the client from the perspective of the constructed self—and neglect or ignore what is always true in our experience; all that is not dependent on circumstances, a particular perspective, mind set or beliefs.

Therapeutic attempts to 'resource' a client often miss the most fundamental and always available resource: the immutable presence of Being or transpersonal Self. In my inquiries into why this is so, I have come to understand that either this essential Self is not known by the counselor or therapist or they do not know how to help clients come to see this ever-present Self in their immediate experience. One focus of this paper is to explore approaches to psychological and spiritual healing that acknowledge the Self as the healing factor in psychotherapy and approaches to bring this Self or the energy of Wholeness into focus with clients early in the therapeutic process.

3. Theoretical Models for Self-Exploration: Internal Family Systems and Nondual Wisdom

Some models of psychotherapy and psychospiritual healing and addiction recovery models are built upon the concept or understanding of the Self, higher self, higher power, essential self, or true nature, among its many names. This section explores the psychospiritual therapeutic model of *Internal Family Systems* (Schwartz and Sweezy 2020) and a combination of the spiritual traditions of the Direct Method or Path (Atmananda Krishna Menon 2009), from the eastern nondual wisdom of Advaita Vedanta, and aspects of Kashmir Shaivism, as two possible approaches that might help clients recognize the Self, as it helped me in my recovery. These are often referred to as the inward and outward-facing paths, respectively, as taught by spiritual teacher Rupert Spira (2017a), which also has a background in the spiritual teachings of Francis Lucille (2006) and Jean Klein (2006). We will also look at how some psychotherapists have integrated nondual wisdom into their therapy practice. For simplicity, henceforward, Internal Family Systems will be referred to as IFS and the Advaita Vedanta and Kashmir Shaivism traditions from the perspective of the teachers and authors mentioned will be referred to as the nondual understanding or nondual wisdom. As the focus is a discussion on the healing factor of the transpersonal Self, this will not be an exhaustive theoretical discussion of the two psychological and spiritual models through which the Self is explored—Internal Family Systems and spiritual nondual wisdom—but a brief description is necessary to understand the approaches to accessing, healing and living from the Self.

3.1. Internal Family Systems

While many psychotherapy approaches make no mention of a self beyond a psychologically, culturally or socially constructed one, one approach in particular, Internal Family Systems, turns attention toward a transpersonal self, and in fact, derives all therapeutic benefit from the standpoint of this often-overlooked Self (Schwartz and Sweezy 2020). The IFS model brings traditional systems thinking—a mental model that promotes the idea that the component parts of a system will act differently when isolated from its environment or other parts of the system (Weinberg 2001)—into the inner psychological realm and conceptualizes and relates to individuals as human systems that make use of "structure, boundaries, positive and negative feedback, homeostasis, and degrees of embeddedness and constraint" that work within principles of "balance, harmony, leadership and development" (Schwartz and Sweezy 2020, p. 26) with which one can assess a human system.

IFS therapy is a mindfulness-based approach to understanding the psychological system that synthesizes two main paradigms: the idea of the plural mind—that we consist of many different psychological parts—and a human systems model, inviting therapists and clients to relate to all levels of the human system. IFS's approach is non-pathologizing, viewing individuals through a holistic and humanistic lens, and seeing people as innately having all the resources they need, rather than consisting of a collection of deficits or having disease. A basic premise of IFS is that "people have an innate drive toward and wisdom about their own health" (Schwartz and Sweezy 2020, p. 26) and it follows that when people are having chronic problems, they are constrained from using their innate resources and strengths due to imbalances, polarization of inner psychological parts of themselves, problems with Self leadership or burdened development as a result of trauma (Schwartz and Sweezy 2020). This 'inner system' consists mostly of unconscious desires, distortions, and agendas called "parts," which can be differentiated from the Self, the seat of consciousness, an "entity that is described and approached in many different ways in spiritual traditions around the world" (Schwartz and Falconer 2017, p. 44) and is characterized by qualities such as presence, clarity, calm and curiosity (Schwartz and Sweezy 2020).

'Parts' are autonomous mental systems within the psychic system that are like subpersonalities with their own abilities, desires, views and range of emotions. From the IFS perspective, every person contains an inner tribe of people that take on extreme roles, or burdens, and who, if released from these roles by a process known as 'unburdening' are likely to discover their full potential (Schwartz and Sweezy 2020). The IFS system consists of parts (subpersonalities) of the individual, that include: Exiles—parts who have been exploited, rejected/abandoned in external relationships and then judged by other parts of the system; Manager parts, who fear the extremity of Exiles and 'lock them up' by employing various strategies to keep them out awareness; and Firefighter parts who are the system's last defense, called upon when Exiles get through the defenses of the Managers and they employ extreme behavior to distract from or suppress the Exile's emotional reactions, which can include addictions or abuse of all kinds including extreme behavior such as self-cutting or stealing (Schwartz and Sweezy 2020).

While everyone has these subpersonalities, Janina Fisher (2017), who uses the IFS model extensively in her work with trauma survivors, describes the brain's innate capacity to split or compartmentalize (fragment) as an ingenious adaptive response to abuse and neglect. In order to survive and maintain some sense of ourselves as 'good,' we reject the abused self as bad and identify it as 'not me' or the Exile (Fisher 2017). This splitting and self-hatred continue long after the traumatic event is over and, while fulfilling the purpose of surviving and adapting to intolerable circumstances, it comes at the cost of "disowning their most vulnerable and wounded selves" (Fisher 2017, p. 19). To ensure this continued dissociation, other parts, the Managers and Firefighters, come into the intrapsychic world, and together, these often-polarized parts form the ecology of the inner system (Schwartz and Sweezy 2020). The Self is independent of the subpersonalities, or the system, and does not hold an extreme position. Fisher (2017) explains that "Self refers to innate qualities possessed by all human beings in undamaged form no matter how much trauma or abuse they have experienced" (p. 8), which include creativity, courage, calm, clarity, confidence and commitment. Healing in IFS is the outcome of discovering these innate qualities as an antidote to the painful experiences suffered by exiled child parts. This healing comes through in what IFS calls "Self leadership"—a process by which those with access to the Self are able to help the parts unburden by listening, understanding and being present with their parts (Schwartz and Sweezy 2020).

The contribution of IFS to my own healing and to the field of psychology is considerable. The therapeutic benefit is mostly dependent on the client's 'access' to Self, and, as such, one of the potential deficiencies of this approach is the possibility that a client might not be able to unblend or separate out these psychological parts from the transpersonal Self in order to engage in Self leadership and to benefit from this modality. For this reason, a spiritual approach borrowing from the nondual wisdom traditions can complement this modality, both in the beginning, as one turns attention toward that which is essential to oneself, and toward the end, when the psychological ego construct is integrated into the wholeness of Being.

3.2. The Nondual Inward- and Outward-Facing Paths and the Original Split

Some spiritual and religious traditions have the concept of the split from God or divinity. In the nondual perspectives, this split is understood to be a belief in separation from wholeness (Krishnamurti 1969) and characterizes what I would describe as my existential wound, which was accompanied by confusion and longing—the undercurrent upon which the swells of addiction and depression arose. In psychological terms, this might be viewed as the first or original attachment wound, and can be understood as the human predicament discussed in vast numbers of philosophies and religions and depicted in art, story, music and poetry.

This wound in myself is what led me into the inquiry into my essential Self or wholeness, and to discover the potential therapeutic benefits of this broader understanding of Self. From this perspective, this apparent separation is not from birth, but is psychologically developmental. It is not actual, but an acquired belief that occurs normally and naturally as we differentiate ourselves from our mothers and the world, and identify with our bodies and individual minds as we start seeing ourselves as existing *inside* the body and the world as existing *outside* the self/body. This lost connection with the true nature of Self can be understood as a natural consequence of being a manifest localized point of human perspective. (For more information on living organisms as dissociated alters of cosmic consciousness, surrounded by its thoughts, please see Kastrup 2018)

Spira (2017b) explains that as this natural separation process progresses, "the seed of the ego of a separate self that lies dormant in the infant, and that until now has been a process of individuation, begins to crystallize into a discrete entity, which identifies itself as the body-mind" (p. 38). He goes on to say that this gradual process of a child establishing their identity as a separate individual is a natural and essential part of development and would lead to psychological problems if not properly concluded. What can cause suffering later in life is not the child's natural process of individuation, but the conceptualization of herself as an entity living inside and as the body. In this model of development, ego as a *process* is replaced by ego as an *entity*, and in most cultures all further development is built upon the understanding of our self as that separate ego entity.

From this theoretical perspective, the deepening of this natural and developmental imagined split might occur through adverse early life experiences that reinforce this sense of separation and create an environment in which a child feels they must further identify with and then subsequently cut off parts of themselves to survive, and is in my view, the root of psychological suffering. The construction of a mental model of separate self, or ego, that must be constantly maintained, built up, and defended is the inevitable consequence of this split. Individual personhood and a functional sense of self in the world are necessary and healthy as a process, and a temporary identification with that process is natural. However, an enduring belief that one is contained within, and defined by that mental or psychological construction, as a separate self-entity, in this view, can result in insecurity and anxiety because that construct is inherently *not secure*, as the 'contents' (thoughts, perceptions, sensations, and feelings) that form and maintain it are continually changing. Due to our natural inclination toward that which is true to our nature, the tendency is to rid ourselves of this insecurity and anxiety by either building up this insecure self, or to rid ourselves of it through a myriad of coping behaviors, not limited to addictions and compulsions of all kinds.

A progression of the developmental differentiation process could include a felt sense of expanding beyond identification with body and mental processes (Spira 2017b) as we see through the objects of sensations, perceptions, feelings and thoughts to *that which* senses, perceives, feels and thinks; and further, toward simply sensing, perceiving, feeling and thinking and the simple knowing or awareness of these experiences. We can 'have' and use an ego construct, but as Wilber (1998) explains, "one is no longer exclusively identified with that self" (p. 31). We can experience and understand that construct as a process within awareness and not as an entity or self.

The extent to which the perceived existential separation or split is reinforced through rejection, shaming, neglect, injustice, abuse or other psychological harm in our early environment is the extent to which we suffer. This suffering can be lessened and eventually alleviated as awareness is brought to the misunderstanding of this perceived separation. Similarly, the extent to which caregivers of children are aware of their own wholeness or Self energy and bring those qualities of Self, such as presence, clarity, openness and love to developing children, is the extent to which those children recognize their innate wholeness of Self and its qualities. I have come to see that when our childhood environment, our caregivers or our communities, perpetuate a sense of separation (both their own and their child's) through the pathways of *lack* (deficiency or incompleteness) and *fear* (of abandonment, death, and rejection), this leads to a deepening sense of separation from the world and a further identification with and fragmentation of the psyche, as described by Schwartz and Sweezy (2020) Internal Family Systems model. When caregivers (or counselors) bring to the child (or client) their own Self energy and know themselves and others as whole in reality, embodying the qualities of true security, love, effortless compassion, openness, and allowing, they implicitly and explicitly foster the child's innate sense of wholeness. Children in this type of environment grow to see the shared beingness with others and the world, which profoundly impacts their experience of life and influences their interactions and relationships with the world and others. Their Self is leading them internally and externally.

This is the broader existential context that was missing for me in my therapy and that in later therapy helped bring a universal and timeless understanding and meaning of life for me. This understanding brought my psychology into context in a way that greatly supported my therapeutic work. I have come to see that when we feel like we are coming apart, we are right on script, we are not doing it wrong, it is deeply and utterly human. It is the cut from the source of ourselves that happens to us all in millions of unique ways. Some of us have had life experiences that have made that cut deeper, but that is not a problem. Whether it is a hairline fracture or a canyon, it is still only an *apparent* separation. It is not any harder to close an imaginary fracture than it is to close an imaginary chasm, as there is not anything in actuality to close. Healing, from this perspective, is whichever path and however much time it takes for the mind and body to catch up to this truth. Those with the imaginary chasms might take longer to see, and more importantly, feel this truth than those with subtle fissures, and may need more support and perhaps multiple pathways to this felt understanding. Approached from the understanding of wholeness, just like the labyrinth's path to center, all roads are the one path home.

3.2.1. The Nondual Vedantic Inward-Facing Path and the Nature of Self

The nondual wisdom that is discussed in these sections is based on the direct path of self-knowledge of *Advaita Vedanta* or the inward-facing path and the aspects of *Kashmir Shaivism* called the outward-facing or Tantric Path imparted by Rupert Spira (2014). See Appendix B for further information on Kashmir Shaivism and Advaita Vedanta.

The inward-facing path taught by Rupert Spira is rooted in the Vedantic tradition of the Direct Method or Path advocated by modern spiritual teachers such as Nisargadatta Maharaj [1973] (2012), Ramana Maharshi ([1948] 2008) and Atmananda Krishna Menon (Pillai 2019; Atmananda Krishna Menon 2009), in which the mind turns its attention away from objective experience towards its own essence or reality (Spira 2016a, 2016b, 2017a, 2017b). It is 'direct' because it does not require years of preparation, study, meditation, practices, or purification of the mind or body to recognize the essence or reality of the Self (Spira 2016c). The direct path does not imply any particular amount of time; much like a direct flight, there are no diversions or plane changes, but the amount of time it takes to get from one 'destination' to another depends on how far one seemingly is from the destination when the journey commences. Again, like the labyrinth, there is only one path, but it could be windy, turn back on itself, or be long or short. In this regard, ultimately, there is no wrong way to go.

Advaita means 'not two' in Sanskrit (*ad-vaita*) or nondual, which is to say that absolute reality and the world of appearances, or the relative world, are 'not two' (Spira 2017b). From this perspective, in reality, there are no subjects and objects, "much as a mirror and its reflections are not separate, or an ocean is one with its many waves" (Wilber 1998, p. 12). The fundamental truth of reality is whole. The Vedas are the sacred scriptures of India and 'Vedanta' is translated as the "end of the Vedas' or the last teaching (Spira 2017b). It is the last place the individual mind can go, the 'last stop' before Self recognition, which in this understanding is considered 'beyond' the finite or limited mind. Advaita inward contemplation is the turning of the attention away from the contents of objective experience (thoughts, feelings, perceptions, sensations) toward the source from which it has arisen. It is in this giving up or turning around that we cease being preoccupied with our suffering and gradually become more interested in the nature of the one who suffers.

This curiosity toward that with which experience is known, leads to self-inquiry and an understanding of our essential Self: pure objectless awareness (Spira 2017a). In the Direct Path, simple awareness is both the path and the goal, or as Spira (2017a) explains, "Being aware is simultaneously the subject that knows, the process of knowing and the object that is known" (p. 66). As the inquiry deepens by exploring the nature of awareness (limitless and timeless and, therefore, not divided), the relative qualities of love, peace, clarity, and intelligence or wisdom move from the background to the foreground of relative experience. Through a process of self-inquiry in which we investigate our immediate experience to verify what is not essential to our Being (through a process called in Sanskrit *net neti*—'not this, not that') and to verify what is true about the nature of Being (asking inner questions, such as "Can anything be experienced outside of awareness?'), we often come to see that we have mistakenly identified ourselves, our Being, with the limits and destiny of the body. We can also then begin to recognize our true nature as the transcendent Self, unlimited (without form) and ever present.

3.2.2. The Outward-Facing Tantric Path: Healing from and Aligning with Self

In *Being Aware of Being Aware* (Spira 2017a), Spira explains that the inward-facing path is only, at best, half the journey. Once we recognize in our *direct* experience the essence of the irreducible nature of the Self it is necessary to face 'outwards' again—toward objective experience, the world and relationships—facing any feelings of separation (fear and lack), becoming aware of behavior, thoughts, and feelings that arise from this belief of separation, and "realigning the way we think and feel, and subsequently act, perceive and relate, with our new understanding" of our wholeness (Spira 2017a, p. 10). Knowing one's essential self as the transcendent nature of awareness, through direct experience, without sensing and understanding its *immanence*—that this awareness pervades all knowledge and experience—can lead to what Spira calls "a fragile alliance" between our essential nature and all objects and others, "manifesting as denial or rejection of embodied life in the world" (Spira 2017a, p. 11). This may become a means through which a sense of further separation or fragmentation from life and the world manifests itself.

The transcendent nature of Self or aware presence is not dependent on qualia or phenomenal experience, as is evident in the experience of simply being aware of being aware; however, awareness is intrinsic to perceptions, sensations, and thoughts (Spira 2017a). If investigated in our experience, it becomes obvious that all that can be known can only be known through thinking, sensing and perceiving (Spira 2016c), which is only known by awareness. It follows that far from being separate from our essential nature as awareness, the world, others, and our bodies—anything that can be experienced—are made of awareness. The gap between subject and object is closed by welcoming all experience, including intolerable feelings, into our Self without agenda, much in the way the Self befriends scared or protective parts in IFS, and brings those fragmented parts back into the Self. In this way, what previously felt separate from us integrates and dissolves into our Being. Through embodied awareness and closing the perceived gap between Self and the world, objective experience now shines with the light of awareness, rather than eclipsing the Self (Spira 2017b). Spira (2016c) describes this intimacy between Self and the world saying, "The world becomes my body." Yet, despite understanding ourselves and the world to be nondual—not in reality separate—the appearance of multiplicity and diversity remains. We live in apparent duality while knowing, and more importantly, feeling ourselves, others, and the world to be one, whole, our true Self.

4. Nothing Lacking, Already Whole: Innate Psychological Health

An important factor in this particular way of looking at the Self and healing, as seen from the IFS model and particularly from the nondual direct path, is that we are essentially whole and have access to well-being and psychological health *now*. What commonly obfuscates this truth is attention to and sole identification with mutable experience, whether it is appearances in the outside world or an overlay of mental, emotional and psychological patterns (IFS parts and their burdens) added to our already whole and innate well-being. The result is the appearance of fragmentation, polarization and brokenness, and the accompanying pain of a sense of separation. In essence, these parts are created as a result of not fully knowing our wholeness (frequently as a result of our early separation-promoting experiences) and then these parts create further fragmentation that reinforces this feeling in a self-perpetuating system. The view that well-being is innate and undamaged by our experiences is somewhat of an expansion on Humanistic psychology, whereby a person is seen to have the capacity to overcome problems, make free choices, and actualize themselves (APA Dictionary of Psychology n.d.). Instead of seeing these as pathways to wholeness, this perspective views these as the natural effects and expressions of knowing deeply that we are *already* whole. In other words, we overcome problems, make free choices and actualize ourselves, not to *become* whole, but as an expression of the wholeness that we already are.

IFS has as a main premise that human nature is essentially and already whole, and thus, is naturally inclined toward health and well-being. Schwartz and Sweezy (2020) compare the positive view of human nature, that is an important aspect of IFS therapy, with the more negative view in developmental psychology's attachment theory, which posits that our basic nature is a result of the parenting we receive during critical periods of early development (Bowlby 1988); if we did not receive 'good enough' parenting during these critical periods, we will "remain broken until we have some kind of corrective reparenting experience from a therapist or significant other" (Schwartz and Sweezy 2020, p. 49). In IFS, the relationship with the therapist in not meant to correct a deficiency in the client's early caretaker relationships in order to advance the client's development, but instead relies upon the relationship to help release the already fully developed and undamaged Self that can naturally regulate and nurture the parts, when they show up in our experience, just as we are equipped to do (Schwartz and Sweezy 2020). Through my own expanding understanding of my essential nature, I have come to see more deeply that the parts are not pathological or disordered, but come about as the intelligent system's way of bringing the person closer to the qualities of Self (safety, peace, fulfillment), albeit through ways that may have some destructive or painful results.

In *The Deep Heart: Our Portal to Presence*, Prendergast (2019), a therapist who uses a nondual approach in his practice, challenges the notion that we must work through layers of psychological conditioning before we can encounter what is essential to us: "There are no preconditions for experiencing our true nature, the true nature that is always available as the background awareness to and core of every experience" (Prendergast 2019, p. 28). For this reason, glimpses of our essential Self can happen at any moment. In this way, the Self is not 'becoming' nor is it attained, created or developed, but is always present and is an expansion of and *includes*, but is not limited to, the ego process and all other aspects and parts. There is nothing to do to discover the Self other than notice the presence of ourselves, which lies beneath the coloring of experience that often focuses our attention on the overlays of our conditioned patterns within our experience.

We can trace our way back to the source of those patterns through various therapeutic or contemplative means. Once even the barest glimpse of our essential Self is recognized, various psychotherapeutic approaches can be undertaken to help heal those other aspects of ourselves that need transformation, while the process is being led and informed by Self. During this process, the client can start to recognize that these protective aspects (the Managers in IFS) are tasked with protecting, and thus maintaining, a sense of a self-entity, that in reality is a process (involving thought, feelings, sensations, images, memory, etc.) that has been identified with. These therapeutic approaches can include depth therapy, parts work, somatic work, expressive arts, or any other therapy that is appropriate for that particular individual. In essence, therapy involves the Self guiding the various aspects of the mind/psyche and body to catch up with what the Self already knows—that we are already whole, but for the thoughts and feelings that arise on behalf of the misunderstanding and belief that we are not.

4.1. Glimpses Beyond the Limits of the Acquired Self: A Deeper Look at Self

The Transpersonal Self goes by many names: Soul, Great Heart, Presence, Atman, Wholeness, True Nature, Higher Power, Authentic Self, Wise Self, Unconditioned or Universal Mind. From the perspective of nondual wisdom, the Self or true nature is you at your most essential. However, what is that exactly? When posed with the question, 'who are you?' one will often describe the very surface layers of identification that might include autobiographical, cultural, racial, or relational information about ourselves, or we describe our personal traits, preferences, habits, mood tendencies, physical or mental characteristics. Some of these qualities are genealogical or biological, but mostly, these are acquired traits that we might call the biographical self—the aspects of ourselves conditioned through experience and cultural contexts. We often describe not so much 'who' but 'what we are like.' In other words, we describe relative and mutable qualities and identifications in the presence of a changing environmental context within a framework of time and space.

By focusing on the recognition and uncovering of the transpersonal Self, the intention is not to minimize or disregard personal, cultural, biographical or historical identities—all of these give our experience of self a richness and depth—but rather to temporarily shift focus to the background of these shifting identifications to better connect with our ground of Being. Who is it that is reading and understanding these words right now? Without referring to memory, including learned concepts, transient states of mind, feelings or projections of the future, how would you describe yourself? In other words, we are not asking what it *feels like* to be you and not *what you think* about you, but what is left after everything that is not essential to you is 'removed', so-to-speak. These are the questions asked and the answers discovered through the direct experience of the individual in the direct path of nondual understanding.

Through considering these questions and searching for the answers in our direct experience, we find that our 'beingness' or awareness seems to be *self-evident* by the very fact that the question, 'who are you?' can even be heard, understood, and reflected upon. That which hears, understands and reflects is who we are at our most essential. We seem to be present and aware even as the question is asked, before 'thought' searches for the answer. In *Presence: Volume I*, Rupert Spira (2016a) states simply, "I may not know *what* I am, but I know *that* I am" (p. 3). The knowledge "I am" seems to be a human given, albeit an overlooked one. From the nondual perspective, Spira (2016b) establishes the primacy of the presence and awareness as the true Self, and often refers to the Self as the presence of awareness. When we say "I feel sad", or "I am tired" it is that which is aware of these experiences that is what we refer to as "I". Our Self, presence or awareness is "the most intimate fact of experience" (Spira 2016b, p. 2). It is simply the knowing of our own Being and is the "primal and essential ingredient of experience", (p. 2) which makes all experience possible and knowable.

In IFS parts therapy, the Self is who we are independent of the development of and occlusion by the parts. The parts of the psyche that came into experience through adaptation to our environment are added to who we are essentially. Schwartz and Sweezy (2020) describe the dual nature of Self as either an active inner leader or an expansive boundaryless state of mind, likening it to the duality of light in quantum physics, whereby photons sometimes act like particles and sometimes like waves. Unlike the nondual traditions that generally see the Self or aware presence not as an entity, object or thing, the IFS perspective views the Self (like the quantum particle) as an aspect that can behave like an entity, available to interact with the parts to hear perspectives, to problem solve and to nurture, but (like a wave) is also transcendent and at one with the universe. In IFS, one can attain a shift in identification with the burdened parts to an understanding of oneself as the essence of Self or Being, which is what most spiritual traditions call enlightenment (Schwartz and Sweezy 2020).

4.2. The Qualities of Self: Recognizing Self Essence

The healing properties of the Self are known through one's relative experience in various ways that can become easily recognizable. According to Prendergast (in Prendergast et al. 2003), the Self is presence and can be described as *Being* that is aware of its own aware presence, and describes the effects a transcendent Self has on others as contagious: "When we are in the Presence of an individual who has awakened from the dream of 'me' [the ego], we can sense an unpretentiousness, lucidity, transparency, joy and ease of being" (p. 5). From the nondual understanding of the transpersonal Self as *Awareness*, the Self is objectless; that is, it is aware of objects but is not itself an object; it is noumenal and not phenomenal (Lucille 2006).

Awareness is known as a lack of disturbance, which is felt in the relative sense as peace; an absence of resistance, that is, therefore, inherently allowing; and as wholeness, lacking nothing, and is therefore felt as happiness, contentment or fulfillment. Another way of describing Awareness is as the *absence* of qualities stemming from separation (rooted in lack, conflict and fear), and described in their positive, they are happiness, peace, love, and openness (Spira 2016b). When we know ourselves as Awareness, we experience this relatively as clarity, understanding, wisdom, compassion, and true security; we feel safe in all our experience. This is not to say that we do not feel sadness, loss, or anger, but these feelings tend to have a different quality in the allowing and peaceful presence of Awareness. They do not arise on behalf of securing the insecure separate self. There is an absence of feeling like the sadness or anger is harming or taking something away from us and they find their proper expression and positive action, if needed, from a place of clarity.

From the IFS perspective, Self is the seat of consciousness and its qualities include those of a good leader: compassion, creativity, perspective, curiosity, confidence, and acceptance (Schwartz and Sweezy 2020). Kelly (Schwartz and Kelly 2018) describes the 11 'i's' of Self Essence as invisible, intelligent, innate, is, indestructible, infinite, impersonal, immediate, illumined, ineffable, and inspired. Self Essence does not change or grow, it just is. Self Essence cannot be hurt or destroyed and is "the authentic fundamental nature of who you are, which is felt as an awake awareness" (Schwartz and Kelly 2018). According to Schwartz and Sweezy (2020), a client whose parts are willing to differentiate, or separate out from the Self, describe feeling calm, light, centered and a sense of well-being and exhibit confidence and demonstrate openheartedness. These are the qualities that are needed for strong Self leadership.

4.3. Who Knows the Self?

In the ordinary meaning of the word, self is usually equivalent to the ego (which, according to Schwartz, is a collection of manager parts); however, in this discussion, the Self is more akin to Jung's Self archetype, which is "paradoxically *not* oneself" (Stein 1998, p. 152) and is closer in connotation to the Indian Upanishads designation of the higher personality or *atman* and is symbolic of unity or wholeness (Stein 1998). However, according to Jung, this wholeness is not completely achievable, since "the polarities and opposites resident in the self are forever generating more and new material" (in Stein 1998, p. 158). I agree with this only if one is identified with the polarities and parts within the psychological system. The ego will never know the Self because it is defined as *not being the ego* or more accurately, the ego is split from the Self and therefore *seemingly* not it. If we know ourselves only as a collection of self-concepts and images, the Self will be eclipsed. Only Self can know the Self. Wholeness only knows wholeness.

As Klein (2006) explains, "The ego cannot 'know' itself because it identifies with what it thinks, feels, experiences" (p. 9). By 'know itself' what is meant is the *nature* of itself or the *essence* of itself, i.e., the Self. In my own experience, the discovery that I am not limited to the objects in my experience resulted in the subtle and ordinary recognition of Self, dissolving the apparent ego or self-concept. According to Schwartz and Sweezy (2020), the parts *do* get to know the Self, but I would like to offer a slightly different perspective from my own experience through my nondual understanding and my work with IFS. I noticed that the parts do not really 'know' the Self, but rather begin to know themselves *as the Self* (not separate from the whole). As the Self permeates the parts with its aware light, it appears that the parts are 'knowing' the Self, but what is really happening is that the parts are transforming *into knowing* (awareness), or into the Self. Or the Self is turning the parts into itself. Upon fully integrating, it becomes obvious that the parts never existed apart from the Self at all. As the nondual 12-step recovery advocate, Paul Hedderman, depicts so accurately, instead of trying to add more paint to the canvas, "...something's going to bleed out from the other side . . . . You're going to know on the level of Being" (Hedderman 2019, p. 6). The knowing light shines through, turning what *cannot know* into *knowing* itself. What I did not realize throughout most of my therapy was that the very search for myself from the point of view of what I *conceived of* myself was what was perpetuating the seeming separation from Self and in fact reaffirmed that something was missing and needed to be supplied from outside of myself ('myself' in this case, the ego, collective parts, psyche or finite mind). The search was adding more paint to the canvas creating a thick cover that was obscuring the fact that *something else* was bleeding through from the other side. The self-luminating light of awareness.

5. Essentially Whole, Relatively Wounded: Parts and the Separate Self

Although we all have access to our essential Self at all times, this does not mean that we do not also have other psychological aspects that are in our experience. We experience the effects of patterns of psychological, mental and emotional activity, seen collectively, in some nondual traditions, as the conditioned mind, separate self, or ego states. In IFS these show up in our experience as Exiles, Managers and Firefighter parts that 'take over' the system and seem to cut off from or obscure the Self. In the nondual understanding, much of what we experience is conditioned mental, emotional and sensory/feeling patterns that revolve around a core belief that the self is a fragment, separate from the world and others and in need of defense and aggrandizement.

It might be helpful to see the Self aspect as the vertical formless dimension outside of time and space (in ever-present now) and the psychological aspects evolving on the horizontal, temporal, developmental plane through which our psychological experiences unfold. Nondual Awareness adds a depth dimension to any of the existing schools of psychology and can positively influence therapy through psychotherapists' own Self awareness. While the concept of nondual awareness has already been incorporated horizontally into the Transpersonal Psychology framework, its main effect occurs 'vertically' as therapists deepen their intimacy with Self (Prendergast et al. 2003). Both IFS and spiritual nondual therapeutic modalities bring this vertical dimension of wholeness to the client's awareness as the basis for further psychotherapeutic work, orienting the client toward their wholeness and bringing that essential wholeness to their relatively wounded and fragmented parts.

5.1. The Missing Self: Identifying with the System in IFS

One might ask, if we are essentially always whole and therefore naturally at peace and fulfilled, why is this not experienced by everyone in every moment? In the IFS model, one reason clients sometimes cannot find or sense Self is not from a lack of desire or ability, but because Self is not an "it" and is therefore often overlooked. Self is not an object that can be seen, heard, touched, smelled, tasted or known by thought. It is not an emotion, image, belief, thought, sensation, or even energy. "Trying to know Self with thought is like using our eyes to try to hear music" (Schwartz and Kelly 2018). The parts (often with extreme feelings or perspectives) overshadow the Self, especially if trauma or abuse was experienced. The parts become blended with the Self, an experience in which a part takes over a person's seat of consciousness (Self), which occurs "along a continuum so that the Self can remain present with some blending or be obscured completely with full blending" (Schwartz and Sweezy 2020, p. 281). In trauma-related responses, a part might hijack the body and completely obscure the Self (Fisher 2017) to such an extent that the only perspective available is that of a scared part. If Self is obscured and the parts are polarized, the inner life can be very conflictual and confusing, sometimes bordering on chaos. I came to see my own polarized parts as a kind of "autoimmune self", where parts of me attacked other parts they thought should not be there; the parts not recognizing that they are all part of the same whole. All of this inner conflict arises to defend or subdue something that does not exist apart from the activity that sustains it. Like the quiet and still eye of the storm, the self that is being protected or exiled is a memory, made of the same wind and rain of mental and emotional activity that created it, and when the storm settles down, all that is left is the eye or "I" of Self.

Overlooking True Nature or the Veiling of Awareness

The knowing of ourselves as aware presence is so simple and obvious, and so apparently insignificant that it is usually overlooked or not noticed. Who is it that fails to notice? Spira (2016b) explains that the Self *cannot* fail to know itself, just as the sun cannot fail to illuminate itself: "It is only *thought* that imagines our Self is not known and that something else, like a body, mind or world, is known" (p. 5). With this thought, our Self appears to contract inside the body and mind, and as a result, "intimacy is veiled, love is lost and seeking begins" (p. 5). The Self still knows only the intimacy of our Being, so it is only from the perspective of *thought*, or the inside "separate self," and never from the true Self, that this veiling occurs.

From this perspective, the overlooking and forgetting of our most intimate Being initiate almost all our thoughts, feelings, activities and relationships and turn out to be the source of unhappiness. However, it is not our Being that overlooks itself—our Being is who we *are*, not something we *do*; it is obscuring thought substantiated by feelings that results in the veiling or loss of the knowing of our Self as it truly is and makes it seem that our Self is something other than the presence of Awareness. Spira (2016a) proclaims that "the history of humanity, on both the individual and the collective scales, is the drama of this loss of our true identity and the subsequent search to regain it" (p. 5).

In addition, a belief forms that our Being resides in, is made of, and is limited to the body and mind. This belief is divided in two parts: a separate inside subject—the self that knows, feels or perceives—and a separate outside object, other or world that is known, felt or perceived. The belief that aware presence is synonymous with and limited to the body and shares its characteristics is responsible for the veiling or forgetting of our true identity of infinite aware presence. This veiling is a powerful illusion, an illusion that gives rise to the belief in an inside separate self and is the root of many more beliefs that are examined in the inward-facing path (Spira 2017a). The consequences of the veiling of our true presence by the belief in a separate, limited, fragmented self, is the cause of all internal suffering and outer conflict in the world.

5.2. *A Combined IFS/Nondual Interpretation of the Overlooking Self*

My nondual understanding informs my view of this veiling of Self through IFS work and I have a somewhat different view through my work with both. In IFS, rather than the protective managers preserving the *Self* (wholeness) per se, the protectors are protecting *the exiles*—those parts deemed unworthy, unsafe, or dangerous by the finite (personal) mind—which, constitute the 'separate self" activity, based on the belief in an illusion of separation. These parts are the result of identifying with traits, or patterns of thought and feeling, judged by the system/mind as dangerous, on some level, to survival.

From a nondual perspective, these parts would be considered resistance or aversion, often compounded by failures of safety in the family or environment. These parts are 'exiled' or seemingly separated from the whole Self and contribute to the *felt sense of and belief in separation* as well as the resulting sense of insecurity that veils the light of Self Awareness, our essential Self. The protectors/Managers (in nonduality, insecure and fearful thoughts and resulting behaviors) operate *on behalf of* these exiles or sense of a separate self. In reaction to the insecurity or fear that arises, Managers also try to *build up, secure,* or *maintain* this separate insecure self. All of this activity results in the further obscuring or veiling of the Self, which Schwartz and Sweezy (2020) describe as the 'pushing out' of Self by protectors, and maintaining the 'system'.

5.3. The Importance of Contacting and Accessing the Self Early in Therapy

From my own experience and personal observations as well as conversations with people who have founds limits to healing in conventional psychotherapy, the contribution of identifying and having a *felt understanding* of the essential Self is vast, immediate, and can greatly facilitate the therapeutic process; softening defenses and saving often months or years of ruminating and getting stuck in egoic stories. The recognition of Self as the presence of awareness expands the vertical dimension into the ideas presented by IFS or other therapies that have a plural mind perspective by exploring the creation of an apparent separate self, constructed by identifying with thoughts and feelings that have a root in aversion and lack (seeking and resisting). The interpretation of and subsequent identification with the seeking/resisting thoughts and feelings lead to what IFS would call exiled parts that constitute the felt sense of separation or fragmentation and contributes to the overshadowing or the veiling of Self.

I believe that this expanded view of IFS therapy brings the psychological aspects into a broader context beyond the study of the psyche. This investigative and contemplative approach coupled with the embodied and intimate tantric practices offer an alternative for those who do not want to, or cannot, do IFS parts therapy in the current model. The implications of this feeling-based understanding have profound effects on how we act, behave, and see the world, ourselves and others, and it liberates energy for creative action. From this view, the consequences of failing to bring the Self into the light of awareness is further polarization, the proliferation of fragmented parts, inner and outer conflict, and a deepening sense of separation, loneliness, and alienation from Self, life, and the world.

Innate Wholeness: Why it Matters

Many, but not all, therapies are based on concepts of pathology, correcting personality deficits or fixing problematic aspects of a person's thinking, and supplying missing experiences often with the goal of helping them cope or restoring functionality in a society that is, quite often, dysfunctional. Some are indeed geared toward these goals with the underlying assumption that 'something is wrong' and needs to be corrected, developed or supplied. To be clear, when a person comes to therapy they are often not functioning well and lots of things appear dysfunctional. The 'already whole' perspective is not suggesting that nothing should change, rather it rests very deeply on the humanistic understanding that the qualities and resources one needs are readily available at all times. This is not to say that skills do not need to be learned, new ways of communicating or behaving are not acquired, patterns changed, and mental, emotional and behavioral habits reconditioned, but the client relies on their innate wisdom to guide them to the resources they need and their intuition about what they need when options are available. Self-guidance in healing IS the healing: Wholeness takes the hand of what is broken and leads her back to the wholeness of Self.

In this way, clients come to see that they have always had these resources and that the ways their system protects them comes from a deep intelligence and love of Self. This is not trying to convince a client to love parts of themselves that they do not (or that other 'parts' do not) or 'seeing what is good' in all the bad—it is seeing that they have always been operating perfectly based on a certain perspective or understanding (through the point of view of child parts or the separate self or ego). Their entire Self *is designed* to lead them back to themselves, back to their essential Self and their innate qualities. Their Self has been hiding in plain sight and they only need to 'get eyes for it' to see what has always been true. This understanding and Self-attunement brings a relaxing of defensive parts as the presence of Self is felt and known. This allows for the deeper layers of feelings to show up and for the client to feel safe. I see this as a paradigm shift, a reorientation that has the power to change the experience of the mental maze into one of a labyrinth of liberation.

6. Conclusions

This inquiry has led me to the conviction that the Self is the center of healing in any therapeutic model or modality, whether it is acknowledged as such, called by another name, or conceived differently, such as a 'capacity to heal' or a quest for wholeness, inner wisdom, or even referred to as the biological effects, such as 'rewiring the brain.' Both IFS and the nondual wisdom traditions hold that the wholeness of the transpersonal Self is self-evident, inherently undamaged, can be accessed readily with willingness and openness, and self-healing. This understanding of Self naturally moves us in the direction of remedying inner and outer injustice with love and openness and is the ultimate presence for attachment for the inner parts and outer relationships (Schwartz and Sweezy 2020).

Nondual wisdom points us to the original wound of the apparent splitting off from the fabric of wholeness, the flow of life, and the shared beingness with everything and everyone. With an ever deepening and never-ending exploration we find that as we are not separate from the world, and that while bodies can be hurt, become sick or injured and eventually die, and finite minds are limited, we know and feel ourselves as not two, not separate, and in this way, we come to know that there is not me and other, us and them, or me against the world; and ultimately, as such, we are ultimately safe everywhere.

This kind of healing is not limited to personal psychological or spiritual healing and does not just affect the client and her immediate relationships. Coming to know the Self as the ground of being through self-inquiry, unburdening the parts, or any other means, allows the activity of mind or ego to drop off or dissipate, allowing the Self's qualities of clarity and courage to radically shift our perspective (Schwartz and Sweezy 2020). As Schwartz says, "Having been released from the optical delusion that we are all separate, we see injustice clearly, we fear for our environment, and we are oriented to take action" (Schwartz and Sweezy 2020, p. 54). We become less ego-centric and more "socio- and species-centric, bio-and earth-centric" (Schwartz and Sweezy 2020, p. 54) from having a clear awareness of our interconnectedness. Self-led action and communication tends to be more effective in the world because such qualities as compassion, clarity and calm often touch the Self in others, whereas action from polarized parts (power-seeking, righteousness, or caretaking) conflict with one another and lead to burnout and cynicism in the long-run.

With the Self leading the way, we find that the awareness of our interconnectedness leads to social and environmental action, according to our individual resources and abilities (Schwartz and Sweezy 2020). With our deepening knowledge of our Self and openness to all parts that arise, we find that our actions, thoughts, feelings and relationships no longer serve the demands of an insecure separate self. Rather our inner and outer lives align with our felt knowledge of shared being and carry with them a universal clarity and power that guides us and includes all. With the consistent felt understanding of the collapse of self and other into one and the recognition that our ground of being is love, our unburdened individual selves are energized and free to act in ways consistent with that love for all beings, in manners that are uniquely suited to each individual.

Throughout my life, I sought healing, wholeness, fulfillment, and happiness in many directions both spiritual and psychological, but it always felt like I was terrifyingly walking a tightrope 1000 miles above the ground, and with each spiritual practice or therapy intervention, I was thrown a tether or sometimes just a thread. I would hang on to it as long as I could, feeling temporarily less wobbly and more secure, but would eventually drop it or it would fray and I would be left on my own, balancing on a tightrope, impossibly high from the ground. It was not until I truly felt my spiritual essence/true nature, the internal golden thread, that in one eternal moment, I saw with utmost clarity that I had always and only *ever* been just inches from the ground—and in that instant, I simply stepped off the tightrope into the infinite ground of Being. I have been here ever since and this is the ground upon which I open myself to life and to others.

Funding: This research received no external funding.

Conflicts of Interest: The author declares no conflict of interest.

Appendix A

Definitions and Terms

- (The capital 'S') Self: transpersonal or essential Self.
- In a general sense, I am using the definition of *transpersonal* found in the APA Dictionary of Psychology within the definition of 'transpersonal psychology': Transpersonal refers to the concern with ends that transcend personal identity and individual, immediate desires (APA Dictionary of Psychology n.d.). I am speaking of that which goes beyond the beliefs of what we think or conceptualize as ourselves as well as the felt sense of those beliefs and self-concepts.
- I use the words *wholeness, true nature, awareness* and *Self* synonymously to represent the *essential Self*.
- Essential Self: Whatever it is that knows or is aware of all experience and does not appear and disappear in experience.
- Functional self: Ego, or sense of localization that gives rise to agency, personal will, autonomy, and identification with a limited body and finite mind.
- The system (in IFS): The organization or the process of mental and emotional processing, meaning making, interpretation, belief making. In parts language, they are exiles, managers, firefighters (Schwartz and Sweezy 2020).
- Psyche/mind: The activity of mind in its totality, including all types of thinking, imagining, and conceptualizing and the internal logic of this mental processing. I use the words 'psyche' and "mind" interchangeably and sometimes use it to mean 'the system.'
- Ego: The self, particularly the conscious sense of self (Latin, "I"). In its popular and quasi-technical sense, ego refers to all the psychological phenomena and processes that are related to the self and that comprise the individual's attitudes, values, and concerns (APA Dictionary of Psychology n.d.)[with which one identifies with].
- Separate self: An activity of thinking, feeling, acting, perceiving and relating on behalf of an imagined, temporary, finite consciousness.
- Object: Anything that can be known: thoughts, feelings, perceptions, sensations. (Also: objects of experience: all that we are aware of.)
- Perceiving: to become aware of through the senses (Merriam-Webster.com Dictionary n.d., accessed on 3 September 2021).
- Psychological self: A subject or personal identification with the system of psychological processes, defenses, and various mental processes. Acquired self: Autobiographical self, based on history, memory, preferences and dislikes, based on experience, learning, conditioning and psychological patterning.
- Illusion: A real object of experience, the reality of which is not what it appears to be.

Appendix B

Resources and Further Reading
Internal Family Systems: https://ifs-institute.com/ (accessed on 2 September 2021).
Rupert Spira: https://rupertspira.com/ (accessed on 2 September 2021).
Francis Lucille: https://francislucille.com/ (accessed on 2 September 2021).
Kashmir Shaivism: https://iep.utm.edu/kashmiri/ (accessed on 2 September 2021).

References

APA Dictionary of Psychology. n.d.a. Transpersonal Psychology. Available online: https://dictionary.apa.org/transpersonal-psychology (accessed on 22 June 2020).
APA Dictionary of Psychology. n.d.b. Humanistic Psychology. Available online: https://dictionary.apa.org/humanistic-psychology (accessed on 27 August 2020).
APA Dictionary of Psychology. n.d.c. Ego. Available online: https://dictionary.apa.org/ego (accessed on 17 June 2020).
Atmananda Krishna Menon. 2009. *Notes on Spiritual Discourses of Srīātmānanda*, 2nd ed. Edited by Tṛipta Nitya. Salisbury: Non-Duality Press & Stillness Speaks, vol. 1.
Bowlby, John. 1988. *A Secure Base: Parent-Child Attachment and Healthy Human Development*. New York: Basic Books.

Brenner, Gail. 2018. *Suffering Is Optional: A Spiritual Guide to Freedom from Self-Judgment & Feelings of Inadequacy*. Oakland: Reveal Press.
Daniels, Michael. 2002a. The Transpersonal Self: 1. A Psychohistory and Phenomenology of the Soul. Available online: http://www.transpersonalscience.org/Papers/daniels02d.pdf (accessed on 28 August 2021).
Daniels, Michael. 2002b. The Transpersonal Self: 2. Comparing Seven Psychological Theories. Available online: https://psychicscience.org/Papers/daniels02b.pdf (accessed on 28 August 2021).
Fisher, Janina. 2017. *Healing the Fragmented Selves of Trauma Survivors Overcoming Internal Self-Alienation*. New York: Routledge Press—Taylor and Francis Group.
GreekMythology.com. 2021. Ariadne. GreekMythology.com Website. Available online: https://www.greekmythology.com/Myths/Mortals/Ariadne/ariadne.html (accessed on 21 July 2020).
Hedderman, Paul. 2019. *The Incomplete Works of Paul Hedderman, Volume I: On Having Never Left*. Independently Published.
Jung, C. G. 1970. *The Collected Works of C.G. Jung*. Princeton: Princeton University Press, vol. 17. First published 1954.
Kastrup, Bernardo. 2018. The universe in consciousness. *Journal of Consciousness Studies* 25: 125–155.
Kingsley, Jenny. 2010. Musing and meandering through labyrinths and mazes. *The Art Book* 17: 90–92. [CrossRef]
Klein, Jean. 2006. *I am*. Edited by Emma Edwards. Oakland: Non-Duality Press.
Krishnamurti, J. 1969. *Freedom from the Known*. Edited by Mary Lutyens. London: Gollancz.
Life, David. 2007. See More Clearly by Practicing Drishti. Available online: https://www.yogajournal.com/yoga-101/philosophy/the-eye-of-the-beholder (accessed on 28 August 2007).
Lucille, Francis. 2006. *The Perfume of Silence*. Temecula: Truespeech Productions.
Nisargadatta Maharaj. 2012. *I Am That: Talks with Sri Nisargadatta Maharaj*. Edited by Sudhakar S. Dikshit. Translated by Maurice Frydman. Durham: Acorn Press.
Maharshi, Ramana. 2008. *Who am I?: The Teachings of Bhagavan Sri Ramana Maharshi*. Tamil Nadu: Sri Ramanasramam.
Merriam-Webster.com Dictionary. n.d. Perceive. Available online: https://www.merriam-webster.com/dictionary/perceive (accessed on 3 September 2021).
Pillai, Narayana N. 2019. *Atmananda Krishna Menon: Direct Path to Realization 'I'-Principle. Chattampi Swami Archive Project*. Trivandrum: Centre for South Indian Studies.
Prendergast, John J., Peter Fenner, and Sheila Krystal. 2003. *The Sacred Mirror: Nondual Wisdom & Psychotherapy*. St. Paul: Paragon House.
Prendergast, John J. 2019. *The Deep Heart: Our Portal to Presence*. Boulder: Sounds True.
Schwartz, Richard C., and Robert Falconer. 2017. *Many Minds, One Self: Evidence for a Radical Shift in Paradigm*. Oak Park: Trailheads.
Schwartz, Richard C., and Loch Kelly. 2018. Accessing and Living from Self. IFS Institute online Course. Available online: http://courses.ifscircle.com/self/ (accessed on 11 November 2019).
Schwartz, Richard C., and Martha Sweezy. 2020. *Internal Family Systems Therapy*. New York: The Guilford Press.
Spira, Rupert. 2014. *The Light of Pure Knowing: Thirty Meditations on the Essence of Non-Duality*. Oxford: Sahaja Publications.
Spira, Rupert. 2016a. *Presence, Volume I: The Art of Peace and Happiness*. Oxford: Sahaja Publications.
Spira, Rupert. 2016b. *Presence, Volume II: The Intimacy of all Experience*. Oxford: Sahaja Publications.
Spira, Rupert. 2016c. *Transparent Body, Luminous World: The Tantric Yoga of Sensation and Perception*. Oxford: Sahaja Publications.
Spira, Rupert. 2017a. *Being Aware of Being Aware*. Oxford: Sahaja Publications.
Spira, Rupert. 2017b. *The Nature of Consciousness*. Oxford: Sahaja Publications.
Stein, Murray. 1998. *Jung's Map of the Soul: An Introduction*. Chicago: Open Court.
Welwood, John. 1983. *Awakening the Heart: East/West Approaches to Psychotherapy and the Healing Relationship*. Boston: Shambhala.
Weinberg, Gerald M. 2001. *An Introduction to General Systems Thinking*. New York: Dorset House Publishing.
Wilber, Ken. 1998. *The Essential Ken Wilber: An Introductory Reader*. Boston: Shambhala.

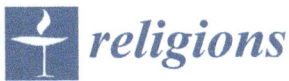

Article

Do Involvement in Alcoholics Anonymous and Religiousness Both Directly and Indirectly through Meaning in Life Lead to Spiritual Experiences?

Marcin Wnuk

Department of Psychology, Adam Mickiewicz University in Poznań, 60-568 Poznań, Poland; marwnu@amu.edu.pl

Abstract: Spirituality is a key element of Alcoholics Anonymous (AA) recovery. However, little is known about the potential religious and secular sources of spiritual experiences in AA fellowship. The aim of the study was to verify if in a sample of AA participants, meaning in life mediates the relationship between their religiousness and spiritual experiences, as well as between their involvement in AA and spiritual experiences. The study sample consisted of 70 Polish AA participants, and the following tools were used: the Alcoholics Anonymous Involvement Scale (AAIS); Santa Clara Strength of Religious Faith Questionnaire (SCSORFQ); Purpose in Life Test (PIL); two one-item measures regarding frequency of prayer and Mass attendance; and the Daily Spiritual Experiences Scale (DSES) duration of AA participation, which was positively related to involvement in addiction self-help groups and religiousness. Involvement in AA and religiousness were positively related to meaning in life, which in turn positively correlated with spiritual experiences. This research indicated that in a sample of AA participants, finding meaning in life partially mediates the relationship between religiousness and spiritual experiences, as well as fully mediating the relationship between involvement in AA and spiritual experiences. The theoretical and practical implications are discussed.

Keywords: Alcoholics Anonymous; religiousness; involvement in self-help groups; meaning in life; spiritual experiences; mediator variable

Citation: Wnuk, Marcin. 2021. Do Involvement in Alcoholics Anonymous and Religiousness Both Directly and Indirectly through Meaning in Life Lead to Spiritual Experiences? *Religions* 12: 794. https://doi.org/10.3390/rel12100794

Academic Editors: Bernadette Flanagan and Noelia Molina

Received: 31 July 2021
Accepted: 17 September 2021
Published: 23 September 2021

Publisher's Note: MDPI stays neutral with regard to jurisdictional claims in published maps and institutional affiliations.

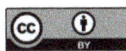

Copyright: © 2021 by the author. Licensee MDPI, Basel, Switzerland. This article is an open access article distributed under the terms and conditions of the Creative Commons Attribution (CC BY) license (https://creativecommons.org/licenses/by/4.0/).

1. Introduction

According to the literature on alcohol-dependent individuals, involvement in Alcoholics Anonymous (AA) is related to positive outcomes such as sobriety (Zemore 2007; Kaskutas et al. 2003), lower likelihood of relapse (Sheeren 1988), fewer psychiatric severity and depressive symptoms (Galanter et al. 2012), and lower anxiety (Galanter et al. 2012). Recent longitudinal studies have indicated that the AA attendance indirectly, through improving individuals' spirituality, decreased alcohol consumption (usually through sobriety; Kelly et al. 2011; Krentzman et al. 2013; Tonigan et al. 2013; Zemore 2007). Besides involvement in AA, another source of spirituality among AA members is religiousness (Pardini et al. 2000; Lyons et al. 2011; Richard et al. 2000). Despite the fact that they may present religious skepticism, most AA participants identify themselves as spiritual but not religious (McClure and Wilkinson 2020). In comparison to participants of other therapeutic programs for alcohol addiction, AA members also significantly more frequently declare that spirituality is not the same as religiousness (Atkins and Hawdon 2007).

According to Kurtz and White (2015), it is reasonable to distinguish between two groups of participants within AA fellowship: religious spirituality followers and secular spirituality followers. These two groups, which differ in attitude toward spirituality, reflect two different means of spiritual growth in self-help groups, with the first based on religiousness and the second on AA involvement. In the first group, religion can be a framework for having a meaning-oriented system (Silberman 2005), leading to spiritual growth. In the second group, the source of a framework for a meaning-oriented system that facilitates spiritual experiences can be the AA philosophy (Alcoholics Anonymous 2001). Little is known about the mechanisms through which involvement in AA and religiousness influence the spiritual experiences of AA participants. In particular, in addiction literature, a lack of precise, well-established definitions for spirituality and religiousness have led to some misunderstandings, as has using them interchangeably (Kelly 2017).

Religiousness and spirituality are separate but overlapping constructs, with spirituality being a broader concept than religiousness (Baumsteiger and Chenneville 2015). Spiritual experiences can be results of both religious practices (King et al. 2020) and some secular activities, such as involvement in AA (Krentzman et al. 2017). Spiritual experiences are conceptualized as a feeling God's presence, feeling deep inner peace or harmony, feeling spiritually touched by the beauty of creation, experiencing a connection to all of life, feeling a selfless caring for others and a desire to be closer to God, or being in union with the divine (Underwood 2011).

The aim of this study was to verify two mechanisms leading to AA participants' spiritual experiences. The first one, called religious spirituality, leads to AA participants' spiritual experiences through facilitating finding meaning in life as a result of religiousness. The second one, secular spirituality, offers AA involvement as an antecedent to finding meaning and purpose in life, which in turn positively correlates with spiritual experiences.

2. Literature Review

Both participants who use their own religiousness as a recovery tool and non-religious members who identify themselves as religiously skeptical are involved in AA. The spiritual character of the 12-step program (Kurtz and White 2015; Liisi 1981), a core AA philosophy (Alcoholics Anonymous 2001), has a positive impact on openness to diverse religious affiliations and individuals without religious inclinations. Studies have also proven that the beneficial effect of AA membership is comparable to religion for secular members who define themselves as atheists or agnostic (Tonigan et al. 2002; Winzelberg and Humphreys 1999). Additional research has shown that involvement in AA is positively related to religiousness (Krentzman et al. 2017; Kelly et al. 2011), but some authors have indicated that religious barriers pose difficulties for AA involvement (George and Tucker 1996).

Still, some studies have confirmed that individuals who participate in spiritual and religious activities are more likely to later become affiliated with AA (Kelly and Moos 2003; Emrick et al. 1993). For example, in a study by Krentzman et al. (2017), involvement in AA measured by the Alcoholics Anonymous Involvement Scale positively correlated with private religious practices and positive religious coping. One study of different recovery groups (the 12-step program, Self-Management for Addiction Recovery, Women for Sobriety, and Secular Organizations for Sobriety) also has showed that while the average length of sobriety was similar across groups, spiritual and religious factors were more likely to predict greater program participation among 12-step members than Self-Management for Addiction Recovery or Secular Organizations for Sobriety members (Atkins and Hawdon 2007).

Hypothesis 1 (H1). *In a sample of Polish AA participants, AA involvement is positively correlated with religiousness.*

AA participation differs from AA involvement, but both of these constructs are positively related (Krentzman et al. 2011). AA attendance is a *conditio sine qua non* for AA involvement, but it is not an AA involvement indicator because it does not consist of activities being of AA involvement aspects, such as reading of AA literature, being a sponsor, or having a sponsor (Humphreys et al. 1998). It means not necessarily someone who attends AA meetings for a long period of time must engage in sponsorship, considers himself/herself an AA member, or performs service, although most of the AA participants do this. Previous research has highlighted that involvement in AA has changed positively, but these results are limited to a relatively short period of time, no longer than 6 months (Vederhus et al. 2014; Manning et al. 2012). In a study by Tonigan et al. (2017), a higher percentage of participants with long AA lifetime histories in comparison with participants with short AA lifetime histories reported higher rates of attending AA, considered themselves AA members, had an AA sponsor, and experienced a spiritual awakening in AA.

Longer AA attendance can lead to growing religious commitment of AA participants. According to research by Tonigan et al. (2017), longer duration of AA participation was related to spiritual/religious practices, such as frequency of prayer, meditation, and thoughts about God, which in turn led to decrease in alcohol consumption and an increase in the percentage of days of abstinence. In another study, positive perceptions of God was related in AA membership (Krentzman et al. 2011).

Hypothesis 2 (H2). *In a sample of Polish AA participants, duration of AA participation is positively correlated with involvement in AA and religiousness.*

Besides religiousness (Sørensen et al. 2019; Wnuk 2015), among alcohol-dependent individuals, one of the antecedents of meaning in life is involvement in Alcoholics Anonymous (Montgomery et al. 1995; Tonigan 2001; Carroll 1993; Gomes and Hart 2009; Oakes et al. 2000). Involvement in addiction self-help groups facilitates finding meaning in life for substance-addicted individuals (Montgomery et al. 1995; Tonigan 2001; Carroll 1993; Gomes and Hart 2009; Oakes et al. 2000). For example, among participants of Narcotics Anonymous (NA) in the U.S., involvement in NA predicted their level of purpose in life (DeLucia et al. 2016). In a sample of AA participants from Great Britain, the completion of steps 4 and 5 of the 12-step program, as well as involvement in AA, correlated positively with their existential wellbeing (Gomes and Hart 2009). In turn, finding meaning and purpose in life is an important factor for spirituality among individuals diagnosed with addiction. Indeed, many studies have noted the positive relationship between meaning in life and spiritual experiences among alcohol- and drug-addicted patients (Lyons et al. 2011; Webb et al. 2006; Gutierrez 2019). It means that religiousness and involvement in AA can be factors that indirectly through meaning in life positively influence spirituality of AA, with these two aspects of AA functionality serving as a meaning-oriented system (Silberman 2005) that positively affects spiritual experiences.

On the other hand, some studies have indicated a direct positive relationship between AA religiousness (Pardini et al. 2000; Lyons et al. 2011) and spirituality, as well as between involvement in AA and spirituality. For example, Pardini et al. (2000) found that faith leads to higher self-rated spirituality. Lyons et al. (2011) also noted that the religious spiritual practices of drug-addicted individuals predict their spiritual experiences. Moreover, in two studies conducted by Krentzman et al. (2013, 2017), involvement in AA predicted spiritual experiences of AA participants.

This means that both religiousness and AA involvement can positively influence AA spiritual experiences, both directly and indirectly through meaning in life.

These four mechanisms were tested.

Hypothesis 3 (H3). *In a sample of Polish AA participants, meaning in life mediates the relationship between religiousness and spiritual experiences.*

Hypothesis 4 (H4). *In a sample of Polish AA participants, meaning in life mediates the relationship between AA involvement and spiritual experiences.*

3. Materials and Methods

3.1. Participants

The participants of this study were 70 individuals addicted to alcohol who attended AA meetings in Poland. The participants orally confirmed their consent to take part in the study, and the data were collected via questionnaire between January and June 2014. The questionnaires were distributed by a psychologist during AA meetings and collected at the next meeting after the participants completed them at home. Of the 200 distributed questionnaires, only 70 were returned. This means that the questionnaire return rate was low. This was due to the fact that many participants were absent at the next meeting. Each participant answered "yes" for the question about being diagnosed with alcohol dependence—"Have you ever been diagnosed with alcohol dependence?".

3.2. Measures

3.2.1. Spiritual Experiences

The Daily Spiritual Experiences Scale (DSES) consists of 16 questions, each with 6 points ranging from 1 (*never or almost never*) to 6 (*many times daily*). The more points scored, the greater the respondent's level of spirituality. Depending on the population, the scale's reliability ranges from $\alpha = 0.86$ to 0.95 (Laustalot et al. 2006). The short version of this measure was used for this study, which consists of 6 items.

3.2.2. Strength of Religious Faith

The Santa Clara Strength of Religious Faith Questionnaire (SCSORFQ) consists of 10 items that respondents rate on a 5-point Likert scale from 1 (*strongly disagree*) to 5 (*strongly agree*). Factor analysis confirmed that the questionnaire items make up one dimension that can be called the strength of religious beliefs (Lewis et al. 2001; Wnuk 2017). The scale's reliability has been determined as $\alpha = 0.94$–0.96 (Plante and Boccaccini 1997a, 1997b; Wnuk 2017).

3.2.3. Involvement in AA

The Alcoholics Anonymous Involvement Scale (AAIS) was used to assess the participants' lifetime AA attendance (Tonigan et al. 1996). The AAIS consists of 13 items related to AA attendance and involvement in AA activities. For 9 items, participants respond "yes" or "no". For this study, 6 items were chosen that ask if the participants consider themselves a member of AA, go to 90 meetings in 90 days, celebrate AA birthdays, have and/or are a sponsor, and have had a spiritual awakening. For these questions, participants responded "yes" or "no".

3.2.4. Duration of AA Participation

For the question regarding duration in AA participation, the participants responded with their corresponding number of months in AA.

3.2.5. Meaning in Life

The Purpose in Life Test (PIL) consists of 20 items concerning meaning in life, which subjects respond to by indicating a field on a continuum ranging from 1 to 7, with 7 representing maximum meaning in life and 1 representing the minimum. The score is computed by adding up the responses to all items. The higher the score, the stronger the satisfaction of the respondent's need for meaning in life; the lower the score, the greater the respondent's existential frustration. This test's reliability, when measured as Pearson's r coefficient, was 0.82, and when measured with the Spearman–Brown correction, it was 0.90 (Crumbaugh and Maholick 1964).

3.2.6. Prayer

The scale for measuring how often the participants prayed consisted of never (1), sometimes (2), once a month (3), once a week (4), and every day (5).

3.2.7. Mass Attendance

The participants' Mass attendance was measured on the basis of a 5-point scale consisting of (1) never, with the exception of baptisms, weddings, or funerals; (2) a few times a year; (3) 1–2 times monthly; (4) 2–3 times monthly; and (5) once per week or more.

3.3. Statistical Analyses

All statistical analyses were conducted using IBM SPSS Statistics software (Version 27.0). Structural equation modeling was used to verify the research hypotheses. The structural model was tested by applying path analyses to investigate the relationships among the latent variable of religiousness and the measurable variables, such as AA involvement, meaning in life, duration of AA participation, and spiritual experiences. Religiousness consisted of three indicators: religious faith and two religious practices, such as Mass attendance and prayer. Due to this study's relatively small sample size, the Bollen–Stine bootstrapping method for 5000 samples was used to increase the likelihood of the obtained results' veracity.

The following goodness of fit indicators were used: root mean square error of approximation (RMSEA), the comparative fit index (CFI), goodness of fit index (GFI), and normed fit index (NFI). RMSEA values less than 0.08, and ideally below 0.05, indicated an adequate fit to the data (Browne and Cudeck 1993). Values of 0.90 or greater, and ideally above 0.95, denoted good model fits for the CFI and GFI (Hu and Bentler 1999); in turn, the NFI should exceed 0.90 (Steiger 1990).

4. Results

The research variables descriptive statistics are presented in Table 1. R-Pearson correlation coefficients between research variables are presented in Table 2, while the measurement results of the tested model's goodness of fit indicators are shown in Table 3. Final model was presented at Figure 1.

Table 1. Descriptive statistics in Alcoholics Anonymous sample ($n = 70$).

	Duration of AA Participation	AAIS	SCSORFQ	Frequency of Prayer	Frequency of Mass Attendance	PIL	DSES
Mean	102.76	3.77	39.84	4.18	3.41	108.14	21.37
SD	71.38	1.42	10.30	1.36	1.61	14.84	7.39
Skewness	0.73	−0.53	−1.38	−1.24	−0.35	−0.88	0.76
Kurtosis	0.09	0.47	−1.45	−0.18	−1.59	0.96	0.03
Minimum	1	0	10	1	1	66	5
Maximum	312	6	50	5	5	134	41
Reliability		0.68	0.95	—	—	0.79	0.94

(Source: author's research). AAIS—Alcoholics Anonymous Involvement Scale; SCSORFQ—Santa Clara Strength of Religious Faith Questionnaire; PIL—Purpose in Life Test; DSES—Daily Spiritual Experiences Scale.

Table 2. R-Pearson correlation coefficients between research variables ($n = 70$).

	1	2	3	4	5	6
1. Prayer						
2. Mass attendance	0.61 **					
3. Strength of religious faith	0.72 **	0.76 **				
4. Spiritual experiences	0.52 **	0.58 **	0.77 **			
5. Meaning in life	0.36 **	0.29 *	0.42 **	0.55 **		
6. Involvement in AA	0.24 *	0.20	0.31 **	0.38 **	0.35 **	
7. Duration of AA participation	0.34 **	0.29 *	0.38 **	0.40 **	0.34 **	0.48 **

* $p \leq 0.05$. ** $p \leq 0.01$.

Table 3. Model fit indicators in a sample of Alcoholics Anonymous (*n* = 70).

CMIN/DF	RMSEA	CFI	GFI	NFI	The Bollen–Stine Bootstrapping Method
0.890 (*p* = 0.540)	[0.000 90% (0.000; 0.058)]	1	0.97	0.97	(*p* = 0.914)

(Source: author's research).

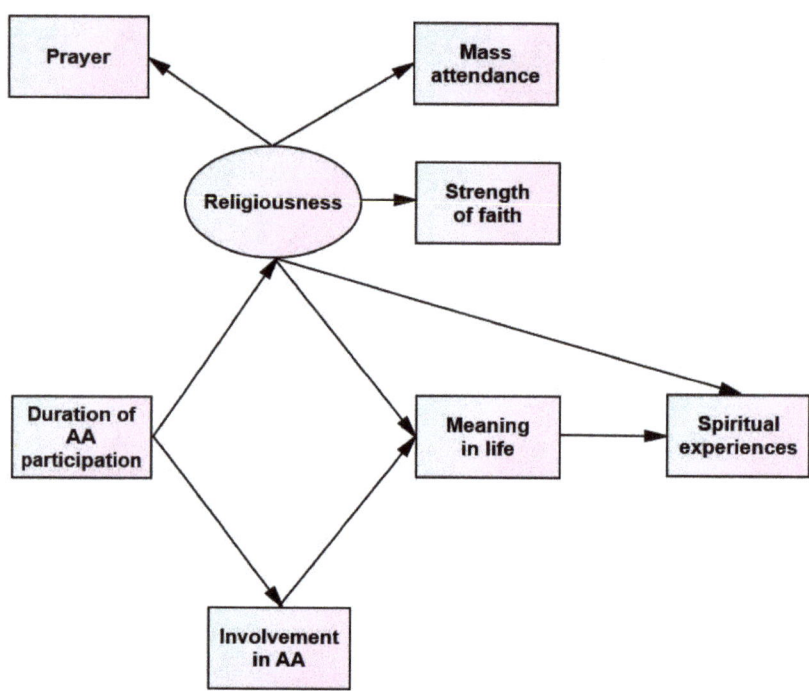

Figure 1. Final model of research. (Source: author's research).

The standardized regression weights for each verified paths, apart of the path between AA involvement and spiritual experiences (CI 95% [−0.122, 0.133], beta = 0.014; *p* = 0.830), were statistically significant. Inconsistent with first hypothesis, the correlation between AA involvement and religiousness (beta = 0.139; *p* = 0.247) was not statistically significant. Additionally, the RMSEA value was less than the ideal 0.05 (Browne and Cudeck 1993), although the CFI and GFI values were greater than the anticipated at 0.95 (Hu and Bentler 1999), and the NFI value was greater than 0.90 (Steiger 1990).

Duration of AA participation predicted both AA involvement (CI 95% [0.264, 0.647], beta = 0.488; *p* < 0.01) and religiousness (CI 95% [0.166, 0.572], beta = 0.391; *p* < 0.01), while it indirectly influenced meaning in life (CI 95% [0.142, 0.373], indirect effect = 0.260; *p* < 0.01) and spiritual experiences (CI 95% [0.157, 0.472], indirect effect = 0.334; *p* < 0.01).

Religiousness was both a predictor of meaning in life (CI 95% [0.131, 0.540], beta = 0.345; *p* < 0.01) and spiritual experiences (CI 95% [0.471, 0.833], beta = 0.677; *p* < 0.01). In addition, religiousness indirectly influenced spiritual experiences (CI 95% [0.024, 0.200], indirect effect = 0.091; *p* < 0.05), as did AA involvement (CI 95% [0.005, 0.169], indirect effect = 0.068; *p* < 0.05).

Meaning in life was also a predictor of spiritual experiences (CI 95% [0.016, 0.486], beta = 0.265; *p* < 0.05).

The tested model explained 42.82% of the variance in the AA members' spiritual experiences.

Religiousness as a latent variable consisted of three observed religious indicators: strength of religious faith, frequency of prayer, and frequency of Mass attendance. This religiousness indicators were intercorrelated. Both frequency of prayer and frequency of Mass attendance moderately correlated with spiritual experiences. Correlation between religious faith and spiritual experiences was strong, meaning that these were overlapping constructs. From the other side, this correlation was not too strong (less than 0.8) to admit that these are the same constructs or that these are indicators that measure the same construct. Additionally, religiousness as a latent variable was only moderate, not being strong predictor of spiritual experiences, despite the fact that strength of religious faith was the strongest observed indicator of religiousness as a latent variable.

Moreover, differences in relationships between observed religiousness indicators and involvement in AA, as well as religiousness as a latent variable and involvement in AA, were noticed. Frequency of prayer and the strength of religious faith were positively related to involvement in AA, but frequency of Mass attendance was not correlated with involvement in AA. Furthermore, religiousness as a latent variable was not statistically significantly correlated with involvement in AA.

5. Discussion

The aim of this study was to explore the potential influence of AA participants' religiousness and AA involvement to find meaning in life as a predictor of their spiritual experiences. In this model, both religiousness and AA involvement served as potential sources of a meaning-making-oriented framework as an element that facilitates spiritual experiences. However, the hypothesis predicting a positive correlation between religiousness and AA involvement was not confirmed because the relationship between the two variables was not statistically significant. These results are not consistent with previous research (Krentzman et al. 2017), indicating religiousness and AA involvement as related variables that are engaged in the spiritual process. This inconsistency can be explained by differences in research samples, distinct socio-cultural contexts, the use of different measures of religiousness, cross-sectional as opposed to longitudinal research design, and the fact that only six items from the original AAIS were used here.

However, the most important factors that determined this difference seemed to be duration of AA participation and abstinence duration, which differed significantly between these studies. It is also possible that in the first stage of the recovery process, involvement in AA is related to religiousness, because of the restoration of this sphere of life that was neglected prior to sobriety. Another important factor that could decide upon the lack of this correlation was religiousness as a latent variable, which consisted of three observed indicators. Two of these indicators, found by R-Pearson coefficient, were positively related to involvement in AA, but one of them was not. It means that frequency of prayer and strength of religious faith were positively correlated with involvement in AA, but frequency of Mass attendance and religiousness as a latent variable were not correlated with involvement in AA. On the other side, it is difficult to predict if in the model, only one indicator of religiousness as an observed variable, such as strength of religious faith or frequency of prayer, would lead to statistically significant correlations between them and involvement in AA. To verify these assumptions, we tested two additional models. The first one was strength of religious faith as an observed variable instead of religiousness as a latent variable, and the second one was frequency of prayer as an observed indicator of religiousness. In both cases, there were no statistically significant correlations between strength of religious faith and involvement in AA, as well as between frequency of prayer and involvement in AA, despite the fact that both of these models were well fitted to the data.

Meanwhile, the hypothesis regarding AA membership as a positive predictor of AA involvement as well as religiousness was confirmed. This means that for alcohol-addicted individuals from Poland, longer duration of AA participation is positively related to AA involvement and religious practices, as well as strength of religious faith. These results are consistent with previous research that emphasized that AA participation longer than 6 months is positively related to AA involvement (Vederhus et al. 2014; Manning et al. 2012). As in the study by Krentzman et al. (2011), religiousness was correlated with duration of AA participation. These results have confirmed that AA membership facilitates both AA involvement and religiousness, and these two factors are important elements in the spiritual process based on self-help group participation in Poland.

The hypotheses regarding the mediating role of meaning in life in the relationships between Polish AA participants' involvement in AA or religiousness and spiritual experiences were confirmed, but with one exception. In reference to relationships between religiousness, meaning in life, and spiritual experiences, religiousness predicted spiritual experiences both directly and indirectly through meaning in life. Involvement in AA influenced spiritual experiences only indirectly via meaning in life.

The achieved results were mostly consistent with extant research and have suggested that involvement in self-help groups and religiousness facilitate finding meaning in life for alcohol-addicted individuals (Wnuk 2015; Montgomery et al. 1995; Tonigan 2001; Carroll 1993; Gomes and Hart 2009; Oakes et al. 2000), which in turn leads to more frequent spiritual experiences (Lyons et al. 2011; Webb et al. 2006; Gutierrez 2019). It is worth noting that the direct effect of religiousness as a predictor of spiritual experiences was much greater than its indirect effect. This is attributable to religion and the AA philosophy being two different meaning-oriented systems (Silberman 2003, 2005) that allow alcohol-dependent individuals to improve their spirituality through finding purpose and meaning in life as a result of committing to self-help groups or increasing their faith and religious practices. These two spiritual mechanisms are thus parallel to and independent of each other.

Following Kurtz and White's (2015) implications, the first mechanism, secular spirituality, has its roots in AA involvement, and the second, religious spirituality, has its source in religious commitment. Both of these mechanisms can be used parallelly with religiously inclined AA participants as well as religiously sceptic AA members. Even religiously skeptical members of AA can restore their religiousness or experience religious conversion because of AA participation.

Longer duration of AA participation is correlated with greater AA involvement and religious commitment. Religion and AA membership both serve alcohol-dependent individuals in participating in self-help groups as frameworks to perceive, experience, and explain life events through the prism of life philosophy. The two frameworks also offer examples from religious and self-help fellowships to model attitudes in the social learning process (Bandura 1986). Ultimately, they allow AA participants to understand the history of their life; facilitate building a new identity; integrate difficult and painful life events; and make life easier as something coherent, predictable, and controllable. Using Frankl's (1992) *tragic optimism* metaphor, both religious commitment and AA involvement support alcohol-addicted individuals as they transform their tragic and painful situation caused by alcohol dependence into something meaningful. Both religion and the AA philosophy can deliver ultimate life meaning, supporting finding of purpose in life in every situation, especially those most complicated, painful, and difficult to manage (Frankl 1992). Independent of whether religion or AA philosophy lead to AA participants finding meaning in life, the final result of this process is spiritual growth, as reflected in the AA participants' spiritual experiences. Both the secular and religious mechanisms leading to spiritual experiences through finding meaning in life seem to be involved in Neff and MacMaster's (2005) "spiritual transformation". On the basis of social learning (Bandura 1986), the spiritual transformation process includes not only an increased meaning in life, but also, for example, changing perceptions of God, openness to forgiveness, and improved self-acceptance. According to Kurtz and White (2015), AA participants can achieve spiritual growth in two different ways, depending on their attitude towards religion. Notably, non-religious or religiously skeptical AA participants can use secular support, such as involvement in AA, on the way to spiritual growth, and still experience similar benefits to the AA religiously inclined members, which can achieve this purpose on the basis of religious commitment (Tonigan et al. 2002; Winzelberg and Humphreys 1999). They can also use religious methods to achieve this goal.

This research yields some theoretical and practical implications. We confirmed two independent spiritual mechanisms based on secular and religious factors (involvement in AA and religiousness) that indirectly led to spiritual experiences among Polish AA participants by increasing meaning in life. Additionally, this study has indicated that these mechanisms are results of AA membership. Longer duration in AA was also related to both more AA involvement and greater religiousness, which in turn indirectly led to the participants' more frequent spiritual experiences through finding meaning in life.

From a practical point of view, practitioners, therapists, and counselors can suggest patients with an alcohol addiction to join AA self-help groups as well as partake in religious practices or develop their faith as a potential way to find meaning in life and thus facilitate spiritual growth. For religiously skeptical individuals, creating therapeutic programs and interventions using elements of the AA philosophy as a probable meaning-oriented system, which can lead to spiritual experiences, may work better. For religiously inclined patients, these therapeutic programs should consist of factors connected to religion and faith as a potential way to improve finding meaning in life and spiritual growth.

6. Limitations and Future Research

The conducted research has some limitations. First of all, the generalizability of achieved results is limited only to Roman Catholic AA participants from Poland. The research participants' mean sobriety duration was also relatively long, and the data did not encompass their relapse history and other addictions or diseases that could potentially have influenced their treatment. Additional research is needed to investigate the confirmed model among representatives of other religious denominations, agnostics and atheists, other races, AA members without stable sobriety, and in other cultural contexts.

The sample study was relatively small as well, and the bootstrapping method was used as a good solution in case of *normally distributed* variables. Using a larger research sample, which would also include alcohol-dependent individuals who recently started their AA participation and do not yet have stable sobriety, is recommended. A larger sample could also permit the verification of, for example, sex and other addictions or diseases as moderators between research variables. Further, it is important to verify whether the presented recovery model could be employed for other self-help groups dedicated to both substance and behavioral addictions, such as drugs, gambling, sex, and work.

One of the measures used, namely, the Alcoholics Anonymous Involvement Scale, had reliability coefficient slightly below the acceptable level, which is 0.7. This was probably caused by specificity of AA fellowship in Poland and cultural differences. For example, being a sponsor or having a sponsor is not a common phenomenon among Polish AA participants.

From the methodological point of view, it is worth noting that participation in the research was a very selective process because the questionnaire returning rate was low. The conducted study had a cross-sectional, not longitudinal, design. The cross-sectional research model provides the possibility of interpreting the direction of identified relationships between variables, although not from a causation perspective. For more complexity, however, other potential predictors of meaning in life should be incorporated, as should other religious variables (Sørensen et al. 2019) such as religious orientation or religious coping. This research used one latent variable, meaning that the results can only be interpreted as associations, which could differ from connections between observed variables. Finally, future studies could examine strictly observed and not latent variables in order to show the precise relationships between observed variables and verify whether the patterns of associations regarding latent variables are the same.

Funding: This study was funded by author sources.

Institutional Review Board Statement: Ethical review and approval were waived for this study, due to non-potential harming influence.

Informed Consent Statement: Informed consent was obtained from all subjects involved in the study.

Data Availability Statement: The data presented in this study are available on request from the corresponding author. The data are not publicly available due to privacy of the participants.

Conflicts of Interest: The author declares no conflict of interest.

References

Alcoholics Anonymous. 2001. *Alcoholics Anonymous: The Story of How Many Thousands of Men and Women Have Recovered from Alcoholism*, 4th ed. New York: Alcoholics Anonymous World Services.

Atkins, Randolph G., and James E. Hawdon. 2007. Religiosity and participation invmutual-aid support groups for addiction. *Journal of Substance Abuse Treatment* 33: 321–31. [CrossRef] [PubMed]

Bandura, Albert. 1986. *Prentice-Hall Series in Social Learning Theory. Social Foundations of Thought and Action: A Social Cognitive Theory*. Englewood Cliffs: Prentice-Hall, Inc.

Baumsteiger, Rachel, and Tiffany Chenneville. 2015. Challenges to the conceptualization and measurement of religiosity and spirituality in mental health research. *Journal of Religion and Health* 54: 2344–54. [CrossRef]

Browne, Michael W., and Robert Cudeck. 1993. Alternative ways of assessing model fit. In *Testing Structural Equation Models*. Edited by Kenneth A. Bollen and J. Scott Long. Newbury Park: Sage, pp. 136–62.

Carroll, Stephanie. 1993. Spirituality and purpose in life in alcoholism recovery. *Journal of Studies on Alcohol* 54: 297–301. [CrossRef] [PubMed]

Crumbaugh, James C., and Leonard T. Maholick. 1964. An experimental study in existentialism: The psychometric approach to Frankl's concept of noogenic neurosis. *Journal of Clinical Psychology* 20: 200–7. [CrossRef]

DeLucia, Christian, Brandon G. Bergman, Danette Beitra, Hillary L. Howrey, Stephanie Seibert, Amy E. Ellis, and Jessica Mizrachi. 2016. Beyond Abstinence: An examination of psychological well-being in members of Narcotics Anonymous. *Journal of Happiness Studies* 17: 817–32. [CrossRef]

Emrick, Chad D., J. Scott Tonigan, Henry Montgomery, and Laura Little. 1993. Alcoholics Anonymous: What is currently known? In *Research on Alcoholics Anonymous: Opportunities and Alternatives*. Edited by Barbara S. McCrady and William R. Miller. Piscataway: Rutgers Center of Alcohol Studies, pp. 41–76.

Frankl, V. Emil. 1992. *Man's Search for Meaning: An Introduction to Logotherapy*, 4th ed. Translated by I. Lasch. Boston: Beacon Press.

Galanter, Marc, Helen Dermatis, and Courtney Santucci. 2012. Young People in Alcoholics Anonymous: The role of spiritual orientation and AA member affiliation. *Journal of Addictive Diseases* 31: 173–82. [CrossRef]

George, Anita A., and Jalie A. Tucker. 1996. Help-seeking for alcohol-related problems: Social contexts surrounding entry into alcoholism treatment or Alcoholics Anonymous. *Journal of Studies on Alcohol* 57: 449–57. [CrossRef]

Gomes, Kevin, and Kenneth E. Hart. 2009. Adherence to recovery practices prescribed by Alcoholics Anonymous: Benefits to sustained abstinence and subjective quality of life. *Alcoholism Treatment Quarterly* 27: 223–35. [CrossRef]

Gutierrez, Daniel. 2019. Spiritus contra spiritum: Addiction, hope, and the search for meaning. *Spirituality in Clinical Practice* 6: 229–39. [CrossRef]

Hu, Li-Tze, and Peter M. Bentler. 1999. Cutoff criteria for fit indexes in covariance structure analysis: Conventional criteria versus new alternatives. *Structural Equation Modeling* 6: 1–55. [CrossRef]

Humphreys, Keith, L. Ann Kaskutas, and Constance Weisner. 1998. The Alcoholics Anonymous Affiliation Scale: Development, reliability, and norms for diverse treated and untreated populations. *Alcoholism, Clinical and Experimental Research* 22: 974–78. [CrossRef] [PubMed]

Kaskutas, Lee Ann, Norman Turk, Jason Bond, and Constance Weisner. 2003. The role of religion, spirituality and Alcoholics Anonymous in sustained sobriety. *Alcoholism Treatment Quarterly* 21: 1–16. [CrossRef]

Kelly, John F. 2017. Is Alcoholics Anonymous religious, spiritual, neither? Findings from 25 years of mechanisms of behavior change research. *Addiction (Abingdon, England)* 112: 929–36. [CrossRef] [PubMed]

Kelly, John F., and Rudolf Moos. 2003. Dropout from 12-step self-help groups: Prevalence, predictors, and counteracting treatment influences. *Journal of Substance Abuse Treatment* 24: 241–50. [CrossRef]

Kelly, John F., Robert L. Stout, Molly Magill, J. Scott Tonigan, and Maria E. Pagano. 2011. Spirituality in recovery: A lagged mediational analysis of alcoholics anonymous' principal theoretical mechanism of behavior change. *Alcoholism, Clinical and Experimental Research* 35: 454–63. [CrossRef]

King, Pamela E., Jennifer M. Vaughn, Yeonsoo Yoo, Jonathan M. Tirrell, Elizabeth M. Dowling, Richard M. Lerner, G. J. Geldhof, Jacqueline V. Lerner, Guillermo Iraheta, Kate Williams, and et al. 2020. Exploring religiousness and hope: Examining the roles of spirituality and social connections among salvadoran youth. *Religions* 11: 75. [CrossRef]

Krentzman, Amy R., Elizabeth Robinson, Brian E. Perron, and James A. Cranford. 2011. Predictors of membership in Alcoholics Anonymous in a sample of successfully remitted alcoholics. *Journal of Psychoactive Drugs* 43: 20–26. [CrossRef]

Krentzman, Amy R., James A. Cranford, and Elizabeth Robinson. 2013. Multiple dimensions of spirituality in recovery: A lagged mediational analysis of Alcoholics Anonymous' principal theoretical mechanism of behavior change. *Substance Abuse* 34: 20–32. [CrossRef]

Krentzman, Amy R., Stephen Strobbe, J. Irene Harris, Jennifer M. Jester, and Elizabeth Robinson. 2017. Decreased drinking and alcoholics anonymous are associated with different dimensions of spirituality. *Psychology of Religion and Spirituality* 9: S40–S48. [CrossRef]

Kurtz, Ernest, and William L. White. 2015. Recovery Spirituality. *Religions* 6: 58–81. [CrossRef]

Laustalot, Fleetwood V., Sharon B. Wyatt, Barbara Boss, and Tina McDyess. 2006. Psychometric examination of the Daily Spiritual experiences Scale. *Journal of Cultural Diversity* 13: 162–67.

Lewis, Christopher Alan, Mark Shevlin, Conor McGuckin, and Marek Navrátil. 2001. The Santa Clara Strength of Religious Faith Questionnaire: Confirmatory Factor Analysis. *Pastoral Psychology* 49: 379–84. [CrossRef]

Liisi, Sasi K. 1981. *Twelve Steps and Twelve Traditions*. New York: Alcoholics Anonymous World Services, Inc.

Lyons, Geoffrey C. B., Frank P. Deane, Peter Caputi, and Peter J. Kelly. 2011. Spirituality and the treatment of substance use disorders: An exploration of forgiveness, resentment and purpose in life. *Addiction Research & Theory* 19: 459–69.

Manning, Victoria, David Best, Nathan Faulkner, Emily Titherington, Alun Morinan, Francis Keaney, Michael Gossop, and John Strang. 2012. Does active referral by a doctor or 12-Step peer improve 12-Step meeting attendance? Results from a pilot randomised control trial. *Drug and Alcohol Dependence* 126: 131–37. [CrossRef]

McClure, Paul K., and Lindsay R. Wilkinson. 2020. Attending substance abuse groups and identifying as spiritual but not religious. *Review of Religious Research* 62: 197–218. [CrossRef]

Montgomery, Henry A., William R. Miller, and Scott J. Tonigan. 1995. Does Alcoholics Anonymous involvement predict treatment outcome? *Journal of Substance Abuse Treatment* 12: 241–46. [CrossRef]

Neff, J. Alan, and Samuel A. MacMaster. 2005. Spiritual mechanisms underlying substance abuse behavior change in faith-based substance abuse treatment. *Journal of Social Work Practice in the Addictions* 5: 33–54. [CrossRef]

Oakes, K. Elizabeth, John P. Allen, and Joseph W. Ciarrocchi. 2000. Spirituality, religious problem-solving, and sobriety in Alcoholics Anonymous. *Alcoholism Treatment Quarterly* 18: 37–50. [CrossRef]

Pardini, Dustin A., Thomas G. Plante, Allen Sherman, and Jamie E. Stump. 2000. Religious faith and spirituality in substance abuse recovery. Determining the mental health benefits. *Journal of Substance Abuse Treatment* 19: 347–54. [CrossRef]

Plante, Thomas G., and Marcus Boccaccini. 1997a. Reliability and validity of the Santa Clara Strength of Religious Faith Questionnaire. *Pastoral Psychology* 45: 429–37. [CrossRef]

Plante, Thomas G., and Marcus T. Boccaccini. 1997b. The Santa Clara Strength of Religious Faith Questionnaire. *Pastoral Psychology* 45: 375–87. [CrossRef]

Richard, Alan J., David C. Bell, and Jerry W. Carlson. 2000. Individual religiosity, moral community, and drug user treatment. *Journal for the Scientific Study of Religion* 39: 240–46. [CrossRef]

Sheeren, Mary. 1988. The relationship between relapse and involvement in alcoholics anonymous. *Journal of Studies on Alcohol* 49: 104–6. [CrossRef]

Silberman, Israela. 2003. Spiritual role modeling: The teaching of meaning systems: Comment. *International Journal for the Psychology of Religion* 13: 175–95. [CrossRef]

Silberman, Israela. 2005. Religion as a meaning system: Implications for the new millennium. *Journal of Social Issues* 61: 641–63. [CrossRef]

Sørensen, Torgeir, Peter la Cour, Lars Johan Danbolt, Hans Stifoss-Hanssen, Lars Lien, Valerie DeMarinis, Heidi Frølund Pedersen, and Tatjana Schnell. 2019. The sources of meaning and meaning in life questionnaire in the Norwegian context: Relations to mental health, quality of life, and self-efficacy. *International Journal for the Psychology of Religion* 29: 32–45. [CrossRef]

Steiger, James H. 1990. Structural model evaluation and modification: An interval estimation approach. *Multivariate Behavioral Research* 25: 173–80. [CrossRef]

Tonigan, J. Scott. 2001. Benefits of Alcoholics Anonymous attendance: Replication of findings between clinical research sites in Project MATCH. *Alcoholism Treatment Quarterly* 19: 67–77. [CrossRef]

Tonigan, J. Scott, Elizabeth A. McCallion, Tessa Frohe, and Matthew R. Pearson. 2017. Lifetime Alcoholics Anonymous attendance as a predictor of spiritual gains in the Relapse Replication and Extension Project (RREP). *Psychology of Addictive Behaviors: Journal of the Society of Psychologists in Addictive Behaviors* 31: 54–60. [CrossRef]

Tonigan, J. Scott, Gerard J. Connors, and William R. Miller. 1996. Alcoholics Anonymous Involvement (AAI) scale: Reliability and norms. *Psychology of Addictive Behaviors* 10: 75–80. [CrossRef]

Tonigan, J. Scott, Kristina N. Rynes, and Barbara S. McCrady. 2013. Spirituality as a change mechanism in 12-step programs: A replication, extension, and refinement. *Substance Use & Misuse* 48: 1161–73.

Tonigan, J. Scott, William R. Miller, and Carol Schermer. 2002. Atheists, agnostics and Alcoholics Anonymous. *Journal of Studies on Alcohol* 63: 534–41. [CrossRef]

Underwood, G. Lynn. 2011. The Daily Spiritual Experience Scale: Overview and results. *Religions* 2: 29–50. [CrossRef]

Vederhus, John-Kåre, Christine Timko, Oistein Kristensen, Bente Hjemdahl, and Thomas Clausen. 2014. Motivational intervention to enhance post-detoxification 12-Step group affiliation: A randomized controlled trial. *Addiction (Abingdon, England)* 109: 766–73. [CrossRef] [PubMed]

Webb, R. Jon, Elizabeth Robinson, Kirk J. Brower, and Robert A. Zucker. 2006. Forgiveness and alcohol problems among people entering substance abuse treatment. *Journal of Addictive Diseases* 24: 55–67. [CrossRef] [PubMed]

Winzelberg, Andrew, and Keith Humphreys. 1999. Should patients' religiosity influence clinicians' referral to 12-step self-help groups? Evidence from a study of 3018 male substance abuse patients. *Journal of Consulting and Clinical Psychology* 67: 790–94. [CrossRef]

Wnuk, Marcin. 2015. Determining the influence religious-spiritual values on levels of hope and the meaning of life in alcohol co-dependent subjects receiving support in self-help groups. *Journal of Substance Use* 20: 194–99. [CrossRef]

Wnuk, Marcin. 2017. A Psychometric Evaluation of the Santa Clara Strength of Religious Faith Questionnaire among Students from Poland and Chile. *Pastoral Psychology* 66: 551–62. [CrossRef]

Zemore, Sarah E. 2007. A role for spiritual change in the benefits of 12-step involvement. *Alcoholism, Clinical and Experimental Research* 31: 76s–79s. [CrossRef]

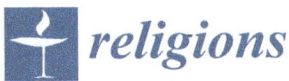

Article

Climate Change, Addiction, and Spiritual Liberation

Margaret Bullitt-Jonas [1,2,3]

1. Missioner for Creation Care, Episcopal Diocese of Western Massachusetts, Springfield, MA 01103, USA; margaretbj@aol.com
2. Missioner for Creation Care, Southern New England Conference, United Church of Christ, Framingham, MA 01702, USA
3. Creation Care Advisor, Episcopal Diocese of Massachusetts, Boston, MA 02111, USA

Abstract: Climate scientists have sounded the alarm: The only way to preserve a planet that is generally habitable for human beings is to carry out a transformation of society at a rate and scale that are historically unprecedented. Can we do this? Will we do this? Drawing on her long-term recovery from addiction and on her decades of ministry as a climate activist, the author reflects on how understanding the dynamics of addiction and recovery might inform our efforts to protect the web of life and to bear witness to the liberating God of love who makes all things new.

Keywords: addiction; recovery; Twelve-Step Program; climate change

Citation: Bullitt-Jonas, Margaret. 2021. Climate Change, Addiction, and Spiritual Liberation. *Religions* 12: 709. https://doi.org/10.3390/rel12090709

Academic Editors: Bernadette Flanagan and Noelia Molina

Received: 4 August 2021
Accepted: 27 August 2021
Published: 1 September 2021

Publisher's Note: MDPI stays neutral with regard to jurisdictional claims in published maps and institutional affiliations.

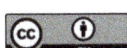

Copyright: © 2021 by the author. Licensee MDPI, Basel, Switzerland. This article is an open access article distributed under the terms and conditions of the Creative Commons Attribution (CC BY) license (https://creativecommons.org/licenses/by/4.0/).

1. An Addict's World

The addict looks away. The addict sees but does not see. She does not want to see. There is nothing to see here. Change the subject.

The addict is empty. She does not have enough. She must be filled. She must be filled right now.

The addict carries out repetitive, compulsive rituals that disconnect her from self, others, Earth, and the sacred.

The addict functions like a machine. She repeats the same behavior over and over, despite its harmful consequences to herself and perhaps to others, too.

The addict is ruthless. She dominates, forces, and exploits. The addict treats everything, including herself, as an It.

The addict is cut off from her body. Who cares what the body wants? She ignores and overrides the body, its wisdom and needs.

The addict is cut off from the rest of the natural world.

The addict lies to herself and she lies to others. (*There is no problem here. Do you see a problem? I do not see a problem*).

The addict is numb. She does not feel.

The addict is self-centered, isolated, and alone.

The addict is used to this. This is normal. This is the way things are. Nothing will ever change.

The addict is powerless. She is trapped. She cannot stop herself. She intends to change, she plans to change, she promises to change, she tries to change. She does not change.

The addict hates herself.

Her life is unmanageable.

2. A Story of Recovery

Writing these words, I conjure up my state of mind forty years ago, when I was gripped by an eating disorder. As a teenager and young adult, I ate compulsively. To compensate for the binges, which I carried out in secret, I ran endless miles, tried every diet under the sun, and fasted for days on end. I made endless vows—this time I would not eat more than I needed; this time I would overcome my cravings—but my vows, however ardently expressed, had no power to set me free. Inevitably, I went back to the box of donuts, or the jar of peanut butter devoured hastily and with the shades drawn, lest anyone see me, lest I see myself.

My drug was food. As any addict knows, addiction distorts and numbs our awareness of the body. In those years of compulsive overeating, I paid little attention to my body's rhythms or needs. Feelings did not matter. So what if I was sad or lonely? So what if I was angry, excited or bored? Whatever I felt, I swallowed it down with food and set out for another grueling run. Was it night-time and was my body eager for sleep? I did not care. I would stay up late, make a tour of the all-night supermarket, and eat until my stomach ached. Was I disappointed and needing to cry, or angry and needing to be heard? Quick—I would pave over those feelings and force some cheese or chocolate down my throat. Was my body aching from the abuse I dished out? Too bad. After a bout of bingeing, I would get up the next morning and go out for a seven-mile run, maybe start another fast or launch another stringent diet. Pummel and punish the body—that was my motto. Clear-cut the forest and move on.

Like every addict who has lost control, I could not stop what I was doing, and I saw no way out. At last, through the grace of God, at the age of thirty, I found a path to recovery. Now almost seventy, I sing the familiar words of the hymn "Amazing Grace"—*I once was lost and now am found*—and look back with gratitude to 13 April 1982, the day I walked into a Twelve-Step meeting and held up the white flag of surrender: *Help. I give up. My life is unmanageable*. I could not fight the battle any longer, for it was a battle I always lost. I needed help beyond myself. I needed a Higher Power. I had to make peace with my body or die (Bullitt-Jonas 1998).

That day was the turning-point of my life, the beginning of a journey to wholeness. One day at a time, I began practicing the Twelve-Step Program of Overeaters Anonymous and dug into the physical, emotional, and spiritual work of reconciling with my body, myself, and the important people in my life. I began to take responsibility for the first bit of nature entrusted to my care—my body. Day by day I began to honor its limits and listen to its needs. I met regularly with a psychotherapist and began to untangle my inner knots. Additionally, I embarked on a spiritual search. Impelled by an intense desire to know what was real, what was lasting, trustworthy, and true, I ventured back into the church I had long ago abandoned and sat in the shadowed back pew so that I could listen from afar. I longed to know who God was, and how to meet God in my own experience. I began to study and practice meditation and prayer.

My mind, it turned out, was as jumpy as water on a hot skillet. I was surprised by the inner racket: worries, memories, regrets, and plans. Arguments, scraps of music, commercial jingles. How could I love God, my neighbor, or myself if I was perpetually distracted? I learned to bring awareness to the breath and to return to the present moment, disciplining my attention so that I could perceive more accurately what was here. As my mind settled down, strong feelings surged through me. Shame, sorrow, anger, yearning—for years, they had been tamped down in my long bout with addiction, but now, here they were, roaring back to life. I sat with the feelings and breathed, learning to give them space and let them be. The feelings ebbed and flowed. They always passed. No one died. In fact, the more I allowed them to come and go, the more spacious I felt, and the more truly alive.

Love kept showing up. When I welcomed everything into awareness, clinging to nothing and pushing nothing away, an unexpected tenderness would eventually rise up from within and gather me up like a child. I went off for a ten-day silent retreat at a meditation center in western Massachusetts. I followed the drill: You sit. You walk. You sit. You walk. That is it. You do nothing but bring awareness to the present moment.

One day I left the retreat house for a walk in the woods. I paid attention to sensations as they came, the feel of my foot on the ground, the sound of birds, the sight of birches, hemlock, and pine. My thoughts lay still. I was nothing but eyes and ears, the weight of each foot, the breath in my nostrils. At one point I stopped walking, overwhelmed by the sense that the whole world was inside me. I was carrying the round blue planet inside my chest. My heart held the world. I cradled it tenderly, weeping with joy.

I did not know it then, but that vision of carrying the world in my heart would become one of the core images to which I would return in prayer in the decades ahead, a place of consolation that renewed my strength for climate activism. Years later, someone gave me a contemporary icon of Christ bending over the world, his arms embracing the planet.[1] I caught my breath in recognition. *Yes, that's right. That's just how it is.*

3. Climate Change and Addiction

Two years after starting my recovery I finished what I was doing, made a swerve, and headed to seminary. I needed to know: Who is the God who just saved my life? I was ordained in the Episcopal Church in June 1988. Not two weeks later, I picked up the New York Times and was startled by its front-page headline, "Global warming has begun (Shabecoff 1988)". NASA climate scientist James Hanson had testified to a congressional committee that scientists were becoming alarmed about the so-called "greenhouse effect" of burning fossil fuels. Human activity—driven by an economy dependent on coal, gas, and oil—was pushing the planet past its limits. The relentless extraction and burning of fossil fuels was polluting the global atmosphere with heat-trapping gasses; therefore, the atmosphere was rapidly heating. Scientists were concerned that the relentless consumption of dirty fossil fuels would disrupt the fragile balance of life. Great suffering lay ahead if we did not change course. We needed to stop what we were doing.

From that day forward, I began to track news about climate change. It became increasingly clear that the society in which I lived was behaving with the reckless abandon of an addict. In the ruthless push to drill oil wells, construct pipelines, blow off mountain-tops, devour forests, and gobble up every last resource of the planet, we are laying waste to the land, air, and water upon which all life depends. The most vulnerable groups—low-income and Black, Brown, Indigenous, and people of color communities—are those hurt first and hardest by the effects of climate change, although even wealthy and privileged communities are beginning to suffer (Sengupta 2021). The resonance with addiction is haunting: as a society and a species we are caught up in highly destructive patterns of over-consumption and we have been unwilling or unable to quit.

In the months after James Hansen's testimony, a question emerged that became the riddle of my life, a question that fuels my vocation as a faith-based climate activist to this day: If God can empower a crazy addict such as me to make peace with their body, is it not possible that God can empower a crazed, addicted humanity to make peace with each other and the body of Earth?

4. The Shock of Climate Change

When I step outside this morning, I smell smoke. Haze blurs the heated air. Plumes of wildfire smoke that traveled thousands of miles across the country have reached us here in New England. With every breath, we inhale the residue of forests burning in western North America. Traces of distant trees that were set ablaze in massive fires sparked by unprecedented drought and heat now line our lungs. We are all connected.

Midway through the tumultuous, scorching summer of 2021, the damage caused by climate change is increasingly visible. Each day brings new reports of extreme heat, drought, fire, and floods. (Extreme precipitation is linked to global warming, because warmer air holds more water and therefore deposits more water when it rains—just as a larger bucket can hold and deposit more water). The American West and Southwest are gripped by megadrought, an extraordinarily brutal and persistent drought which is draining reservoirs, withering fields, and increasing the spread of enormous wildfires. The Pacific Northwest, a usually cool and foggy part of the world, has roasted in record-setting levels of heat. Hundreds of people died in what one expert called "the most anomalous heat event ever observed on Earth".[2] North America is not the only place experiencing record temperatures—so, too, are the Middle East, South Asia, and Russia (Tharoor 2021). Meanwhile, torrential rains have drenched the mid-Atlantic. As much as ten inches of rain fell in southeastern Pennsylvania in under four hours. In China, terrified commuters riding subways stood on seats and clung to poles to avoid floodwaters from record-breaking rains.[3] Flooding recently killed hundreds of people in Central Europe, Uganda, Nigeria, and Italy. Famine stalks Madagascar as a drought tied to climate change dries up waterholes and crops. In Siberia, tens of thousands of square miles of forest are on fire, potentially releasing carbon into the atmosphere from the frozen ground below.

Today's headlines are frightening and stark, and they come in rapid succession. Fossil fuel emissions have disrupted Earth's atmosphere and biosphere even more quickly and dramatically than scientists predicted only a few years ago. If society is an addict dependent on coal, gas, and oil, then the addiction has reached its crisis point: Will we change course or will billions of us die, taking down with us the lives of countless other beings?

In a State of the Union address delivered in 2006, President George W. Bush warned of America's addiction to oil (Bush 2006). Of course, our dangerous relationship with fossil fuels does not function exactly like a substance addiction—we are not busily injecting oil into our veins in an effort to get high or experiencing DTs if access to coal is withdrawn. However, our society and economy—indeed, our whole way of life—does function like a person with a behavioral or process addiction: we are wretchedly, tragically—as a Christian, I would add "sinfully"—continuing to carry out activities that quickly or slowly will kill us and that are already killing countless people and other living beings worldwide. More than one Secretary General of the United Nations has called our present course "suicidal". Another word that comes to mind is "ecocidal". Indeed, a global panel of experts is now drafting a law to make ecocide—widespread destruction of the environment—a crime that can be prosecuted under international law (Saddique 2021; Surma et al. 2021).

5. Denial and Truth-Telling

What insights from the dynamics of addiction and recovery might inform our efforts to save what is left of the web of life and our struggle to preserve a habitable world? Six themes rise to the top: denial and truth-telling; isolation and community; grieving our losses; taking moral responsibility; praying the Serenity Prayer; and urgency, fear, and love.

Let us begin with denial and truth-telling. Built into addictive processes is the addict's insistent refusal or inability to perceive the reality or magnitude of the harm their behavior is causing themselves or others. Denial and minimization are characteristic ways that addicts avoid confronting their problem. As we wrote in *Rooted and Rising: Voices of Courage in a Time of Climate Crisis*, when it comes to facing the truth of climate change (Schade and Bullitt-Jonas 2019, pp. xx–xxi):

> The American public's widespread denial of climate change has had a stunning run. This is understandable, given that most people want to avoid thinking about something as deeply troubling as the Earth's climate crisis spinning out of control. We humans seem to have a built-in knack for delaying as long as possible the recognition of particularly troublesome facts. Some of us even turn denial and avoidance into a fine art. As comedian George Carlin observed, "I don't believe there's any problem in this country, no matter how tough it is, that Americans, when they roll up their sleeves, can't completely ignore".

However, we cannot ascribe the robust denial of climate change among many Americans solely to a supposed national capacity for dodging reality as long as possible. Nor should we assume that the denial of climate change and addiction to oil is a purely internal, mental problem that springs from a disorder in the brain, as one science writer has proposed (Stover 2014). Nor is denial just a "defect of character", to use the language of the Twelve-Step Program—it is actually being generated and amplified by external forces, vested interests that have been hard at work since the late 1980s, spending billions of dollars in a deliberate campaign of disinformation to keep the American public confused about the reality, causes, and urgency of climate change (Oreskes and Conway 2011; Gelbspan 1997; Union of Concerned Scientists 2007).

Today, as Michael E. Mann explains in his masterful new book, *The New Climate War*, because the devastating impacts of climate change are now obvious in the daily news cycle, "the forces of denial and delay ... can no longer insist, with a straight face, that nothing is happening. Outright denial of the physical evidence of climate change simply isn't credible anymore". As a result, fossil fuel corporations and oil-funded governments that continue to profit from our dependence on fossil fuels are shifting tactics to "a softer form of denialism" based on deception, distraction, and delay (Mann 2021, p. 3). This is what Mann calls "the new climate war", and the planet is losing.

Breaking through denial, whether its source be internal or external, is an essential aspect of climate activism. Climate activism faces outward: we have urgent work to do on the streets, in boardrooms, and in the backrooms where decisions are made. Mobilizing an effective, systemic response to the crisis at hand requires contending with political and corporate powers that seek to mire us in denial, distraction, and delay.

However, climate activism faces inward, too, as we reckon with our own layers of denial. You do not need to be a full-fledged climate sceptic who challenges the conclusions of mainstream science to be a person who slips into denial. Kari Marie Norgaard, a Professor of Sociology and Environmental Studies at the University of Oregon, has written helpfully about what she calls "the everyday denial of climate change, (Norgaard 2012)" the way that ordinary people who feel overwhelmed by the climate crisis simply change the subject to more manageable topics rather than face their guilt, fear, and helplessness. She connects this with the work of Robert Jay Lifton and Richard Falk, who studied, in relation to nuclear peril, "the absurdity of the double life": the way that people can live in two realities, being aware, on the one hand, of an enormous existential threat, while desperately clinging, on the other hand, to a pretense of conventional, ordinary reality.

We probably experience this cognitive dissonance in our own lives: although some part of us is aware that climate change looms over everything, we do our best to avoid thinking about it and we keep our focus on the immediate concerns of daily life. Friends of mine confess that even though they know that climate change is real, they do not pay very much attention to it: it is too painful to consider; they prefer to focus on more immediate, manageable concerns. In her brilliant novel, *Weather*, Jenny Offill evokes the difficulty of holding in mind both the close-in immediacy of our intimate, daily lives and the terrifying, large-scale reality of the unfolding climate catastrophe (Offill 2020).

Nevertheless, overcoming personal and collective denial is foundational to the ongoing work of recovering from addiction and creating a more just and sustainable future. As a recovering addict, I know how hard it can be to face, and keep facing, the truth: I remember how, in the early months of recovery, I needed to be reminded multiple times a day that I was a compulsive overeater and that a good day was a day in which I did not hurt myself with food. Unless I stayed in touch with allies in the Twelve-Step Program and unless I used its tools and carried out its Steps, it was simply too easy to slide back into denial and into the "stinking thinking" that led to relapse.

Similarly, as a faith-based climate activist, I must renew my commitment every day to dissolve my denial and to face reality as it is, not as I wish it were. That is not easy. As T.S. Eliot put it, "Humankind cannot bear very much reality (Eliot 1971, p. 118)". Can I make daily space in my mind and heart for the reality of climate change? Can I do something each day to keep myself informed, honor my emotional response, and carry out whatever actions I can that will contribute to healing? Just as an addict must renew her commitment to her own recovery daily, can we who live in an addictive society renew our commitment to overcome denial of the climate crisis daily, and take some action, large or small, that leads to healing?

6. Isolation and Community

The Twelve-Step recovery process is carried out in community. Part of the power of the Twelve-Step model is the candor of its small group sharing: in every meeting, addicts seeking recovery share the truth of their lives and their desire to be sober (or drug-free or abstinent). We encounter each other as equals, because everyone, whether newcomer or old-timer, is in some sense a beginner and as dependent as anyone else on a power beyond themselves. In that circle of sometimes raw self-disclosure, we share our vulnerabilities and our experience, strength, and hope. Addiction is often called a disease of isolation, and by attending meetings, making phone calls, sponsoring and being sponsored, and carrying out acts of service, we gradually learn to find our place in a larger community. If, as Ann and Barry Ulanov so aptly put it, "Sin is the refusal to get our feet wet in the ocean of God's connectedness (Ulanov and Ulanov 1982, p. 96)", then the Twelve-Step model of healing in community is a release from sin. We are pulled into a current of connectedness that empowers us to set each other free: I may not be able to stop myself from overeating, but you can help me to stop; you may not be able to stop yourself from overeating, but I can help you to stop. To an addict who has white-knuckled countless lonely, failed attempts to kick the habit, entering the stream of relationships in a Twelve-Step Program can offer what feels like a miracle: buoyed by the support we feel all around us, it becomes much less difficult—perhaps even easy—to stay sober or abstinent, one day at a time. The antidote to addiction is connection.

I have never experienced a Twelve-Step meeting organized around recovery from addiction to fossil fuels or to exploiting the Earth,[4] but I understand the power of relationships to sustain my work as a climate activist. Who are the people to whom I can confess my confusion, fear, grief and outrage about the devastation of Earth and Earth's communities, both human and other-than-human? Who are the people seeking to move through their own despair and into a life of service? Who are the people trying to amend their lives so that they live more gently on the Earth and who inspire me to do the same? Who are the people committed to making sacrifices and taking risks for the sake of keeping fossil fuels in the ground and protecting life as it has evolved on this planet? These are some of the people I want to be close to, because I can learn from them and grow with them. Even if we never sit together in one room, even if they live someplace far away—indeed, even if I never meet them and never even learn their names—they are my circle of support, allies in my own struggle to live in harmony and balance with Earth.

"Don't talk, don't trust, don't feel"—those three core rules of alcoholic and dysfunctional family systems were laid out by Dr. Claudia Black years ago in her seminal book, *It Will Never Happen to Me!*" (Black 1981). Some of the other rules include "don't think" (about what is going on) and "don't question" (what is happening). Whenever we gather to talk honestly about the climate crisis, trust each other with our truth, dare to feel our feelings, think about what is going on, and ask questions about what is happening, we transgress those dysfunctional dynamics and begin to build a more authentic and resilient network of relationships. Simply breaking the silence around climate change—speaking honestly to a friend about one's worry or concern—can be the beginning of release from the paralyzing isolation that tells us that climate change is too big, too frightening, or too political to discuss.

Experiencing the healing power of connections extends to our relationship with the natural world. Just as addicts generally treat their bodies with violence or contempt, so most of us in today's dominant culture were raised to override and ignore the needs of the living world around us. Nature was supposed to be at our beck and call, a limitless resource that human beings were entitled to drain—nothing more than commodities to be bought, sold, processed, consumed, and discarded. Many Westerners are only beginning to acknowledge our deep alienation from the rest of the created order and are only now discovering the deep wisdom of Indigenous traditions and our own mystical traditions, which speak of the essential interconnectedness, sacredness, and mutuality of everything that exists.

Learning to cultivate loving, life-giving relationships with other people and with the other creatures and elements with whom we share the planet is medicine for addiction of every kind.

7. Grieving Our Losses

Facing addiction requires facing grief. Addicts who are beginning their journey of recovery will likely have many losses to grieve, such as a failed marriage, a lost job, a damaged reputation, or estranged co-workers, children, and friends. Furthermore, in relinquishing their drug of choice, addicts are also losing what seemed to be their lover or best friend, the substance or behavior to which they clung—even if they hated it—in order to manage their life. Not only that, when addicts stop using their drug, the feelings that had been suppressed by their compulsive behavior will likely come surging back into awareness: grief, shame, fear, anger, loneliness, confusion, the whole nine yards. Living into recovery, a day at a time, can be an emotionally turbulent process.

Confronting the climate crisis likewise requires acknowledging grief and other painful feelings. Grief is the normal, healthy response to loss, but the dominant culture in which we live does not handle grief well. Many of us tend to sidestep or suppress our grief, fearing that we will look weak, sentimental, morbid, or pathetic. We may also avoid thinking about climate change because we fear being overwhelmed by our emotions. What can we possibly feel in response to the acidifying ocean, the children choking from asthma in our inner cities, the rising seas, the ever-increasing droughts and floods, and the cascade of species being made extinct? Who wants to allow an emotional response to hearing that climate change is already making parts of the world too hot and humid for humans to survive (Mellen and Neff 2021)? Or that unchecked climate change could collapse whole eco-systems quite abruptly, starting within the next ten years (Berwyn 2020)? Or that the natural world is at a far greater risk from climate breakdown than was previously thought (Harvey 2020)? Stunned by the gravity of news such as this, many of us feel helpless and turn away. The scale of the problem feels too big in comparison with our one small life and our limited powers. We might as well cling to business as usual for as long as we can—drive, shop, send the kids to school, earn the promotion, fix supper, check social media—and let someone else handle the bigger problem, maybe the experts or maybe future generations. We might as well stay distracted, busy, and numb. We might as well zone out for as long as possible.

Emotional withdrawal is a natural response to trauma. We are all living in the context of ongoing and accelerating global trauma, even if our corner of the world has not yet borne the full brunt of climate change. It is understandable if we are inclined to anesthetize ourselves and shut down emotionally. However, shutting down is its own form of suffering. As Franz Kafka observed, "You can hold yourself back from the sufferings of the world, that is something you are free to do and it accords with your nature, but perhaps this very holding back is the one suffering you could avoid".

It is easier to release into grief when we feel supported, understood, and upheld. This is where the power of community comes in. Like addicts recovering in the Twelve-Step Program, we do not have to tremble in fear or shed tears alone. A variety of circles have formed in recent years to help participants grapple with the spiritual and existential questions raised by climate emergency and other forms of collective trauma. Among others, they include The Work That Reconnects, based on the teachings of Joanna Macy; Rabbi Jennie Rosen's organization, Dayenu; and Margaret Klein Salomon's Climate Awakening.[5] Psychological and psychiatric associations are increasingly aware of the mental health challenges posed by social and ecological breakdown and are training clinicians to address these issues in their work with clients.[6] Parish leaders also have a golden opportunity to gather members of their congregation for prayerful, small-group conversations about climate change and to create communities of truth-telling that allow the honest expression of pain.

We are blessed that many faith traditions provide tools and rituals for accessing and processing grief. Learning practices of contemplative prayer and meditation can be helpful, because they give traumatized people a technique to calm down, steady the mind, and quiet the nervous system. Contemplative prayer, often defined as "a long, loving look at the real", resonates with the Zen teaching, "Stay present to what's happening". In a time of emotional turbulence and agitation, contemplative prayer can help us cultivate trust and patience. We learn to sit still in the midst of uncertainty, to wait in the darkness, to relinquish our anxious and futile quest to stay in control, and to listen for the inner voice of love. To cite the psalmist: "Be still . . . and know that I am God" (Psalm 46:11).

From out of the stillness, feelings arise that may need expression—even visceral, bodily expressions, such as wailing, stamping, dancing,[7] drumming, and singing. Expressive prayer is essential to articulating grief, whether we do it together or alone. Lament is an ancient form of prayer found in the Psalms, in the prophets, and in the words and actions of Jesus. He wept at the death of Lazarus, he wept over the city of Jerusalem, and he cried out to God on the cross, using the lament of Psalm 22. Lament is not self-pity nor is it simply whining. Lament is a deep outpouring of sorrow to God. Learning how to pray with painful feelings can help us to grow in intimacy with God and to experience solidarity with everyone who suffers (Bullitt-Jonas 2000). Spiritual directors with an awareness of the dynamics of addiction can help the people they guide to explore pathways of prayer that allow the expression of feelings (Bullitt-Jonas 1991).

Lament, especially public lament, can be empowering. Theologians such as Walter Brueggemann (Brueggemann 1978; Sharp 2011, pp. 179–205), drawing on the work of Dorothee Soelle, Jurgen Moltmann, and Abraham Heschel, have brilliantly shown us that lament is the beginning of criticism of an unjust social order. Articulating anguish and experiencing passion—defined as "the capacity and readiness to care, to suffer, to die, and to feel (Brueggemann 1978, p. 41)"—is the enemy of any society built on ignoring the cries of the marginalized and oppressed, the cry of the Earth and the cry of the poor. Lament can end in hope or praise, because in lament we experience the presence of a living, loving, and liberating God. Lament can lead to action, because the more we experience our unshakable union with a love which is stronger than death, the freer we will be to take actions commensurate with the emergency in which we find ourselves.

The climate crisis brings us to our knees. It also brings us to our feet.

8. Taking Moral Responsibility

Basic to the process of recovery in the Twelve-Step Program is taking moral responsibility for one's actions. Addiction is not "a moral issue", if by that we mean that addicts are "weak" or "bad" people without moral principles; in fact, addicts are people with a complex medical disease or condition. However, addiction does have a moral dimension: you cannot be set free from addictive behavior unless you carry out a deep housecleaning. Seven of the Twelve Steps (Steps 4–10) engage recovering addicts in a thorough and ongoing process of growth in moral self-awareness, accountability, and responsibility.

Reckoning with our moral responsibility for contributing to the climate crisis is complex (Jenkins 2008, 2013; Moore and Nelson 2010; Northcott 2007; Rasmussen 1996). Climate change is a justice issue on many levels. For starters, it is an issue of *social and economic* justice, because impoverished individuals, communities, and nations are those who suffer the effects of climate change first and hardest; they are the ones least able to adapt, and the ones least likely to have a seat at the table where policy decisions are made. Climate change is also an issue of *international* justice. As the Union of Concerned Scientists points out, "The world's countries emit vastly different levels of heat-trapping gases into the atmosphere (Union of Concerned Scientists 2008)". Climate change is caused mostly by the wealthy nations—developed countries and major emerging economies lead in total carbon dioxide emissions—but it is the poorer nations which are most vulnerable to its painful effects. The question of international justice becomes even more pointed when considering the per capita consumption of fossil fuels. Saudi Arabia and the United States are tied in first place for the world's highest per capita carbon emissions, far outpacing the per capita outputs of poor nations (Statista 2021). One analysis reviewed public health studies of the effects of burning fossil fuels and concluded that the lifestyles of about three average Americans create enough planet-heating emissions to kill one person (Millman 2021).

Climate change is a matter of *intergenerational* justice, because right now we are stealing a habitable Earth from our children and our children's children. If we continue with business as usual, we will leave a ruined world to those who come after us. No wonder so many members of the Sunrise Movement [8] and so many other young climate activists are angry!

Climate justice is likewise inextricably linked to *racial* justice. In the piercing words of Hop Hopkins, the Sierra Club's Director of Organizational Transformation, "You can't have climate change without sacrifice zones, and you can't have sacrifice zones without disposable people, and you can't have disposable people without racism (Hopkins 2020)".

Perhaps we must speak of *interspecies* justice, as well, because for the first time in the planet's history, a single species, *Homo sapiens,* is in the process of wiping out vast populations of other creatures, and even entire species. Driven by climate change and other pressures of human activities, the world's wildlife populations have plummeted by more than two-thirds in the last 50 years, according to a 2020 report by the World Wildlife Fund (Rott 2020). We are also in the midst of Earth's sixth extinction event. With dismay, scientists are describing what they call a "biological annihilation (Ceballos et al. 2017)". Recognizing that we are now in an emergency that threatens human civilization, one expert commented, "This is far more than just being about losing the wonders of nature, desperately sad though that is . . . This is actually now jeopardizing the future of people. Nature is not a 'nice to have'—it is our life-support system (Carrington 2018)".

To push away the horror—and the responsibility—it might be tempting to shift the blame for the climate crisis onto the generations that preceded us. "After all", we may tell ourselves, "burning fossil fuels began long before I was born; people have been burning fossil fuels since the eighteenth century, when the Industrial Revolution began". However, adults such as me cannot get away with that attempt at moral deflection (which is so characteristic of an addict): more than half of all CO_2 emissions since 1751 were emitted in the last 30 years (Stainforth 2020). That is, in a single lifetime—ours.

Clearly, the climate crisis is not only a scientific, political, economic, or technical issue—it is a moral issue, as well. What if members of a high-carbon, high-consumption society faced our guilt and took Step 4 ("Made a searching and moral inventory of ourselves")? What if we carried out the Steps that follow and took bold, even radical action to address the moral injustice of climate change?

Taking personal responsibility means that each of us does our part to solve the problem. Many of us start reducing our personal and household "carbon footprint". We recycle, we buy less stuff, we eat less meat and move toward a plant-based diet. We do whatever we can afford to do—install solar panels, buy an electric car, eat local, organic foods, upgrade insulation, turn down the heat, use less air conditioning. Taking these kinds of personal steps to reduce our carbon footprint is worthwhile in many ways: they align our lives more closely with our values; they can inspire friends and neighbors to follow suit, making it socially acceptable and morally normative to live more gently on Earth; and they relieve our sense of cognitive dissonance—we know that we are taking action to address an existential crisis. After all, as Lao Tzu said, "A journey of a thousand miles begins with a single step". Making personal changes in lifestyle may be that vital first step on the ramp to more effective action.

However, do not be fooled—if we limit taking personal responsibility simply to changing our lifestyle and consumer choices, we are falling for the lie that individual behavior is enough. It is not. Turning off the lights and driving an electric car may be the right thing to do and make us feel morally "cleaner", but moral action only makes a substantive difference when we join the fight for systemic change. A societal transformation from top to bottom is what is required to avert climate chaos—that is what the world's pre-eminent climate scientists told us in the 2018 report from the U.N.'s Intergovernmental Panel on Climate Change. The only way to do that is to push for collective solutions, to become politically engaged, and to make it politically possible to do what is scientifically necessary to maintain a habitable world.

In the meantime, fossil fuel corporations are working hard to shift responsibility for the damage that their products cause (damage that these companies concealed and denied for decades) to individual consumers. Like drug dealers, they make a fortune by pushing a deadly product and then blame their customers if they buy it and become sick. A fascinating article by Amy Westervelt explains how, for over 100 years, various industries, including tobacco, beverage packaging, guns, and fossil fuels, "have weaponized American individualism, laying the blame for systemic issues at the feet of individual citizens".[9] Westervelt observes that BP "famously invented the ultimate tool for pinning greenhouse gas emissions on individual consumers: the carbon footprint calculator".[10] As she points out:

> This rhetorical framing flourishes not only because it taps into America's individualistic identity, but also because it presents easy solutions: simply buy different things in your own life, walk or bike a bit more, and everything will be fine! It also provides a purity test that no climate activist can possibly pass. It's the perfect setup for oil companies: The problem is consumers, not industry, and no consumer can ever reduce their carbon footprint enough to be a credible critic. (Westervelt 2021)

Framing the climate crisis in moral terms gives us an opportunity to understand that effective moral action includes collective moral action. To be blunt, do not be a consumer, be a citizen.

The scope and speed of the climate crisis require more than personal changes in behavior—they require collective action and a push for policies such as pricing or regulating carbon, eliminating fossil fuels subsidies, providing incentives for clean renewable energy, and ensuring that historically marginalized communities enjoy the benefits of clean energy.

Climate scientists are increasingly concerned that if global warming continues unchecked, the Earth will soon pass so-called "tipping points" beyond which possibly irrevocable disaster will ensue (Harvey and Agencies 2021). Is it possible to create a *social* tipping point that would propel a swift transition to clean energy? According to one study (Otto et al. 2020), providing a moral framework for the climate crisis would contribute to a social tipping point and help activate "contagious and fast-spreading processes" that lead to global decarbonization. Using a term from the field of addiction, the study argues that revealing the moral implications of fossil fuels is an "intervention" that would accelerate a rapid global transformation to carbon-neutral societies. Let us start this addict on the road to recovery.

9. Praying the Serenity Prayer

Like most recovering addicts in the Twelve-Step Program, I frequently turn to the Serenity Prayer: "God, grant me the serenity to accept the things I cannot change, courage to change the things I can, and wisdom to know the difference". Based on a longer prayer by theologian Reinhold Niebuhr, these words have helped countless addicts to search their minds and hearts as they sort out what to hold on to and what to let go, what is theirs to do and what is not. Implicitly, the prayer invites us to rein in our compulsive craving for control and to find peace even in the midst of trouble. It rouses us from passivity and inertia so that we change what we can (and should) change. Additionally, it recognizes that we do not see these things clearly, and need to ask for God's help.

The prayer is immensely useful for everyone concerned about climate change. What is it that I need serenity to accept? What is it that I need courage to change? How do I know which is which? The questions themselves drive me into prayer, and the answers change over time as I listen and learn. I pray for serenity to accept the reality of the climate crisis and the painful manifestations of that crisis which emerge every day—and I find my way to serenity only as I pray my way through outrage, fear, and grief. I pray for courage to change the things I can—and I find that courage only as I keep entrusting my actions to God. I pray for the wisdom to know what is and is not mine to do—and I try to forgive myself when I get that wrong. The Serenity Prayer is pithy, enigmatic, and as pure as prayer comes—it does not give answers; it simply opens a door to God.

We bring into prayer what we know about the world, so it is good to be aware that many internal and external forces are at work, insisting that there is little we can do to slow climate change. I will mention only two. One is external: fossil fuel corporations are eager to amplify our supposed helplessness to quit using their products. They are delighted when "collapse-aware" people throw in the towel and accept that we are doomed, that it's too late to take effective active to stave off climate catastrophe. As Michael Mann explains, "Doomism potentially leads us down the same path of inaction as outright denial of the threat". He adds, "The surest path to catastrophic climate change is the false belief that it's too late to act (Mann 2021, pp. 179, 223)".

A second message that dampens courageous action is internal: without knowing it, we tend to accept an increasingly degraded natural world as normal. It has been called "shifting baseline syndrome" or "sliding baseline syndrome": each generation adapts to worsening circumstances over time, disregarding the abundance that previous generations knew, while peacefully accepting what remains as fine, or to be expected. We slowly adjust to unthinkable circumstances. As David Roberts explains, the scariest thing about global warming is that we could grow accustomed to it—grow used to massive fires, severe flooding, killing levels of heat—and never experience a moment of reckoning. We could sleepwalk our way to catastrophe (Roberts 2020; Campbell 2020).

Humans have been a successful species partly because we are so adaptable, but the capacity to adapt can also be a moral and even mortal liability. I think of the bitter comment uttered by Raskolnikov, the anti-hero of Dostoevsky's *Crime and Punishment*: "Men are scoundrels; they can get used to anything (Dostoevsky 1989, p. 22)!" I also think of the less bitter, but still bracing quote attributed to Thomas Merton: "The biggest human temptation is to settle for too little".

When does our purported serenity to accept the things we cannot change in fact mask our apathy and amnesia? When does serenity camouflage the refusal to care—what Fr. James Keenan calls "the failure to bother to love"? Rabbi Abraham Heschel insisted that "Prayer is meaningless unless it is subversive, unless it seeks to overthrow and to ruin the pyramids of callousness, hatred, opportunism, falsehoods". Subversive prayer breaks through cheap serenity. True serenity springs not from choosing comfort and avoiding conflict, but from the desire to seek only God's will, to abide in God's love, and to carry out what love requires, even when doing so is costly or difficult.

Once upon a time in the United States, people accepted many things as normal—slavery, Jim Crow, child labor, 80-h work weeks, the disenfranchisement of women and African Americans, the indiscriminate use of DDT, and so much more. What awoke them from their "serenity" was the persistent, massive, collective efforts of countless ardent people who were unwilling to settle for so little. What is it that we, too, must refuse to accept as normal? Are we willing to join the movements now rising up around the world—the climate justice movement, the human rights movement, the Indigenous rights movement, and the coalitions—both faith-based and secular—that are pressing to eliminate dirty emissions, restore a safe climate, reverse the sixth mass extinction of species, and create a just society that works for everyone?[11]

10. Urgency, Fear, and Love

People suffering with addiction do not walk casually into a Twelve-Step meeting. We are not there to pass the time. We are not there to virtue signal. We are not there to pass a purity test. We are there to save our lives. Urgency is what drives a person into recovery. We have reached the point of admitting, as the Big Book of Alcoholics Anonymous puts it, that "half-measures availed us nothing"[12]—not launching another diet, not drinking only on weekends, not shooting up just once in a while. We need a thorough makeover, a transformation which is physical, emotional, and spiritual.

Urgency is what today's climate prophets are conveying. Scientists speak with alarm about the very short time we have left in which to safeguard a stable climate; they speak about the urgent need for "rapid and far-reaching (United Nations Sustainable Development Goals 2018)". changes in all aspects of society. We cannot miss the urgency of Greta Thunberg, the Swedish teenager with the round face, straight blonde hair, and fierce, unyielding eyes, who spoke with such intensity to the U.S. Congress, the U.N. COP meeting, and the World Economic Forum, telling the world, telling the adults who failed to take action: "The house is on fire". Our planetary home is on fire. It is going up in flames.

It is a precious moment when an addict listens, grasps the urgency, feels the heat, and makes the decision to choose life. It is a precious moment when an addict admits that their life is unmanageable, that they need help beyond themselves, and that the time has come for decisive action. It is a precious moment when an addict realizes that the old way of life has to die in order for new life to be born. Will our generation be able to look back with gratitude one day and sing "Amazing Grace"?

Fear is what forced me into recovery, and fear may be what forces society to awaken to the climate crisis at last. Given the predicament in which we find ourselves, we have good reason to be afraid. However, fear cannot sustain us over the long haul—only love can do that.

Therefore, I thank God for all the people who are willing to face their fear, to empathize with other people's fear, and to stand together. I thank God for all the people who refuse to turn away from each other or against each other, but who decide instead to turn toward each other, to join forces and join hands. I thank God for the deep message of all the world's religions: we are interconnected with each other and with the web of life.

As an addictive society wakes from its restless, deathly sleep, faith communities can help to restore our capacity to love God and neighbors. In a sermon, D'var Torah, and dharma talk; in prayer groups, worship services, and meditation groups; in pastoral care, outreach, and bold public advocacy, communities of faith and spiritual practice can renew our intention and deepen our capacity to act in loving ways, to respect the dignity of every human being, and to cherish the sacredness of the natural world. Faith communities speak to the heart of what it means to be human. When people are closing their eyes to a crisis or going mad with hatred and fear, only love can restore us to sanity.

We can be more than addicts on a self-destructive path. Additionally, we can be more than chaplains at the deathbed of a dying order. We can be midwives to the new and beautiful world that is longing to be born.

Funding: This research received no external funding.

Institutional Review Board Statement: Not applicable.

Informed Consent Statement: Not applicable.

Conflicts of Interest: The author declares no conflict of interest.

Notes

[1] Robert Lentz, OFM, "Compassion Mandala", https://robertlentzartwork.wordpress.com/2012/06/19/httpswww-trinitystores-comstoreart-productsrlcmm/ (accessed on 27 July 2021).

[2] Christopher Burt, quoted by (Cappuci 2021).

[3] This example and those that follow are cited by (Kaplan and Dennis 2021).

[4] One very interesting initiative that weaves together addiction/recovery, Christian faith, and care for the Earth is EcoFaith Recovery. Based in the Pacific Northwest, EcoFaith Recovery is "a leadership development effort grounded in the Christian tradition and welcoming all who seek recovery from societal addictions to unsustainable ways of life. Our recovery begins as we come out of isolation and rediscover our relatedness to God, ourselves, each other, and the entire earth community of which we are a part". See: http://www.ecofaithrecovery.org/ (accessed on 31 August 2021).

5   https://workthatreconnects.org/, https://dayenu.org/, https://climateawakening.org/ (accessed on 30 July 2021).
6   See, for example, Climate Psychology Alliance https://www.climatepsychologyalliance.org/ (accessed on 31 August 2021) Climate Psychology Alliance North America https://www.climatepsychology.us/ (accessed on 31 August 2021) and Climate Psychiatry Alliance https://www.climatepsychiatry.org/ (accessed on 31 August 2021).
7   In 1992, Joanna Macy brought the Elm Dance to people living in areas that had been poisoned by the Chernobyl disaster. This simple circle dance, now associated with The Work That Reconnect, is intended for all who experience collective trauma, https://workthatreconnects.org/resources/elm-dance/ (accessed on 31 July 2021).
8   The Sunrise Movement is a youth movement to stop climate change and create millions of good jobs in the process, https://www.sunrisemovement.org/ (accessed on 31 August 2021).
9   (Westervelt 2021). In *The New Climate War*, Michael E. Mann addresses this topic in a chapter entitled, "It's YOUR Fault", pp. 63–97.
10 "Calculate and offset your emissions", https://www.bp.com/en_gb/target-neutral/home/calculate-and-offset-your-emissions.html (accessed on 31 August 2021).
11 See, for instance, The Climate Mobilization, Indigenous Environmental Network, 350.org, Poor People's Campaign, Sunrise Movement, Extinction Rebellion, Mothers Out Front, Interfaith Power & Light, GreenFaith, The Shalom Center, Dayenu, and many others.
12 https://www.aa.org/assets/en_us/en_bigbook_chapt5.pdf (accessed on 31 August 2021).

References

Berwyn, Bob. 2020. Unchecked Global Warming Could Collapse Whole Ecosystems, Maybe within 10 Years. April 8. Available online: https://insideclimatenews.org/news/08042020/global-warming-ecosystem-biodiversity-rising-heat-species/ (accessed on 30 July 2021).
Black, Claudia. 1981. *It Will Never Happen to Me!* New York: Ballantine Books.
Brueggemann, Walter. 1978. *The Prophetic Imagination*. Philadelphia: Fortress Press.
Bullitt-Jonas, Margaret. 1991. Spiritual Direction for Adult Children of Alcoholics. *Human Development*. Volume 12, No. 1. pp. 5–10. Available online: https://revivingcreation.org/wp-content/uploads/2014/03/Spiritual-Direction.pdf (accessed on 31 July 2021).
Bullitt-Jonas, Margaret. 1998. *Holy Hunger: A Woman's Journey from Food Addiction to Spiritual Fulfillment*. New York: Vintage Books.
Bullitt-Jonas, Margaret. 2000. Feeling and Pain and Prayer. In *Praying as a Christian: The Best of the Review*-7. Edited by David L. Fleming. St. Louis: Review for Religious, pp. 139–52. Available online: https://revivingcreation.org/wp-content/uploads/2014/03/Feeling-and-Pain-and-Prayer.pdf (accessed on 31 July 2021).
Bush, George W. 2006. State of the Union Address by the President. January 31. Available online: https://georgewbush-whitehouse.archives.gov/stateoftheunion/2006/ (accessed on 27 July 2021).
Campbell, SueEllen. 2020. Recent Pieces on Importance of 'Sliding Baselines'. September 24. Available online: https://yaleclimateconnections.org/2020/09/recent-pieces-on-importance-of-sliding-baselines/ (accessed on 1 August 2021).
Cappuci, Matthew. 2021. Pacific Northwest Heat Wave Was "Virtually Impossible" without Climate Change, Scientists Find. July 7. Available online: https://www.washingtonpost.com/weather/2021/07/07/pacific-northwest-heat-wave-climate/ (accessed on 27 July 2021).
Carrington, Damian. 2018. Humanity has wiped out 60% of animal populations since 1970, report finds. *The Guardian*. October 29. Available online: https://www.theguardian.com/environment/2018/oct/30/humanity-wiped-out-animals-since-1970-major-report-finds (accessed on 31 July 2021).
Ceballos, Gerardo, Paul R. Ehrlich, and Rodolfo Dirzo. 2017. Biological Annihilation via the Ongoing Sixth Mass Extinction Signaled by Vertebrate Population Losses and Declines. *Proceedings of the National Academy of Sciences of the United States of America* 114: E6089–E6096. Available online: https://www.pnas.org/content/114/30/E6089 (accessed on 31 July 2021). [CrossRef] [PubMed]
Dostoevsky, Feodor. 1989. *Crime and Punishment*, 3rd ed. Edited by George Gibian. New York: W.W. Norton & Co.
Eliot, T. S. 1971. "Burnt Norton", in "Four Quartets". In *The Complete Poems and Plays 1909–1950*. San Diego: Harcourt Brace Jovanovich, p. 118.
Gelbspan, Ross. 1997. *The Heat Is on: The Climate Crisis, The Coverup, The Prescription*. Cambridge: Perseus Books.
Harvey, Fiona. 2020. Wildlife destruction not a slippery slope but a series of cliff edges. *The Guardian*. April 8. Available online: https://www.theguardian.com/environment/2020/apr/08/wildlife-destruction-not-a-slippery-slope-but-a-series-of-cliff-edges (accessed on 20 July 2021).
Harvey, Fiona, and Agencies. 2021. IPCC steps up warning on climate tipping points in leaked draft report. *The Guardian*. June 23. Available online: https://www.theguardian.com/environment/2021/jun/23/climate-change-dangerous-thresholds-un-report (accessed on 1 August 2021).
Hopkins, Hop. 2020. Racism Is Killing the Planet. June 8. Available online: https://www.sierraclub.org/sierra/racism-killing-planet (accessed on 31 July 2021).
Jenkins, Willis. 2008. *Ecologies of Grace: Environmental Ethics and Christian Theology*. New York: Oxford University Press.
Jenkins, Willis. 2013. *Future of Ethics: Sustainability, Social Justice, and Religious Creativity*. Washington: Georgetown University Press.

Kaplan, Sarah, and Brady Dennis. 2021. Amid summer of fire and floods, a moment of truth for climate action. *The Washington Post*. July 24. Available online: https://www.washingtonpost.com/climate-environment/2021/07/24/amid-summer-fire-floods-moment-truth-climate-action/ (accessed on 28 July 2021).

Mann, Michael E. 2021. *The New Climate War: The Fight to Take Back the Planet*. New York: Public Affairs, Hachette Book Group, p. 3.

Mellen, Ruby, and William Neff. 2021. Beyond human endurance: How climate change is making parts of the world too hot and humid to survive. *The Washington Post*. Available online: https://www.washingtonpost.com/world/interactive/2021/climate-change-humidity/ (accessed on 28 July 2021).

Millman, Oliver. 2021. Three Americans create enough carbon emissions to kill one person, study finds. *The Guardian*. July 29. Available online: https://www.theguardian.com/environment/2021/jul/29/carbon-emissions-americans-social-cost (accessed on 31 July 2021).

Moore, Kathleen Dean, and Michael P. Nelson, eds. 2010. *Moral Ground: Ethical Action for a Planet in Peril*. San Antonio: Trinity University Press.

Norgaard, Kari Marie. 2012. The Everyday Denial of Climate Change. July 5. Available online: https://thebulletin.org/2012/07/the-everyday-denial-of-climate-change/ (accessed on 28 July 2021).

Northcott, Michael S. 2007. *A Moral Climate: The Ethics of Global Warming*. Maryknoll: Orbis.

Offill, Jenny. 2020. *Weather*. New York: Knopf.

Oreskes, Naomi, and Erik M. M. Conway. 2011. *Merchants of Doubt: How a Handful of Scientists Obscured the Truth on Issues from Tobacco Smoke to Global Warming*. New York: Bloomsbury Press.

Otto, Ilona M., Jonathan F. Donges, Roger Cremades, Avit Bhowmik, Richard J. Hewitt, Wolfgang Lucht, Johan Rockström, Franziska Allerberger, Mark McCaffrey, Sylvanus S. P. Doe, and et al. 2020. Social Tipping Dynamics for Stabilizing Earth's Climate by 2050. Proceedings of the National Academy of Sciences (PNAS). February 4. Available online: https://www.pnas.org/content/117/5/2354 (accessed on 1 August 2021).

Rasmussen, Larry. 1996. *Earth Community, Earth Ethics*. Maryknoll: Orbis.

Roberts, David. 2020. The Scariest Thing about Global Warming (and Covid-19). Vox, Updated December 4. Available online: https://www.vox.com/energy-and-environment/2020/7/7/21311027/covid-19-climate-change-global-warming-shifting-baselines (accessed on 1 August 2021).

Rott, Nathan. 2020. The World Lost Two Thirds of Its Wildlife in 50 Years. We are to Blame. September 10. Available online: https://www.npr.org/2020/09/10/911500907/the-world-lost-two-thirds-of-its-wildlife-in-50-years-we-are-to-blame (accessed on 31 July 2021).

Saddique, Haroon. 2021. Legal Experts Worldwide Draw up 'Historic' Definition of Ecocide. *The Guardian*. June 22. Available online: https://www.theguardian.com/environment/2021/jun/22/legal-experts-worldwide-draw-up-historic-definition-of-ecocide (accessed on 29 July 2021).

Schade, Leah, and Margaret Bullitt-Jonas. 2019. *Rooted and Rising: Voices of Courage in a Time of Climate Crisis*. Lanham: Rowman & Littlefield.

Sengupta, Somini. 2021. 'No One Is Safe': Extreme Weather Batters the Wealthy World. *The New York Times*. July 17. Available online: https://www.nytimes.com/2021/07/17/climate/heatwave-weather-hot.html (accessed on 28 July 2021).

Shabecoff, Philip. 1988. Global Warming Has Begun, Expert Tells Senate. *The New York Times*. June 24. Available online: https://www.nytimes.com/1988/06/24/us/global-warming-has-begun-expert-tells-senate.html (accessed on 27 July 2021).

Sharp, Carolyn J. 2011. A Necessary Condition of a Good, Loud Lament. In *Disruptive Grace*. Minneapolis: Fortress Press, pp. 179–205.

Stainforth, Thorfinn. 2020. *More than Half of All CO_2 Emissions Since 1751 Emitted in the Last 30 Years*. London: Institute for European Environmental Policy, April 29, Available online: https://ieep.eu/news/more-than-half-of-all-co2-emissions-since-1751-emitted-in-the-last-30-years (accessed on 31 July 2021).

Statista. 2021. Wealthy Nations Lead per Capita Emissions. March 1. Available online: https://www.statista.com/chart/24306/carbon-emissions-per-capita-by-country/ (accessed on 1 August 2021).

Stover, Dawn. 2014. Addicted to Oil. *Bulletin of the Atomic Scientists*. May 18. Available online: https://thebulletin.org/2014/05/addicted-to-oil/ (accessed on 28 July 2021).

Surma, Katie, Inside Climate News, and Yuliya Talmazan. 2021. The Push to Make 'Ecocide' an International Crime Takes a Big Step Forward. June 22. Available online: https://www.nbcnews.com/news/world/push-make-ecocide-international-crime-takes-big-step-forward-n1272059 (accessed on 29 July 2021).

Tharoor, Ishaan. 2021. It's the Climate Change, Stupid. June 30. Available online: https://www.washingtonpost.com/world/2021/06/30/climate-change-heat-politics/ (accessed on 27 July 2021).

Ulanov, Ann, and Barry Ulanov. 1982. *Primary Speech: A Psychology of Prayer*. Atlanta: John Knox Press, p. 96.

Union of Concerned Scientists. 2007. Smoke, Mirrors, and Hot Air: How ExxonMobil Uses Big Tobacco's Tactics to 'Manufacture Uncertainty' on Climate Change. July 16. Available online: https://www.ucsusa.org/resources/smoke-mirrors-hot-air (accessed on 28 July 2021).

Union of Concerned Scientists. 2008. Each Country's Share of CO_2 Emissions. July 16 Updated 12 August 2020. Available online: https://www.ucsusa.org/resources/each-countrys-share-co2-emissions (accessed on 31 July 2021).

United Nations Sustainable Development Goals. 2018. Special Climate Report: 1.5 °C Is Possible but Requires Unprecedented and Urgent Action. October. Available online: https://www.un.org/sustainabledevelopment/blog/2018/10/special-climate-report-1-5oc-is-possible-but-requires-unprecedented-and-urgent-action/ (accessed on 2 August 2021).

Westervelt, Amy. 2021. Big Oil Is Trying to Make Climate Change Your Problem to Solve. Don't Let Them. *Rolling Stone*. May 14. Available online: https://www.rollingstone.com/politics/politics-news/climate-change-exxonmobil-harvard-study-1169682/ (accessed on 1 August 2021).

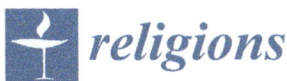

Article

The Effect of Religious Beliefs and Attitudes in Intrinsic and Extrinsic Optimism and Pessimism in Players of Games of Chance

Lisete S. Mónico * and Valentim R. Alferes

Faculty of Psychology and Education Sciences, University of Coimbra, 3000-115 Coimbra, Portugal; valferes@fpce.uc.pt
* Correspondence: lisete.monico@fpce.uc.pt

Abstract: Games of chance usually make people feel a whirlwind of emotions, especially in gambling. While those games depend more on luck than on individuals' skills, optimism should be a distinctive feature. Considering the classic literature of the effects of religiosity on risk behaviors, the issue of the influence of religiosity on optimism in players of games of chance has been less studied, especially when we considered optimism as a multidimensional concept comprising intrinsic and extrinsic optimism and pessimism. Aims: To analyze the effect of religious beliefs and attitudes in optimism and pessimism dimensions in players of games of chance and gambling. Method: The sample consists of 271 recurring players of games of chance and gambling, who answered a questionnaire composed of measures of religious beliefs and attitudes, optimism, pessimism, and estimates of future occurrences, evidencing good psychometric properties. Results: Players are moderately religious and more optimistic than pessimistic, estimating a chance of 36% of highly unlikely desirable events. The structural model showed an overall influence of religious beliefs and attitudes higher on optimism ($R^2 = 44\%$) than on pessimism ($R^2 = 5\%$). However, the distinction between intrinsic and extrinsic optimism has shown that the players anchor their optimism in different kinds of beliefs. Extrinsic desirable events, like winning the lottery, were more predicted by religious beliefs and attitudes in comparison with intrinsic desirable events. Inversely, religious beliefs and attitudes tend to predict more intrinsic pessimism in comparison with intrinsic optimism. Conclusions: Optimism is not a one-dimensional construct, should be analyzed considering the dichotomies of optimism/pessimism and intrinsic/extrinsic. In recurring players of games of chance and gambling, religious beliefs and attitudes predicted more optimism than pessimism, being more associated with extrinsic than intrinsic desirable events. More intrinsically pessimistic players seem to recur to religiosity to anchor their positive expectations.

Keywords: religious beliefs; religious attitudes; optimism; pessimism; players of games of chance

Citation: Mónico, Lisete S., and Valentim R. Alferes. 2022. The Effect of Religious Beliefs and Attitudes in Intrinsic and Extrinsic Optimism and Pessimism in Players of Games of Chance. *Religions* 13: 97. https://doi.org/10.3390/rel13020097

Academic Editors: Bernadette Flanagan and Noelia Molina

Received: 28 September 2021
Accepted: 14 January 2022
Published: 20 January 2022

Publisher's Note: MDPI stays neutral with regard to jurisdictional claims in published maps and institutional affiliations.

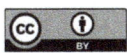

Copyright: © 2022 by the authors. Licensee MDPI, Basel, Switzerland. This article is an open access article distributed under the terms and conditions of the Creative Commons Attribution (CC BY) license (https://creativecommons.org/licenses/by/4.0/).

1. Introduction

When we think about players of games of chance and gambling, the idea of optimistic people comes to mind. Games of chance usually make people feel a whirlwind of emotions, especially in gambling. Whereas those games depend more on luck than on individuals' skills, optimism should be a distinctive feature.

Whenever a person plays, they have at least a glimmer of hope that they can win. Following this reasoning, players should be optimists or, at least, more optimistic than pessimists. Most of the literature shows that people, in general, perceive their future as being happier than the future of other people, believing that they are more likely to experience desirable situations and less likely to experience undesirable ones (Mens et al. 2021).

Considering that all areas of life are mediated by aims, the behavior of individuals is determined by the self-regulatory mechanisms adopted with a view to achieving them.

Predictions based on the theory of social comparison (Festinger 1954) would not give optimism its general character (Carver and Scheier 2001; Mónico 2021). Furthermore, in the course of the life cycle, the emergence of adversities is practically inevitable, and the difficulty in overcoming them may lead individuals to pessimism (Swann et al. 1987). In the case of players of games of chance and gambling, the times they lost a game or a bet are very frequent, and the reasoning concerning the chances of winning should point to low probabilities. For Carver and Scheier (1982, 2012), optimism enters into self-regulation when people, despite anticipating obstacles to achieving certain goals, maintain the belief that they will be successful (Armor and Taylor 1998; Scheier and Carver 1992). The aim of this paper is to analyze if and how optimism can be anchored in religious beliefs and attitudes in players of games of chance and gambling.

Classic is the idea that religion instigates, among other functions, normative behavior. However, the investigation that religion can promote optimism has been less studied, especially when we considered optimism as a multidimensional concept comprising intrinsic and extrinsic optimism and pessimism. It is not uncommon to observe situations in which players of games of chance resort in some way to their religiosity, believing that it will help them to win. In Portugal, some research has identified a positive association between religiosity and optimism (Mónico 2012a, 2013a, 2013b; Mónico and Alferes 2019; Mónico et al. 2016). Classic authors also pointed some connections between religiosity and some dimensions of psychological capital (e.g., W. James, Freud, Weber, Durkheim, Allport; Mattis et al. 2004). It is interesting to explore this relationship, especially if and how players anchor their optimism in their religiosity, and to what extent optimism and pessimism dimensions are associated with a perception of greater probability of occurrence of desirable events and the prevention of the undesirable ones.

2. Background

2.1. Religiosity and Religious Beliefs and Attitudes

It is understood that religiosity, or religious culture (Sitzmann and Campbell 2021), is the individual level of commitment to beliefs, doctrines, and practices of some religion (Barker and Warburg 1998; Mookherjee 1994). Counterpart expression of religious experience (Geerts 1990) concerns the extent to which an individual believes, follows, and practices a religious doctrine, considering its two regulating poles: beliefs and rites. In the classic work of (James [1902] 1985), religiosity is defined as "the feelings, acts, and experiences of individual men in their solitude, so far as they apprehend themselves to stand in relation to whatever they may consider the divine" (p. 34). This can be introduced either in a traditional way, in a formal and non-reflective way that follows the customs, or in an individual way, looking for answers to questions, needs, ideas, and ideals (Grom 1994).

People's religiosity is highly influenced by culture (Sitzmann and Campbell 2021), religious practices, and motivations. Within and between religious groups, the nature and intensity of beliefs are extremely variable (Ávila 2003; Mónico 2011; Pargament 1997). Multiple surveys have been carried out with the aim of ascertaining the extent to which people hold religious beliefs (Hinde 2010). However, the meaning of the expression "I believe" becomes controversial and difficult to ascertain (Gellner 1992). The boundaries that distinguish faith and belief are not clear. Moreover, spirituality is independent of any religion or belief system, considered as a complex multi-dimensional and multi-cultural concept (Mónico and Margaça 2021).

Although it has different meanings (Fowler 1995; Hood 1995; Pargament 1997; Wulff 1997), the construct of faith is indistinguishable from that of other attitudes . Focusing on the reasoning and dynamic process of elaboration, faith is seen as an adherence of the mind founded on arguments that do not constitute a rigorous demonstration (...), a mental attitude that includes both a commitment and a free adhesion" (p. 92).

Argyle (2000) equates faith with an attitude that, as a favorable or unfavorable disposition, expressed in words and/or behavior (Eagly and Chaiken 1998), can be divided into the classical cognitive, emotional, and behavioral components. Hinde (2010) highlights the supernatural focus of religious beliefs, as they involve unusual beings, entities, and experiences, encompassing counter-intuitive pretensions and complex concepts, not fully intelligible and often controversial or inconsistent. In fact, religious beliefs are not constrained to the possibility of empirical materialization (Haught 1995), are established by authority, by consensus, or by both (Fowler 1995; Lawson and McCauley 1990), and they are supported by social consent and traditions (Brown 1988). Thus, we understand the tendency in modern western societies to consider religious beliefs as mere opinions or attitudes, as opposed to empirical beliefs seen as knowledge. However, we are in line with McGuire's (2002) conception, which considers that both beliefs—religious and empirical—constitute "knowledge" for the individual who believes in them, being real in their consequences and outlining the experiences and actions of the individual.

The double meaning of religious beliefs and attitudes is pointed out by the classic work of Dittes (1969), when he states that the individual believes in a supernatural or superhuman objective reality, however, based on the subjectivity of the psychological conditions of human beings. According to the author, for a religious individual, believing is not a way of facing the world and the future, but a relationship with a being/entity through symbolic actions, supported by reports and representations of the divine and inspiring rules of conduct.

2.2. Optimism and Pessimism

Optimism. The scope of optimism is represented in the literature by two interrelated concepts: the positive expectations for the future (Domino and Conway 2001; Erthal et al. 2021) and the tendency to believe that the world is the "best of all possible worlds" (Gillham et al. 2001, p. 53). "Optimists are people who expect good experiences in the future. Pessimists are people who expect bad experiences" (Carver and Scheier 2001, p. 31). Thus, "optimism is seen as a cognitive feature (a goal, an expectation, a belief or a causal attribution) about the desired and perceived as successful future" (Barros 2004, p. 101). The tendency towards the positive, the expectation of obtaining good results and the explanation attributed to the negative events characterize, in general, optimism, detected in areas of life as distinct as health, professional or academic achievement, interpersonal relationships, and security (Buunk 2001; McKenna 1993; Mónico 2013a, 2021; Mónico et al. 2016; Weinstein 1987). The conceptual definitions are directed towards positive expectations, usually generalized and stable (Mónico 2011, 2021), linked to two key brain areas: the anterior cingulate cortex (ACC—imagination of the future and self-referential information procession) and the inferior frontal gyrus (IFG—response inhibition and handling with important cues). ACC action was positively associated with trait optimism and with the estimations of positive events, and IFG with behavioral measures of optimistic propensity (Erthal et al. 2021).

Pessimism. The nature and intensity of beliefs related to the failure to reach the intended goals, essentially in situations of adversity, constitutes an identifier of people's level of pessimism (Mónico 2013c). Absolute or dispositional pessimism refers to generalized expectations of the occurrence of negative events, for the individual, or the tendency to expect unfavorable life outcomes (Kruger and Burrus 2004). A state of pessimism leads to the undertaking of reduced efforts in the achievement of the goals, especially when pessimism is a dispositional trait (Scheier and Carver 1985). The stable tendency to maintain negative expectations about own results reveals a pessimistic trait (Carver and Scheier 2001), consistently influencing expectations throughout situations.

As we find unrealistic optimism in people (Weinstein 1980, 1987), Kruger and Burrus (2004) call attention to the existence of unrealistic pessimism. This type of pessimism occurs for very rare desirable events (e.g., living after 100 years), characterized by the lower expectations of these events for the person, compared to other individuals. In addition to the evidence of comparative optimism, Chambers et al. (2003) propose the existence of a comparative pessimism, detected in desirable and unusual situations, although also in undesirable and common events. The concept of defensive pessimism was proposed by Cantor et al. in the mid-eighties and represents a cognitive strategy that individuals use to prepare for stress-inducing situations (Norem and Cantor 1986), differing from the attributional style defensive of Seligman (Gillham et al. 2001; Seligman 2006) and the pessimism-trait advocated by Carver and Scheier (2001). The question is whether it is always adaptive to expect the best (Carver and Scheier 2001).

Optimism, pessimism, and gambling. Some of the literature has been devoted to studying the relationship between optimism and gambling. Gibson and Sanbonmatsu (2004) found that optimistic players were more likely to have positive gambling expectations and report maintaining these expectations following losses, in comparison with pessimistic players. They also indicated money as the main motivation for gambling. After poor gaming performance, the pessimistic players tend to decrease more their betting and expectations, when compared to optimists. These last players, after losing, recalled more wins than do pessimistic players.

Intrinsic vs. extrinsic optimism and pessimism. In this paper, we consider the distinction between intrinsic and extrinsic optimism and pessimism (Mónico 2011, 2012b, 2013c). Intrinsic optimism refers to the expectation that good future experiences depend on their own personal skills and extrinsic optimism to the conviction that the good results will prevail due to situational factors, not having the elderly control over these factors (luck, chance).

A basic premise of optimism anchored in internality beliefs is the expectation that desirable occurrences will happen via assignment of causality to factors internal to the individual, personal, and dependent of himself. Inversely, individuals with optimism based on externality beliefs believe that their positive events will be determined by situational factors, external and not controllable by themselves, caused by others, or determined by luck or by chance.

Applying the concept of internality and externality to pessimism, we found the same reasoning. As the locus of control (Rotter 1990), we consider that the continuum which goes from extreme optimism to extreme pessimism is permeated by internality or externality beliefs, and the anticipation of positive (optimism) or negative (pessimism) outcomes can be attributed to internal or external individual factors. Thus, by internality optimism, we consider the expectation that good future experiences depend on their own personal skills. Externality optimism refers to the conviction that good results will prevail due to situational factors, with the elderly control not having over these factors, like luck or chance (Mónico 2011, 2012b, 2013c). In this research, in addition to measures of optimism and pessimism based on conventional authors, we operationalized optimism and pessimism based on the estimation of the occurrence of certain events in the respondent's life, both positive and negative, based either on intrinsic or extrinsic factors.

3. Method

3.1. Sample

The sample consisted of 271 Portuguese recurring players of games of chance and gambling, 186 (68.6%) being male and 85 (31.4%) male, with an average age of 41.50 years-old (SD = 14.97; age range: 16–87 years), M_{age} = 42.72 (SD = 15.55) for males and M_{age} = 38.85 (SD = 13.32) for females. Regarding education, 44 (16.2%) participants completed 4 years of education, 72 (26.6%) 9 years of education, 93 (34.3%) 12 years of education, and 62 (22.9%) completed higher education. The majority of the participants were married (n = 166, 61.3%), 83 (30.6%) is single, 17 (6.3%) divorced, and 4 (1.5%) are widowed (1 missing-value).

In total, 58 players (21.4%) lived in the countryside, 73 in a suburban area (26.9%), and 139 in urban areas (51.3%) (1 m:L:ssing-value, 0.4%); 259 belonged to Portugal Continental (95.6%), 62 (22.9%) to the north of the country, 169 (62.4%) to the central region, 21 (7.7%) to Lisboa and Vale do Tejo, 5 (1.8%) to the Alentejo, 2 (0.7%) to the Algarve, and 12 (84.4%) to Portuguese islands Madeira and Azores. With regard to the professional situation of the respondents, the majority were employed (n = 225, 83.0%), with diverse occupations, followed by students (n = 32, 11.8%) and retired (n = 14, 5.2%).

3.2. Data Analysis

All the analysis was performed by using the statistical program SPSS and AMOS (IBM Corp. 2020). Skewness and kurtosis values indicate a normal distribution, |Sk| < 1.30 and |Ku| < 1.73 (−0.562 < Sk < 0.807 and −0.592 < ku < 0.683 for the composite scores).

Exploratory Factor Analysis (EFA) was performed with SPSS by Principal Component Analysis (PCA), VARIMAX rotation (Kaiser's normalization), given that we expected independent factors. The PCA assumptions were tested through the sample size (ratio of 5 subjects per item and at least 100 participants; Gorsuch 2015), the normality and linearity of the variables, factorability of R, and sample adequacy (Tabachnick and Fidell 2019). Reliability was calculated by Cronbach's alpha (Nunnally and Bernstein 2010). The score of 0.80 was taken as a good reliability indicator (Urbina 2014), and 0.60 as acceptable (DeVellis 2012).

For the analysis of variance (ANOVA) and multivariate analysis of variance (MANOVA), the assumptions of independence of observations and homogeneity of error variance and covariance matrices of the dependent variables were checked. Post hoc Tukey HSD tests were performed for pairwise multiple comparisons.

Structural equation modeling was carried out with IBM AMOS and the maximum likelihood estimation method. The goodness of fit was analyzed using CMIN/DF (normed chi-square), NFI (normed fit index), CFI (comparative fit index), and RMSEA (Root Mean Square Error of Approximation) (Kline 2016; Schumacker and Lomax 2016).

Internal consistency was assessed by Cronbach's alpha coefficient (Nunnally and Bernstein 2010), both for the global scale and their dimensions. Despite reliability coefficients higher than 0.70 being considered acceptable for convergence and reliability, we have based on Nunnally and Bernstein (2010) and DeVellis (2012) for reliability in each dimension. Mean scores were calculated based on the average of items in each factor.

A probability of 0.05 for the Type I error was considered for all the inferential statistics.

3.3. Materials

A survey was carried out using a self-administered questionnaire composed of the Religious Beliefs and Attitudes Scale, the Optimism and Pessimism Scale, and a sociodemographic questionnaire.

3.3.1. Religious Beliefs and Attitudes Scale

This scale was built and validated by Mónico (2011) with a larger sample of Portuguese citizens. It is composed of 13 multiple-choice items (from 1 = totally disagree to 5 = totally agree). The PCA performed with this sample (see Table 1) pointed to a one-factor solution responsible for 79.74% of the total variability and good reliability (α = 0.96, see Table 1).

3.3.2. Optimism and Pessimism Scale

The *Optimism and Pessimism Scale* were adapted from the literature (Barros 1998; Scheier et al. 1994; Schweizer and Koch 2001; Snyder et al. 1991) and Wiseman (2006). The 12 multiple-choice items, answered from 1 (strongly disagree) to 5 (strongly agree), were analyzed through a PCA (see Table 2), emerging two independent factors with acceptable reliability: *Optimism* (7 items, α = 0.71) and *Pessimism* (5 items, α = 0.66).

Table 1. *Religious Beliefs and Attitudes Scale* (RBAS: mean scores (M), standard-deviations (SD), factorial loadings (s), commonalities (h^2), and Cronbach's internal consistency coefficient (α) for the one-dimension solution.

Items			M	SD	s	h^2
[DEUS_36]	[RBA1]	I believe God hears my prayers.	3.46	1.32	0.88	0.77
[DEUS_13]	[RBA2]	In moments of happiness, I believe it was God who helped me.	3.44	1.31	0.88	0.78
[DEUS_19]	[RBA3]	I feel that God protects me from the adversities of life.	3.32	1.27	0.90	0.81
[DEUS_24]	[RBA4]	I need God's help to make important decisions in my life.	2.93	1.36	0.87	0.76
[DEUS_40]	[RBA5]	Everything I am and everything I hope to be I owe to God.	2.93	1.29	0.85	0.72
[DEUS_34]	[RBA6]	I usually thank God for the happiness of my life.	3.49	1.32	0.85	0.73
[DEUS_32]	RBA7	When I have a problem, I get closer to God.	3.34	1.26	0.79	0.62
[DEUS_28]	RBA8	The universe was created by God.	3.42	1.44	0.77	0.59
[DEUS_31]	RBA9	I trust what God has destined for me.	3.38	1.30	0.86	0.74
[DEUS_37]	RBA10	I believe that God will reward me for my current sufferings.	3.26	1.28	0.78	0.60
[DEUS_58]	RBA11	Without faith in God, I would lose the strength to fight.	3.08	1.35	0.79	0.63
[DEUS_39]	RBA12	Lately, my belief in God has increased.	2.95	1.28	0.77	0.59
[DEUS_21]	RBA13	I trust God more than myself to overcome problems.	2.41	1.25	0.70	0.49
		TOTAL KMO = 0.97; Bartlett's test: χ^2 (78) = 3082.28 ($p < 0.001$); α = 0.960	3.16	1.39		

Table 2. PCA of the *Optimism and Pessimism Scale*: Descriptive statistics (M and SD), factorial loadings (s) of the rotatex component matrix (F1, F2), commonalities (h^2), eigenvalues, shared variance, and Cronbach's alpha.

			M	SD	F1 (s)	F2 (s)	h^2
		F1: Optimism					
7.44	IO1	I vigorously pursue my goals.	3.86	0.84	**0.67**	−0.04	0.45
7.29	IO2	I always find a solution to a problem.	3.45	0.83	**0.65**	0.05	0.43
7.53	IO3	I have a lot of confidence in myself.	3.97	0.80	**0.61**	−0.14	0.38
7.26	IO4	No task is too difficult for me.	3.17	0.93	**0.59**	0.05	0.35
7.62	IO5	I am always optimistic about my future.	3.63	0.92	**0.57**	−0.33	0.43
7.41	IO6	I can think of many ways to get out of trouble.	3.63	0.86	**0.55**	0.02	0.31
7.23	IO7	I overcome even the most difficult problems.	3.57	0.84	**0.55**	−0.02	0.30
		F2: Pessimism					
7.20	IP1	I rarely expect things to go my way.	2.51	1.07	−0.04	**0.72**	0.52
7.17	IP2	When life is going well, I am afraid that there will soon be some adversity.	2.91	1.18	0	**0.65**	0.43
7.22	IP3	If something can go wrong for me, it sure will happen.	2.36	0.98	−0.01	**0.64**	0.41
7.35	IP4	I rarely hope that good things will happen to me.	2.46	1.08	−0.01	**0.61**	0.37
7.61	IP5	In difficult situations, I am always expecting the worst.	2.65	1.09	−0.17	**0.61**	0.40
		Eigenvalues			2.76	2.00	
		% of explained variance			23.01	16.71	
		Cronbach's α			0.71	0.66	

3.3.3. Estimation of Future Desirable Events Scale

We considered the estimation of 11 future desirable events, measured from 0 to 100%, adapted from Wiseman (2006). The PCA performed identified two dimensions with good reliability (see Table 3): *Intrinsic desirable events* (6 items, α = 0.83) and *Extrinsic desirable events* (5 items, α = 0.77).

Table 3. PCA of the *Estimation of Desirable Events scale*: Descriptive statistics (M and SD), factorial loadings (s) of the rotatex component matrix (F1, F2), commonalities (h^2), eigenvalues, shared variance, and Cronbach's alpha.

	From 0% to 100%, Please Indicate the Percentage That Best Represents the Possibility of Occurrence of This Event in Your Life ...	M (%)	SD	F1 (s)	F2 (s)	h^2
	F1: Intrinsic desirable events (probability 0–100%)					
IDE1	Having harmony in the family.	75.26	24.78	**0.84**	0.08	0.72
IDE2	Being reciprocated in a romantic relationship.	73.19	27.71	**0.80**	−0.02	0.65
IDE3	Living happily.	70.74	25.46	**0.79**	0.29	0.70
IDE4	Get lucky in life.	58.14	26.55	**0.61**	0.48	0.60
IDE5	Be strong/have courage.	64.53	26.92	**0.58**	0.32	0.44
IDE6	Overcoming my biggest difficulty.	54.01	26.28	**0.49**	0.35	0.36
	F2: Extrinsic desirable events (probability 0–100%)					
EDE1	Become a millionaire.	40.65	32.63	0.11	**0.81**	0.67
EDE2	Win the lottery.	45.02	35.44	0.18	**0.78**	0.65
EDE3	Be famous.	20.90	26.75	0.14	**0.65**	0.45
EDE4	A miracle happens in my life.	41.59	27.28	0.14	**0.65**	0.44
EDE5	Be admired by other people.	31.96	31.44	0.28	**0.55**	0.38
	Eigenvalues			4.52	1.52	
	% of explained variance			28.04	26.90	
	Cronbach's α			0.83	0.77	

3.3.4. Estimation of Future Undesirable Events Scale

We also asked participants for the estimation of 14 future undesirable events, measured from 0 to 100%, adapted from Wiseman (2006). The PCA performed identified two dimensions with good reliability (see Table 4): *Intrinsic desirable events* (6 items, α = 0.83) and *Extrinsic desirable events* (5 items, α = 0.77).

Table 4. PCA of the *Estimation of Undesirable Events Scale*: Descriptive statistics (M and SD), factorial loadings (s) of the rotatex component matrix (F1, F2), commonalities (h^2), eigenvalues, shared variance, and Cronbach's alpha.

	From 0% to 100%, Please Indicate the Number (in Percentage) That Best Represents the Possibility of Occurrence of This Event in Your Life ...	M (%)	SD	F1 (s)	F2 (s)	h^2
	F1: Extrinsic undesirable events (probability 0–100%)					
EUE1	Having a serious chronic illness.	45.24	28.09	**0.86**	0.09	0.75
EUE2	Having a malignant disease (eg., cancer).	46.0	29.4	**0.86**	0.26	0.80
EUE3	Having a cardiovascular disease (eg., heart attack, stroke).	42.9	28.0	**0.78**	0.22	0.66
EUE4	Dying soon.	38.3	28.0	**0.66**	0.29	0.52
EUE5	Going through difficult times in life.	46.60	26.57	**0.62**	0.38	0.52
EUE6	Having a serious accident (eg., driving, at work).	43.1	28.0	**0.60**	0.39	0.52
EUE7	Losing the love of your life (through death, divorce, separation).	38.1	30.9	**0.54**	0.36	0.42
	F2: Intrinsic undesirable events (probability 0–100%)					
IUE1	Not achieving what I idealize.	34.70	24.63	0.19	**0.73**	0.57
IUE2	Not being able to fulfill my duties.	28.73	25.76	0.30	**0.67**	0.54
IUE3	Having bad luck in life.	36.64	26.91	0.30	**0.66**	0.53
IUE4	Losing hope/becoming a pessimist.	24.08	23.63	0.15	**0.66**	0.46
IUE5	Having a worse life than others.	26.90	25.02	0.13	**0.63**	0.41
IUE6	Go into depression.	28.89	28.01	0.39	**0.63**	0.55
IUE7	Trying to commit suicide.	8.33	19.17	0.25	**0.51**	0.33
	Eigenvalues			6.23	1.35	
	% of explained variance			44.49	9.66	
	Cronbach's α			0.88	0.82	

3.3.5. Belief in God and Level of Religiosity

Two simple multiple-choice questions were included in the survey: "Do you believe in God" (1 = I never believed; 2 = I don't believe it, but I already believed; 3 = Now I believe but I didn't believe before; 4 = I always believed) and "Do you consider yourself a religious person?" (Likert scale, from 1 = not religious to 5 = very religious).

3.4. Procedures

The questionnaires were administered by the author and a team of students as part of a research work of the curricular unit of Research Methods of a faculty from the University of Coimbra. The authors of this study provided training in survey data collection and ethical standards. Each student was invited to collect responses from one recurring player of games of chance and gambling (eligibility criteria). Participants were contacted by these students in person, by e-mail, or by telephone, and a date was agreed for the delivery of the questionnaire. Responses were anonymous and delivered in sealed envelopes, delivered by the research team. Anonymity and confidentiality of all participants and their personal answers were ensured for ethical reasons and to avoid biases in their answers.

The questionnaire began with an explanation of the study, clear instructions and guarantee of anonymity and confidentiality of answers, the voluntary nature of participation, and informed consent. The inclusion criterion was to be a recurring player of games of chance and gambling.

4. Results

According to Table 5, the majority of players believe in God ($M = 3.58$) but do not consider themselves significantly religious ($M = 2.73$). They showed moderate scores in the *Religious Beliefs and Attitudes Scale* ($M = 3.26$) and are more optimistic ($M = 3.61$) than pessimistic ($M = 2.58$), $t(270) = 18.20$, $p < 0.001$. On average, players estimate chances of 66% of intrinsic desirable events (e.g., having harmony in the family, living happily, overcoming the biggest difficulty) and fewer probabilities of occurring extrinsic desirable events ($M = 36\%$; e.g., become a millionaire, win the lottery, be famous), namely highly unlikely desirable events, $t(270) = 24.08$, $p < 0.001$. Inversely, the average estimation of extrinsic undesirable events (e.g., dying soon, losing love, having a serious accident, going through difficult times) is higher than the estimation of intrinsic undesirable events (e.g., not achieving idealization, not being able to fulfill duties, losing hope, etc.), $t(270) = 15.98$, $p < 0.001$.

The overall influence of religious beliefs and attitudes on optimism was positive although weak ($r = 0.14$, shared variance of $R^2 = 1.96\%$), as well as with pessimism ($r = 0.20$, $R^2 = 4.0\%$). The relationship between religious beliefs and attitudes was higher with the probability of extrinsic desirable events ($r = 0.27$), indicating that the higher the level of religious beliefs, the more the person believes in the probability of occurrence of extrinsic desirable events (namely, become a millionaire, win the lottery, be famous, a miracle happens in life, and be admired by other people) with a proportion of shared variance of 7.29%. The association of this dimension of optimism it was also positive with the belief in God ($r = 0.17$), and the level of religiosity ($r = 0.19\%$), although with lower magnitude (shared variances of 2.89% and 3.61%, respectively).

The probability of extrinsic desirable events showed positive correlations with the probability of both extrinsic and intrinsic undesirable events ($r = 0.32$ and 0.23, $R^2 = 10.24\%$ and 5.29% of shared variance). Extrinsic optimism was more correlated with religious beliefs and attitudes in comparison with intrinsic optimism ($r = 0.27$ vs. $r = 0.20$, $R^2 = 7.29\%$ vs. $R^2 = 4.0\%$). Religious beliefs and attitudes seems to be similarly correlated with extrinsic and intrinsic pessimism events ($r = 0.20$ and 0.18, $R^2 = 4.0\%$ and 3.24% of shared variance).

Table 5. Descriptive statistics (min, max, Mean, SD) and intercorrelation matrix.

	Min.	Max.	Mean	SD	1	2	3	4	5	6	7	8	9
1. Religious Beliefs and Attitudes Scale (1 to 5 points)	1.08	5.00	3.26	1.00	1	0.14 *	0.23 **	0.20 **	0.27 **	0.20 **	0.18 **	0.71 **	0.69 **
2. Optimism (1 to 5 points)	2.14	5.00	3.61	0.52		1	−0.15 *	0.27 **	0.27 **	0.00	−0.13 *	0.08	0.10
3. Pessimism (1 to 5 points)	1.00	4.40	2.58	0.71			1	−0.09	0.07	0.26 **	0.34 **	0.16 **	0.04
4. F2: Intrinsic desirable events (probability 0–100%)	0.50	100.00	65.98	19.28				1	0.52 **	0.25 **	0.11	0.14 *	0.16 **
5. F Extrinsic desirable events (probability 0–100%)	0.07	100.00	36.02	22.32					1	0.32 **	0.23 **	0.17 **	0.19 **
6. Extrinsic undesirable events (probability 0–100%)	0.00	100.00	42.87	21.69						1	0.66 **	0.07	0.00
7. Intrinsic undesirable events (probability 0–100%)	0.00	100.00	26.90	17.22							1	0.10	0.00
8. Do you believe in God (1 to 4 points)	1.00	4.00	3.58	0.88								1	0.58 **
9. Do you consider yourself a religious person? (1 to 5 points)	1.00	5.00	2.73	0.90									1

* $p < 0.05$; ** $p < 0.01$.

Considering the specificity of the association between the global score of the *Religious Beliefs and Attitudes Scale* and the probability of winning the lottery or becoming a millionaire, we found a significant positive score just for winning the lottery ($r = 0.15$, $p = 0.015$), although the effect size is low ($R^2 = 2.25\%$ of shared variance). Furthermore, the correlation between the global score of the *Religious Beliefs and Attitudes Scale* and the probability of becoming a millionaire is not significant ($r = 0.09$, $p = 0.016$).

The influence of Education level was tested, considering four levels: 1 = until 4 years of school; 2 = until 9 years of school; 3 = until 12 years of school; and 4 = more than 12 years of school. An ANOVA (general linear model) was performed, taking Education as Independent Variable and the Religious Beliefs and Attitudes as the first Dependent Variable. We found an effect size of Education of 9.4%, $F(3, 267) = 9.20$, $p < 0.001$, $\eta_p^2 = 0.094$, $(1-\beta) = 0.996$. The post hoc tests Tukey HSD identified higher religious beliefs and attitudes in participants with fewer years of school. The effect of Education concerning the dimension *Optimism* was non-significant, $F(3, 267) = 1.87$, $p = 0.136$, $\eta_p^2 = 0.021$, $(1-\beta) = 0.481$. Considering *Pessimism* dimension, a significant difference was found, with an effect size of 6% [$F(3, 267) = 5.69$, $p = 0.001$, $\eta_p^2 = 0.060$, $(1-\beta) = 0.946$], due to the higher levels of pessimism in players with fewer years of education in comparison with players with higher education (mean difference of 0.45 and of 0.39 with 4 and 9 years of education, respectively, $p < 0.01$). For the *Estimation of Future Desirable Events Scale*, the MANOVA performed did not show any significant effect size for Education, Wilks' lambda = 0.960, $F(6, 532) = 1.84$, $p = 0.087$, $\eta_p^2 = 0.021$, $(1-\beta) = 0.690$. At last, for the *Estimation of Undesirable Events Scale*, the MANOVA showed a slight effect size for Education (2.4%), Wilks' lambda = 0.953, $F(6, 532) = 1.84$, $p = 0.047$, $\eta_p^2 = 0.024$, although with low observed power, $(1-\beta) = 0.766$. Attending to these results, we did not consider education level as covariate in the model.

The structural model of the influence of religious beliefs and attitudes (*Religious Beliefs and Attitudes Scale*, *belief in God*, and *level of religiosity*) on individuals' optimism and pessimism is shown in Figure 1. For the *Optimism* construct, we considered the items of the Optimism scale, as well as the items evaluating the probability of intrinsic and extrinsic desirable events. For the *Pessimism* construct, we considered the items of the Pessimism scale and the items evaluating the probability of intrinsic and extrinsic undesirable events. The fit index CMIN/DF = 1.94 obtained indicated a good model fit. With respect to the RMSEA, we found the 0.059 value (90CI of 0.055 to 0.062), considered as an acceptable fit indicator, as well as the NFI = 0.71 and the CFI = 0.84 scores. This model indicates that the religious beliefs and attitudes had a higher influence on the players' optimism ($R^2 = 44\%$ of explained variance, $\beta = 0.66$, $p < 0.001$) in comparison with the players' pessimism ($R^2 = 5\%$, $\beta = 0.23$, $p = 0.034$). Briefly, religiosity (religious beliefs and attitudes in our model), showed an effect of 44% in the prediction of optimism and only an effect of 5% in the prediction of pessimism.

The differentiation between intrinsic and extrinsic optimism and pessimism allows us to go further in the influence of religious beliefs and attitudes. The *Optimism and Pessimism Scale* was considered a measure of intrinsic optimism (F1-Optimism) and intrinsic pessimism (F2-Pessimism). Two additional structural models were built, one for optimism and another for pessimism.

Considering the structural model for *Optimism* (see Figure 2), two dimensions were considered: *Intrinsic Optimism* (operationalized with a latent variable composed of the *Optimism* factor of the *Optimism and Pessimism Scale* and the dimension F1-Intrinsic desirable events of the *Estimation of Future Desirable Events Scale*) and *Extrinsic Optimism* (latent variable composed of the *dimension F2-Extrinsic desirable events* of the *Estimation of Future Desirable Events Scale*). *Religious beliefs and attitudes* explain 12% of Intrinsic *Optimism* (R^2 0.12; $\beta = 0.34$, $p = 0.056$), 5% of *Extrinsic undesirable events* ($R^2 = 0.05$, $\beta = 0.22$, $p = 0.008$), and 3.5% of *Intrinsic undesirable events* ($R^2 = 0.035$, $\beta = 0.065$ direct effect + $\beta = 0.177$ indirect effect). We obtained good fit indices for this model considering CMIN/DF=1.90, NFI = 0.831, and CFI = 0.912, and an acceptable fit attending to RMSEA = 0.058.

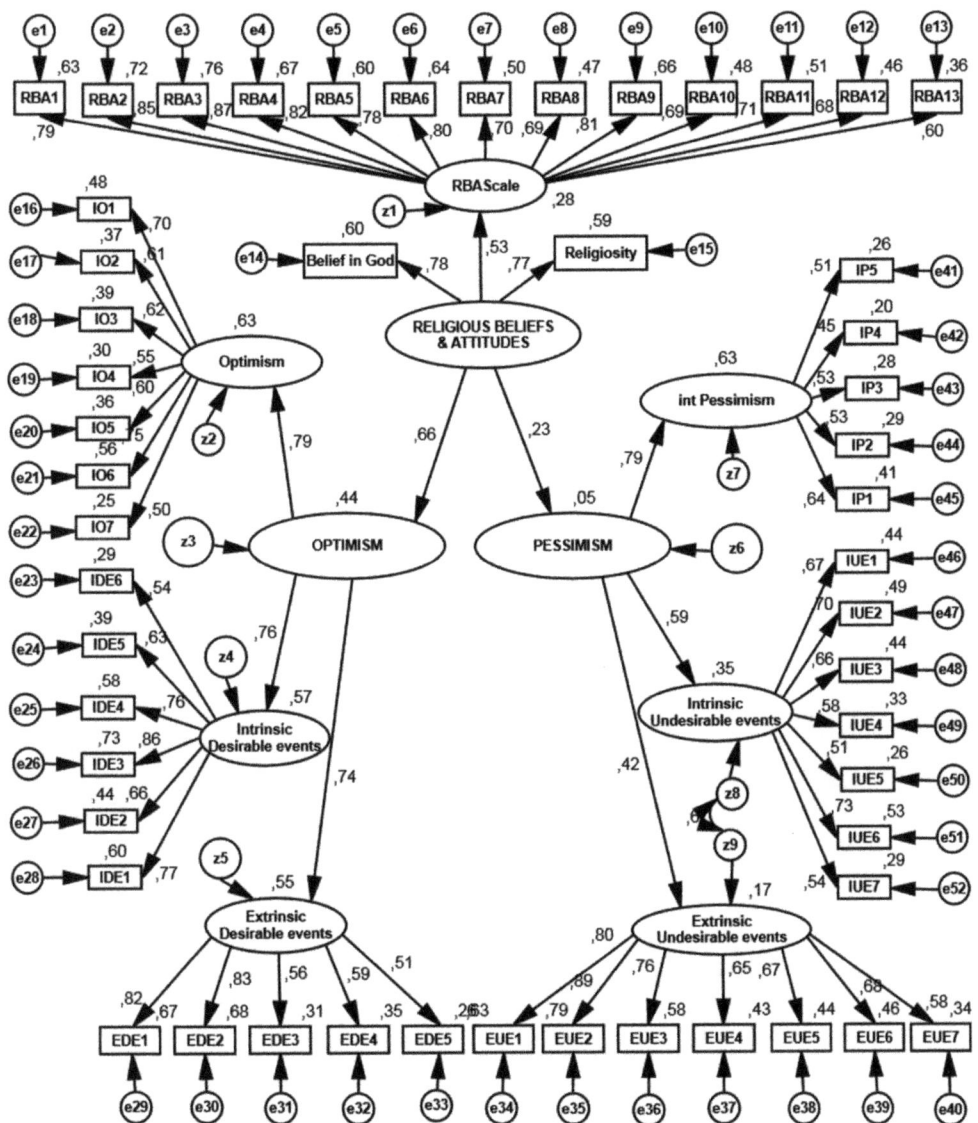

Figure 1. Influence of religious beliefs and attitudes on players' optimism and pessimism: Standardized regression coefficients and proportions of explained variance of the estimated structural model.

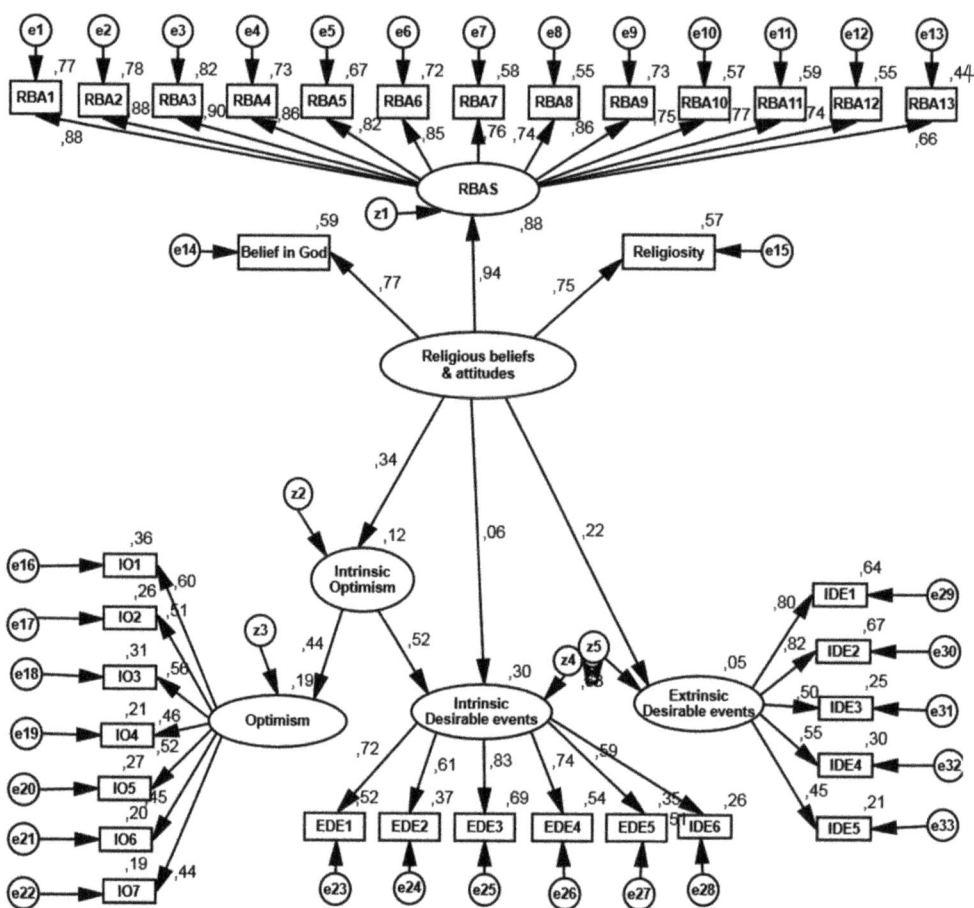

Figure 2. Influence of religious beliefs and attitudes on players' intrinsic and extrinsic optimism: Standardized regression coefficients and proportions of explained variance of the estimated structural model.

Attending to the structural model for *Pessimism* (see Figure 3), two dimensions were also considered: *Intrinsic Pessimism* (operationalized with a latent variable composed of the *Pessimism* factor of the *Optimism and Pessimism Scale* and the dimension F1-*Intrinsic undesirable events* of the *Estimation of Future Undesirable Events Scale*) and *Extrinsic Pessimism* (latent variable composed of the dimension F2-Extrinsic undesirable events of the *Estimation of Future Undesirable Events Scale*). *Religious beliefs and attitudes* explain 13% of *Intrinsic Pessimism* ($R^2 = 0.13$, $\beta = 0.37$, $p = 0.053$), 3.24% of *Extrinsic undesirable events* ($R^2 = 0.0324$, $\beta = 0.18$, $p = 0.008$), and 1.88% of Intrinsic undesirable events ($R^2 = 0.0188$, $\beta = 0.065$ direct effect + $\beta = 0.137$ indirect effect). We obtained good fit indices for this model considering CMIN/DF = 1.85, NFI = 0.840, and CFI = 0.919, and an acceptable fit attending to RMSEA = 0.056.

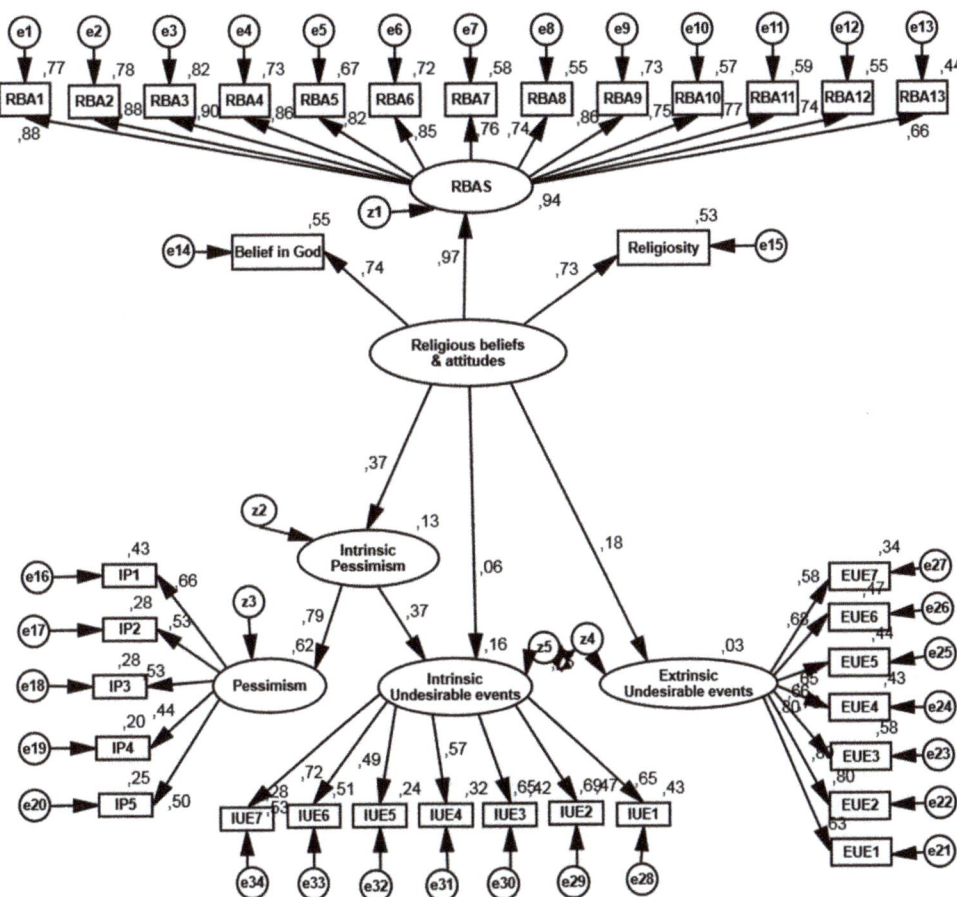

Figure 3. Influence of religious beliefs and attitudes on players' intrinsic and extrinsic pessimism: Standardized regression coefficients and proportions of explained variance of the estimated structural model.

5. Dicussion and Conclusions

Human beings are characterized by a permanent awareness that they are individualized beings, with their own existence distinct from others. Considering the circumstances of each situation, individuals tend to be more or less optimistic. Given the nature of optimism and the fact that it has always been considered a positive, strong, and general distortion in self-benefit (Armor and Taylor 1998; Carver and Scheier 2001; Domino and Conway 2001; Scheier and Carver 1985, 1992), with this research we aimed to understand the agentic features of this construct in the religiousness of game players of chance and gambling.

"Optimism is seen as a cognitive feature (a goal, an expectation, a belief or a causal attribution) about the desired and perceived as successful future" (Barros 2004, p. 101), entailing an involvement with the uncertainty factor. The data collected from the players of our sample enable us to ascertain to what extent dealing with risk is associated with optimism, as well as to what extent religiosity acts as a catalyst for this optimism in situations of games of chance and gambling.

Many studies have shown that, in general, people have expectations of positive results for their own lives. Widely known for optimism, this phenomenon was found in a variety of situations, in samples of all ages and different cultures, Western and non-Western. It is consistent over time and, despite some specificities, during the events.

In this research, the constructs of optimism and pessimism emerged as distinct, tending to be independent rather than inversely related. However, players were more optimistic than pessimistic and more likely to estimate intrinsically desirable events (e.g., living happily, overcoming the biggest difficulty) in comparison with extrinsically desirable events (e.g., becoming a millionaire, being famous).

Considering the nature of optimism and the fact that it has always been characterized as a generalized and robust phenomenon (Domino and Conway 2001), in general terms, we can say that, in addition to people perceiving their future as being more positive than the from others (believing that they are more likely to experience desirable situations and less likely to experience undesirable events) in a variety of circumstances, and compared to those others, they believe they are superior. Given the very low probabilities of winning the lottery or other games of chance, this self-serving bias may explain the high probabilities that players of our sample indicated of winning the lottery (45% in our sample). In circumstances where any kind of evidence—objective in nature or via social comparison—indicates poor probabilities of personal success, such as winning the lottery, individual beliefs play a key role in maintaining the levels of idiosyncratic optimism (Mónico 2011, 2021; Perloff and Fetzer 1986). Among these beliefs, this research was dedicated to those of a religious nature, due to the lack of studies on the religiosity–optimism interconnection, especially in players of games of chance and gambling. Our results show a positive influence of religiosity on optimism.

Given the unpredictability of the situations, individuals are led to develop adaptive strategies in order to maintain or recover the perception of control, including the creation of illusory beliefs of control (Taylor and Brown 1999). Such beliefs are positively associated with subjective well-being and the ability to adjust to threatening and unpredictable situations (for instance, Diez-Esteban et al. 2019, found an influence of the religious backgrounds on corporate risk-taking); these situations are controlled by cognitive strategies, characterized by patterns of religious, political, and/or technological control beliefs. In fact, several studies with people living in an uncontrollable threat situation show that those who show signs of greater psychological well-being and better adjustment to the threat situation are the ones who have developed illusions of control over this threat. Those who have these secondary control schemes automatically activate them in threatening situations, reducing the insecurity and anxiety of the situation and, in this way, restoring the feeling of well-being.

A considerable part of individuals' religiosity satisfies control needs and, in the specific case of the games of chance and gambling, can act as an illusion of control. McCullough and Willoughby (2009) present six key propositions that interrelate religion, self-regulation, and self-control: "(a) that religion can promote self-control; (b) that religion influences how goals are selected, pursued, and organized; (c) that religion facilitates self-monitoring; (d) that religion fosters the development of self-regulatory strength; (e) that religion prescribes and fosters proficiency in a suite of self-regulatory behaviors; and (f) that some of religion's influences on health, well-being, and social behavior may result from religion's influences on self-control and self-regulation" (p. 69).

Divided into the ideological, intellectual, consequential, and ritualistic dimensions (Glock and Stark 1965), religiousness as a propeller of the optimism in players has become the outline of this research. In general, we can conclude that religious beliefs and attitudes are positively associated with optimism in these kinds of players. However, and surprisingly, results show as well a positive association with pessimism, although with a lower effect size. It seems that both optimism and pessimism are evident in these types of players and that they estimate an increased probability of occurrence of positive events but also of negative events. In fact, despite the optimism levels in players of games of chance of our sample, they also presented higher probabilities for undesirable events, especially for extrinsic undesirable events (approx. 43% in our sample), like having a serious chronic or malignant disease or having a serious accident. These results seem to indicate that players of games of chance estimate increased probabilities of both positive and negative events occurring in their lives, supporting the idea that optimism and pessimism are independent constructs. Indeed, research concerning pessimism and, in particular, comparative pessimism (Kruger and Burrus 2004; Taylor and Shepperd 1998) refute the omnipresence of the optimistic trait. Desirable unusual and common undesirable occurrences encourage pessimism, which leads us to deduce that optimism is not a phenomenon as robust and widespread as the literature seems to show (Mónico 2011, 2021). Our results are in line with this finding, or rather, that individuals who are very optimistic towards some situations can also be very pessimistic concerning other situations.

Searching for an interpretation for these results, in recent decades researchers in positive psychology have come to recognize self-regulation as an important aspect of the self, such as resilience, adaptation to adversities (Barros 2004; Brown 1987; Higgins et al. 1999), or even spiritual and religious development (McCullough and Boker 2007; Pargament and Mahoney 2021). We consider that individuals can use beliefs and religious behaviors as a self-regulatory mechanism, which confers them some stability and promotes optimism. As McCullough and Boker (2007) state, "To some extent, spiritual and religious changes may also be caused by self-regulation processes that are intrinsic to individual functioning" (p. 385). The importance that each one gives religion is, in some way, regulated by the functioning of an internal orientation system that seeks to achieve internal balance.

Additionally, the distinction between intrinsic and extrinsic optimism in our sample has shown that the players anchor their optimism in different dimensions of beliefs. The belief that faith or a given way of connecting to the sacred or the divinity(s)—in short, spirituality (Barros 2000; Mónico 2021)—helps the individual to achieve the desired optimism, believing that they can win. The belief in the spiritual, integrated into the intrinsic dimension of the Allportian sense of religious experience (Allport 1966) depends, however, on an external factor: the action of the divine in the subject. In our research, we complement with the attribute of extrinsic the optimism that is based on factors external to oneself (i.e., the belief that the desired results are dependent on a supernatural will or intervention); on the other hand, we base intrinsic optimism when it refers to the positive disposition or attitude that the good results are directly dependent on the individual's aptitudes (Carver and Scheier 2014).

People tend to perceive the world as controllable, revealing the perception of control over the surrounding environment as a need for each individual (Wegener and Bargh 1998). If it is a truism to mention that human beings are faced daily with the unexpected in their environment, perhaps it is not to say that control beliefs, among which we highlight those of a religious scope, are inscribed in the skills developed by each individual with a view to adaptation to the environment (Taylor and Brown 1999). According to McCullough and Willoughby (2009), religiosity constitutes a means of activating self-control and, as evidenced by Buchanan and Seligman (1995), each person may be situated on a continuum that distances from extreme internality to externalities. By integrating this dichotomization in the individual cognitive style regarding the modes of information processing in relation to positive future expectations, we can elaborate for optimism a line of reasoning analogous to the one established for the locus of control (Rotter 1990)—internal vs. external. We consider that an individual whose optimism (or pessimism) is based on beliefs of internality expects the good (or bad) future experiences to depend on his or her own personal aptitudes (or lack of them); the positive (or negative) expectations they maintain are formulated based on the expected results of personal actions. On the other hand, those whose optimism (or pessimism) is based on external factors tends to maintain the conviction that good (or bad) results will prevail due to situational factors, not exercising control over these factors; in this situations, individual optimism or pessimism is not centered on personal factors but, on the contrary, on factors outside the self such as luck, chance or even the help of some (super)natural entity.

Our results evidence that extrinsic desirable events, like winning the lottery, were more predicted by religious beliefs and attitudes in comparison with intrinsic desirable events. In reverse, religious beliefs and attitudes tend to slightly predict more intrinsic pessimism in comparison with intrinsic optimism. Concluding, our results demonstrate the importance of distinguishing internal causes from external causes in the kind of beliefs underlying optimism and pessimism. We believe that we can find a continuous distribution of optimists and pessimists between the two extremes, that is, between those who base their optimism (or their pessimism) solely on factors of an internal nature and those that cement it entirely on externality.

At last, the present research has some limitations that should be addressed. The variables used in this study allowed us to analyze the effect of religious beliefs and attitudes in optimism and pessimism dimensions in players of games of chance and gambling. Although these outputs relating to religiosity, optimism, and pessimism are positive and promising, it is important to replicate this research by introducing new measures, especially focused on intrinsic and extrinsic optimism and pessimism. In relation to the sample, additional studies should be considered, comparing gamblers with no gamblers. The research can also be extended to other players, differentiating results according to the frequency of playing and introducing control variables like the addition games.

Author Contributions: Conceptualization, L.S.M. and V.R.A.; methodology, L.S.M.; software, V.R.A. and L.S.M.; validation, L.S.M.; formal analysis, L.S.M.; investigation, L.S.M.; resources, L.S.M. and V.R.A.; data curation, L.S.M. and V.R.A.; writing—original draft preparation, L.S.M.; writing—review and editing, L.S.M. and V.R.A. All authors have read and agreed to the published version of the manuscript.

Funding: This research received no external funding.

Informed Consent Statement: Informed consent was obtained from all subjects involved in the study.

Data Availability Statement: The data presented in this study are available on request from the first author, e-mail: lisete.monico@fpce.uc.pt.

Acknowledgments: We acknowledge all the participants in this study, and also the person involved in data collection.

Conflicts of Interest: The authors declare no conflict of interest.

References

Allport, Gordon W. 1966. The religious context of prejudice. *Journal for the Scientific Study of Religion* 5: 457–77. [CrossRef]
Argyle, Michael. 2000. *Psychology and Religion: An Introduction*. London: Routledge.
Armor, David A., and Shelley E. Taylor. 1998. Situated optimism: Specific outcome expectancies and self-regulation. *Advances in Experimental Social Psychology* 30: 309–79.
Ávila, Antonio. 2003. *Para conecer la psicologia de la religion*. Navarra: EVD.
Barker, Eileen, and Margit Warburg. 1998. *New Religions and New Religiosity*. Springfield: Aarhus University Press.
Barros, José H. 1998. Optimismo: Teoria e avaliação. *Psicologia, Educação, Cultura* 22: 295–308.
Barros, José H. 2000. *Psicologia da religião*. Coimbra: Livraria Almedina.
Barros, José H. 2004. *Psicologia Positiva*. Porto: ASA.
Brown, Ann. 1987. Metacognition, executive control, self-regulation, and other more mysterious mechanisms. In *Metacognition, Motivation, and Understanding*. Edited by Franz E. Weinert and Rainer H. Klume. Hillsdale: Lawrence Erlbaum Associates, Publishers, pp. 153–71.
Brown, Laurence B. 1988. *The Psychology of Religion: An Introduction*. London: Hollen Street Press.
Buchanan, Gregory McClell, and Martin E. P. Seligman. 1995. *Explanatory Style*. Hillsdale: Erlbaum.
Buunk, Bram P. 2001. Perceived superiority of one's own relationship and perceived prevalence of happy and unhappy relationships. *British Journal of Social Psychology* 40: 565–74. [CrossRef] [PubMed]
Carver, Charles S., and Michael F. Scheier. 1982. Control theory: A useful conceptual framework for personality-social, clinical and health psychology. *Psychological Bulletin* 92: 111–35. [CrossRef] [PubMed]
Carver, Charles S., and Michael F. Scheier. 2001. Optimism, pessimism, and self-regulation. In *Optimism and Pessimism: Implications for Theory, Research, and Practice*, 1st ed. Edited by Edwards C. Chang. Washington: American Psychological Association.

Carver, Charles S., and Michael F. Scheier. 2012. *Attention and Self-Regulation: A Control Theory Approach to Human Behaviour*. New York: Springer.
Carver, Charles S., and Michael F. Scheier. 2014. Dispositional optimism. *Trends in Cognitive Science* 186: 293–99. [CrossRef] [PubMed]
Chambers, John R., Paul D. Windschitl, and Jerry Suls. 2003. Egocentrism, event frequency and comparative optimism: When what happens frequently is "more likely to happen to me". *Personality and Social Psychology Bulletin* 29: 1343–56. [CrossRef] [PubMed]
DeVellis, Robert. 2012. *Scale Development: Theory and Applications*, 3rd ed. Thousand Oaks: Sage.
Diez-Esteban, José María, Jorge Bento Farinha, and Conrado Diego García-Gómez. 2019. Are religion and culture relevant for corporate risk-taking? International evidence. *Business Research Quality* 22: 36–55. [CrossRef]
Dittes, James E. 1969. The psychology of religion. In *Handbook of Social Psychology*, 2nd ed. Edited by Gardner Lindzey and Elliot Aronson. Reading: Addison-Wesley, vol. 5, pp. 602–59.
Domino, Brian, and Daniel W. Conway. 2001. Optimism and pessimism from a historical perspective. In *Optimism and Pessimism: Implications for Theory, Research, and Practice*, 1st ed. Edited by Edward C. Chang. Washington: American Psychological Association.
Eagly, Alice H., and Shelly Chaiken. 1998. Attitude structure and function. In *Handbook of Social Psychology*, 4th ed. Edited by Daniel T. Gilbert, Susan T. Fiske and Gardner Lindzey. New York: McGraw-Hill, vol. 1, pp. 269–322.
Erthal, Fatima, Aline Bastos, Liliane Vilete, Leticia Oliveira, Mirtes Pereira, Mauro Mendlowicz, Eliane Volchan, and Ivan Figueira. 2021. Unveiling the neural underpinnings of optimism: A systematic review. *Cognitive, Affective, and Behavioral Neuroscience* 21: 895–916. [CrossRef] [PubMed]
Festinger, Leon. 1954. A theory of social comparison processes. *Human Relations* 7: 117–40. [CrossRef]
Fowler, James W. 1995. *Stages of Faith: The Psychology of Human Development and the Quest for Meaning*. San Francisco: Harper and Row.
Geerts, Henri. 1990. An inquiry into the meaning of ritual symbolism: Turner and Peirce. In *Current Studies on Rituals: Perspectives for the Psychology of Religion*. Edited by Hans-Gunter Heimbrock and H. Barbara Boudewijnse. Atlanta: Amsterdam, pp. 19–32.
Gellner, Ernest. 1992. *Postmodernism, Reason, and Religion*. London: Routledge.
Gibson, Bryan, and David M. Sanbonmatsu. 2004. Optimism, pessimism, and gambling: The downside of optimism. *Personality and Social Psychological Bulletin* 302: 149–60. [CrossRef]
Gillham, Jane E., Andrew J. Shatté, Karen J. Reivich, and Martin E. P. Seligman. 2001. Optimism, pessimism, and explanatory style. In *Optimism and Pessimism: Implications for Theory, Research, and Practice*, 1st ed. Edited by Edwards C. Chang. Washington: American Psychological Association.
Glock, Charles Y., and Rodney Stark. 1965. *Religion and Society in Tension*. Chicago: Rand McNally and Co.
Gorsuch, Richard. 2015. *Factor Analysis: Classic Second Edition*. New York: Routledge.
Grom, Bernard. 1994. *Psicología de la religión*. Barcelona: Editorial Herder.
Haught, John F. 1995. *Science and Religion: From Conflict to Conversation*. Mahwah: Paulist Press.
Higgins, E. Tory, Heidi Grant, and James Shah. 1999. Self-regulation and quality of life: Emotional and non-emotional life experiences. In *Well-Being: The Foundations of Hedonic Psychology*. Edited by Daniel Kahneman, Ed Diener and Norbert Schwartz. New York: Russell Sage.
Hinde, Robert A. 2010. *Why God Persist: A Scientific Approach to Religion*. London and New York: Routledge.
Hood, Ralph W. 1995. *Handbook of Religious Experience*. Birmingham: Religious Education Press.
IBM Corp. 2020. *IBM SPSS Statistics for Windows (Version 27.0)*. Windows. Armonk: IBM Corp.
James, William. 1985. *The varieties of Religious Experience: A Study in Human Nature*. Cambridge: Harvard University Press. First published 1902.
Kline, Rex. 2016. *Principles and Practice of Structural Equation Modeling*, 4th ed. New York: The Guilford Press.
Kruger, Justin, and Jeremy Burrus. 2004. Egocentrism and focalism in unrealistic optimism and pessimism. *Journal of Experimental Social Psychology* 40: 332–40. [CrossRef]
Lawson, E. Thomas, and Robert N. McCauley. 1990. *Rethinking Religion: Connecting Cognition and Culture*. Cambridge: Cambridge University Press.
Mattis, Jacqueline S., Dwight L. Fontenot, Carrie A. Hatcher-Kay, Nyasha A. Grayman, and Ruby L. Beale. 2004. Religiosity, optimism and pessimism among African Americans. *Personality and Individual Differences* 34: 1025–38. [CrossRef]
McCullough, Michael E., and Steven M. Boker. 2007. Dynamical modeling for studying self-regulatory processes: An example from the study of religious development over the life span. In *Handbook of Methods in Positive Psychology*. Edited by Anthony D. Ong and Manfred van Dulmen. New York: Oxford University Press.
McCullough, Michael E., and Brian L. Willoughby. 2009. Religion, self-regulation, and self-control: Associations, explanations, and implications. *Psychological Bulletin* 135: 1–25. [CrossRef]
McGuire, Meredith B. 2002. *Religion: The Social Context*, 5th ed. Long Grove: Waveland Press.
McKenna, Frank P. 1993. It won't happen to me: Unrealistic optimism or illusion of control? *British Journal of Psychology* 84: 39–50. [CrossRef]
Mens, Maria G., Michael F. Scheier, and Charles S. Carver. 2021. Optimism. In *The Oxford Handbook of Positive Psychology*, 3rd ed. Edited by Charles R. Snyder, Shane J. Lopez, Lisa Edwards and Susana Marques. Oxford: Oxford University Press.
Mónico, Lisete S. 2011. *Individualização religiosa e otimismo*. Edições Vercial.

Mónico, Lisete S. 2012a. Religiosity and optimism in ill and healthy elderly. *International Journal of Developmental and Educational Psychology* 12: 59–70.
Mónico, Lisete. S. 2012b. Vulnerabilidade, velhice e doença: O efeito da religiosidade no optimismo de internalidade e de externalidade. In *Transição para a reforma/aposentação: Contributos para a adaptação*. Edited by Eduardo Santos, Joaquim A. Ferreira, Ricardo Pocinho, João P. Gaspar and Anabela Ramalho. Viseu: Psicosoma, pp. 55–70.
Mónico, Lisete S. 2013a. Aging, health and disease: The effect of religiosity on the optimism of elderly people. In *Promoting Conscious and Active Learning and Aging: How to Face Current and Future Challenges?* Edited by Albertina L. Oliveira. Coimbra: Imprensa da Universidade de Coimbra, pp. 371–82.
Mónico, Lisete S. 2013b. Religiosity and optimism among Portuguese citizens: The effect of religious identity and the mediation by life satisfaction. *Journal of Psychology and Social Behavior Research* 14: 105–15. [CrossRef]
Mónico, Lisete S. 2013c. Religiosidade e otimismo alicerçado em fatores intrínsecos vs. extrínsecos: Estudo comparativo em idosos doentes e saudáveis. In *Cuidadores de pessoas idosas: Caminhos de mudança*. Edited by Dayse Neri de Souza, Marilia Santos Rua and Helena Jorge Cardoso Teixeira. Aveiro: CIDTFF, pp. 253–60.
Mónico, Lisete S. 2021. *Religiosidade e otimismo: Estudo psicossociológico dos peregrinos ao santuário de Fátima*. Fátima: Edições do Santuário de Fátima, in press.
Mónico, Lisete, Valentim R. Alferes, Maria S. Brêda, Carla Carvalho, and Pedro M. Parreira. 2016. Can religiosity improve optimism in participants in states of illness, when controlling for life satisfaction? *BMC Health Services Research* 163: 123.
Mónico, Lisete, and Valentim R. Alferes. 2019. The Effect of Religious Identity on Optimism across the lifespan. In *Communications in Computer and Information Science*. Edited by José García-Alonso and César Fonseca. Cham: Springer, pp. 359–77.
Mónico, Lisete S., and Clara Margaça. 2021. The Workaholism Phenomenon in Portugal: Dimensions and Relations with Workplace Spirituality. *Religions* 12: 852. [CrossRef]
Mookherjee, Harsha N. 1994. Effects of religiosity and selected variables on the perception of well-being. *The Journal of Social Psychology* 134: 403–5. [CrossRef]
Norem, Julie K., and Nancy Cantor. 1986. Defensive pessimism: "Harnessing" anxiety as motivation. *Journal of Personality and Social Psychology* 51: 1208–17. [CrossRef]
Nunnally, Jum C., and Ira H. Bernstein. 2010. *Psychometric Theory*, 3rd ed. New Delhi: McGraw Hill.
Pargament, Kenneth I. 1997. *The Psychology of Religion and Coping: Theory, Research and Practice*. New York: Guilford Press.
Pargament, Kenneth I., and Annette Mahoney. 2021. Spirituality: The Search for the Sacred. In *The Oxford Handbook of Positive Psychology*, 3rd ed. Edited by Charles R. Snyder, Shane J. Lopez, Lisa Edwards and Susana Marques. New York: Oxford University Press.
Perloff, Linda S., and Barbara K. Fetzer. 1986. Self-other judgments and perceived vulnerability to victimization. *Journal of Personality and Social Psychology* 50: 502–10. [CrossRef]
Rotter, Julian B. 1990. Internal versus external control of reinforcement: A case history of a variable. *American Psychologist* 45: 489–93. [CrossRef]
Scheier, Michael F., and Charles S. Carver. 1985. Optimism, coping, and health: Assessment and implications of generalized outcome expectancies. *Health Psychology* 4: 219–47. [CrossRef]
Scheier, Michael F., and Charles S. Carver. 1992. Effects of optimism on psychological and physical well-being: Theoretical overview and empirical update. *Cognitive Therapy and Research* 16: 201–28. [CrossRef]
Scheier, Michael F., Charles S. Carver, and Michael W. Bridges. 1994. Distinguishing optimism from neuroticism and trait anxiety, self-mastery, and self-esteem: A reevaluation of the Life Orientation Test. *Journal of Personality and Social Psychology* 67: 1063–78. [CrossRef]
Schumacker, Randall E., and Richard G. Lomax. 2016. *A Beginner's Guide to Structural Equation Modeling*, 4th ed. New York: Routledge.
Schweizer, Karl, and Wolfgang Koch. 2001. The assessment of components of optimism by POSO-E. *Personality and Individual Differences* 31: 563–74. [CrossRef]
Seligman, Martin E. 2006. *Learned Optimism: How to Change Your Mind and Your Life*. New York: Vintage.
Sitzmann, Traci, and Elizabeth M. Campbell. 2021. The hidden cost of prayer: Religiosity and the gender wage GAP. *Academy of Management Journal* 64: 1016–48. [CrossRef]
Snyder, Charles R., Cheri Harris, John R. Anderson, Sharon A. Holleran, Lori M. Irving, Sandra T. Sigmon, Lauren Yoshinobu, June Gibb, Charyle Langelle, and Pat Harney. 1991. The will and the ways: Development and validation of an individual-differences measure of hope. *Journal of Personality and Social Psychology* 604: 570–85. [CrossRef]
Swann, William B., John J. Griffin, Steven C. Predmore, and Bebe Gaines. 1987. The cognitive-affective crossfire: When self-consistency confronts self-enhancement. *Journal of Personality and Social Psychology* 52: 881–89. [CrossRef]
Tabachnick, Barbara G., and Linda S. Fidell. 2019. *Using Multivariate Statistics*, 7th ed. Boston: Pearson.
Taylor, Shelley E., and Jonathon D. Brown. 1999. Illusion and well-being: A social psychological perspective o mental health. In *The Self in Social Psychology*. Edited by Roy F. Baumeister. Cleveland: Psychology Press, pp. 43–66.
Taylor, Kevin M., and James A. Shepperd. 1998. Bracing for the worst: Severity, testing, and feedback timing as moderators of the optimistic bias. *Personality and Social Psychology Bulletin* 24: 915–26. [CrossRef]
Urbina, Susana. 2014. *Essentials of Psychological Testing*. Hoboken: Wiley.

Wegener, Daniel M., and John A. Bargh. 1998. Control and automaticity in social life. In *Handbook of Social Psychology*, 4th ed. Edited by Daniel T. Gilbert, Susan T. Fiske and Gardner Lindzey. New York: McGraw-Hill, vol. 1, pp. 446–96.
Weinstein, Neil D. 1980. Unrealistic optimism about future life events. *Journal of Personality and Social Psychology* 39: 806–20. [CrossRef]
Weinstein, Neil D. 1987. Unrealistic optimism about susceptibility to health problems: Conclusions from a community wide sample. *Journal of Behavioural Medicine* 10: 481–500. [CrossRef] [PubMed]
Wiseman, Richard. 2006. *O factor Sorte*. Lisboa: Publicações Dom Quixote.
Wulff, David M. 1997. *Psychology of Religion: Classic and Contemporary*, 2nd ed. New York: John Willey and Sons.

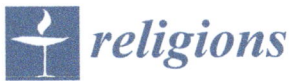

Article

Ontological Addiction Theory and Mindfulness-Based Approaches in the Context of Addiction Theory and Treatment

Paul Barrows * and William Van Gordon

Human Sciences Research Centre, University of Derby, Derby DE22 1GB, UK; w.vangordon@derby.ac.uk
* Correspondence: p.barrows@derby.ac.uk

Abstract: Buddhist-derived interventions have increasingly been employed in the treatment of a range of physical and psychological disorders, and in recent years, there has been significant growth in the use of mindfulness-based interventions (MBIs) for this purpose. Ontological Addiction Theory (OAT) is a novel metaphysical approach to understanding psychopathology within the framework of Buddhist teachings and asserts that many mental illnesses have their root in the widespread mistaken belief in an inherently existent self that operates independently of external phenomena. OAT describes how different types of MBI can help undermine these beliefs and allow a person to reconstruct their view of self and reality to address the root causes of suffering. As well as proving effective in treating many other psychological disorders, MBIs based on OAT have demonstrated efficacy in treating conventional behavioural addictions, such as problem gambling, workaholism, and sex addiction. The goal of this paper is to (i) discuss and appraise the evidence base underlying the use of MBIs for treating addiction; (ii) explicate how OAT advances understanding of the mechanisms of addiction; (iii) delineate how different types of MBI can be employed to address addictive behaviours; and (iv) propose future research avenues for assessing and comparing MBIs in the treatment of addiction.

Keywords: addiction; addiction treatment; Buddhism; mindfulness; ontological addiction

Citation: Barrows, Paul, and William Van Gordon. 2021. Ontological Addiction Theory and Mindfulness-Based Approaches in the Context of Addiction Theory and Treatment. *Religions* 12: 586. https://doi.org/10.3390/rel12080586

Academic Editors:
Bernadette Flanagan and
Noelia Molina

Received: 9 June 2021
Accepted: 27 July 2021
Published: 30 July 2021

Publisher's Note: MDPI stays neutral with regard to jurisdictional claims in published maps and institutional affiliations.

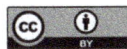

Copyright: © 2021 by the authors. Licensee MDPI, Basel, Switzerland. This article is an open access article distributed under the terms and conditions of the Creative Commons Attribution (CC BY) license (https://creativecommons.org/licenses/by/4.0/).

1. Introduction

Mindfulness is a Buddhist practice that has existed for around 2500 years. Interest in mindfulness has significantly increased over the course of the last four decades; however, given the broad origins of mindfulness within Buddhism and the way it is embedded within concepts that are generally unfamiliar within Western society, definitions and applications encompass a range of meanings (Van Gordon et al. 2015b). Much of the incongruence can be attributed to the way that, in Western society, mindfulness has been secularised and distanced from its Buddhist roots in order to better align with Western values. Thus, while many scholars have adopted a somewhat secular and denatured conceptualisation of mindfulness, others view mindfulness as inseparable from its spiritual roots within Buddhist teachings.

One widely used definition of this former, secularised form of mindfulness has been proposed by Kabat-Zinn, who described mindfulness as "paying attention in a particular way: on purpose, in the present moment, and non-judgementally" (Kabat-Zinn 1994, p. 4). On the other hand, formulations that explicitly embody the spiritual dimension of mindfulness, such as a definition proposed by Shonin and Van Gordon (2016), contextualise mindfulness as "the process of engaging a full, direct, and active awareness of experienced phenomena that is (i) spiritual in aspect and (ii) maintained from one moment to the next" (p. 845). This latter conceptualisation arguably represents a more authentic view of the practise, which highlights important distinctions in the form and function of different types of meditation and ones that are of particular relevance to processes in addiction.

Central to Buddhist teachings are the four noble truths (Chah 2011). The first noble truth is the truth of suffering (Pāli: *dukkha*) or dissatisfaction; the second noble truth is the origin of suffering, which is craving; the third noble truth is the possibility of the cessation of suffering via attaining enlightenment or *nirvana*; the fourth noble truth is that there is a path to *nirvana* via extinguishing craving. In Buddhism, suffering is one of the three marks of existence, or fundamental and inescapable basic truths about the nature of the reality. The other two marks of existence are the truth of the impermanence of all things (Pāli: *anicca*) and the truth that everything, including human beings, are devoid of an inherently existing self (Pāli: *anattā*). Ignorance of these truths (Pāli: *avijjā*) is viewed as the principal mechanism through which the cycle of suffering or dissatisfaction (Pāli: *saṃsāra*) perpetuates. By failing to recognise these truths and allowing our happiness to be contingent on impermanent states and things, we bring about and maintain a cycle of craving, disillusionment, and pain (Chah 2011).

Buddhist practises are therefore concerned primarily with the application of spiritual and meditative principles to understanding and transforming suffering, and key to this is cultivating nonattachment. Cultivating nonattachment in the context of Buddhist practise involves a deeper meditative enquiry into the nature of all phenomena as they arise and pass within the mind. This enquiry is intended to bring about a realisation of the lack of inherent existence not only of the self but of all manifest forms and the interdependence and interconnectedness of all phenomena. These practises are undertaken within the framework of the Noble Eightfold Path in which they are expressed as right view, right resolve, right speech, right conduct, right livelihood, right effort, right mindfulness, and right concentration. These are further organised within a tripartite, "three trainings" (Pāli: *tisikkhā*) principle under which they are classified into those concerned with (i) meditation (right effort, right mindfulness, right meditation); (ii) ethics (right speech, right action, and right livelihood); and (iii) wisdom (right view, right intention) (Van Gordon et al. 2019).

This tripartite division is reflected in the chronological order in which research and subsequent implementation of mindfulness-based interventions (MBIs) have unfolded (Van Gordon et al. 2019, 2020). In the 1980s, there was an examination of mindfulness as a construct and its applications as well as the meditative attentional processes involved (Shonin et al. 2015). This was followed at the turn of the 21st century with a phase in which empathic and ethical awareness predominated in compassion-based and loving-kindness research and practises. In the last few years, however, a third phase has evolved in which wisdom-based practises and their applications have been empirically investigated (Van Gordon et al. 2019). The first of these phases dealt with what have become known as first-generation MBIs (FG-MBIs), while the latter two phases, which more closely embody the practise of mindfulness within a traditional Buddhist framework, are now generally referred to as second-generation MBIs (SG-MBIs) (Van Gordon et al. 2015a).

The use of MBIs has undergone a significant proliferation in evidence-based treatments spanning a wide range of psychological disorders, including mood disorders, anxiety disorders, schizophrenia-spectrum disorders, personality disorders, and substance use disorders (Shonin et al. 2014). Furthermore, in recent years, a novel metaphysical model of psychopathology, Ontological Addiction Theory (OAT), has gained traction that has sought to express and elucidate mental illness within the framework of these Buddhist teachings (Shonin et al. 2016; Van Gordon et al. 2018). The goal of this paper is to (i) discuss and appraise the evidence base underlying the use of MBIs for treating addiction; (ii) explicate how OAT advances understanding of the mechanisms of addiction; (iii) delineate how different forms of MBI can be employed to address addictive behaviours; and (iv) propose future research avenues for assessing and comparing MBIs in the treatment of addiction.

2. First-Generation Mindfulness-Based Interventions in the Treatment of Addiction

Perhaps the most well-known early mindfulness intervention program is the eight-week Mindfulness-Based Stress Reduction (MBSR) developed at the University of Massachusetts Medical School (Kabat-Zinn 1982). This program consists of weekly, group-based classes with a trained teacher lasting around two to two-and-a-half hours supplemented by daily, audio-guided home practise lasting around 45 minutes per day and a day-long mindfulness retreat (Kabat-Zinn 1990). These interventions typically focus on cultivating and maintaining present-moment awareness; this can include breath awareness or awareness of bodily sensations or other perceptual experiences (such as sights and sounds), thoughts, and emotional reactions.

This mindfulness practise has been proposed to involve two main aspects: focused attention and open monitoring (Garland and Howard 2018). The first of these aspects has been termed "bare" attention or "lucid" awareness: a raw, immediate awareness of perceptions, thoughts, and feelings as they impinge upon the mind but unbiased by conceptual thought or judgement (Brown et al. 2007). The second aspect concerns the fact that this watchfulness or lucid awareness must also include an attitude of acceptance and openness even to experiences that may be distressing or difficult. MBSR was initially focused on the treatment of chronic pain and has proven to have positive effects on pain, anxiety, and stress in individuals with chronic disorders (Grossman et al. 2004). However, it has since also been applied to many other clinical and non-clinical populations (Creswell 2017; Ludwig and Kabat-Zinn 2008).

In 2002, a new intervention, Mindfulness-Based Cognitive Therapy (MBCT), was formulated to target depression and relapse in chronic conditions. It combined MBSR with Cognitive Behavioural Therapy (CBT), and findings demonstrate that it has a positive effect on depression, anxiety, and fatigue in people with a range of chronic health conditions (Alsubaie et al. 2017).

Given the growing evidence for the utility of MBIs in effecting wide-ranging improvements in wellbeing, the exploration of mindfulness in the treatment of addictive disorders has come as a natural progression. Similar to depression, addiction is associated with high rates of relapse, and given the role of relapse prevention in MBCT, the structure and methods of MBCT were adapted into similar programs specifically targeting addictive behaviours. For example, programs such as Mindfulness-Based Relapse Prevention (MBRP) and Mindfulness-Oriented Recovery Enhancement (MORE) were tailored to target the mechanisms believed to underlie addiction.

Regarding their impact on the mechanisms of addiction, it is believed that focused attention allows for a grounding of attention onto physical sensations or other sensory awareness, while open monitoring promotes a metacognitive state of awareness in which observation of the contents of awareness is accompanied by a heightened sensitivity to the field of awareness itself as well as the processes that it contains. This can involve a radical reorganisation in attentional processes, memory, and emotion regulation, which, with practise, can effect permanent changes (Garland and Howard 2018).

From a neurological perspective, addiction is now generally understood to be a dysfunction of brain circuitry involved in reward processing and motivation. Bottom-up processes mediated by the basal ganglia area become strengthened by content repeated associations with substance-related reward cues, while top-down executive function processes—mediated by the dorsolateral prefrontal cortex (dPFC), dorsal anterior cingulate cortex (dACC), and parietal cortex—becomes weakened, causing diminished salience of natural reward cues. The *restructuring reward hypothesis* (Garland 2016) states that mindfulness may reduce addictive behaviour by adjusting the balance of salience of rewards away from the valuation of drug-related rewards and cues and back to valuation of natural rewards that were salient before the development of addiction. This occurs by augmenting the capacity of the prefrontal cortex to regulate subcortical networks, modulating activities involved in reward processing, cue reactivity, and stress reactivity (Garland et al. 2017b). This is supported by metanalytic data from neuroimaging studies indicating changes at a neuroanatomical level (Fox et al. 2014), early functional magnetic resonance imaging (fMRI) evidence from a MORE intervention study for smoking cessation (Froeliger et al. 2017), as well as a MORE study targeting opioid use (Garland et al. 2017b).

Garland and Howard (2018) suggest five key mechanisms at play in restructuring reward processing in addiction: (i) enhancing executive functioning; (ii) increasing dispositional mindfulness; (iii) attenuating stress reactivity; (iv) decreasing cue reactivity; and

(v) reduction of thought suppression. This is consistent with a randomized control trial (RCT) examining working memory, selective attention, and decision making with a sample of polysubstance users, which found significant improvements in these measures in the condition which employed mindfulness meditation (Valls-Serrano et al. 2016). Furthermore, in RCTs employing MBRP and MORE, increases in aspects of dispositional mindfulness, such as acceptance, awareness, and nonjudgement, significantly mediated the effects on decreased craving following treatment (Garland et al. 2016; Witkiewitz et al. 2013).

The positive effects of MBIs on addiction may also result from improving response to stress. Several studies examining the impact of MBIs on stress recovery have used heart-rate variability (HRV) as an index of a person's capacity to regulate stress reactivity and recovery. Studies of MBRP interventions for individuals with substance abuse disorders have shown significantly greater increases in HRV responses to stress (Carroll and Lustyk 2018) and significantly attenuated HRV ratio during stress compared to a control group (Brewer et al. 2009). Similarly, another study found significant within-group decreases in cortisol levels (a marker of physiological stress) in smokers taking part in a mindfulness training program (Goldberg et al. 2014).

MBIs might also help by decreasing craving and drug cue reactivity. For example, a study of an MBRP-based intervention resulted in a significantly reduced association between craving and cigarette smoking (Elwafi et al. 2013), and an RCT employing MORE showed significantly reduced attentional bias toward opioid cues (Garland et al. 2017a). In another study, an MBRP for substance use showed significantly reduced associations between postintervention depressive symptoms and craving two months after treatment and predicted reduced substance use at four-month follow-up (Witkiewitz and Bowen 2010). Furthermore, the mediating role of decreased craving was confirmed in a large clinical trial of the effects of a mindfulness-based treatment for smoking abstinence (Spears et al. 2017).

Finally, thought suppression, paradoxically, may actually amplify craving by depleting the very psychological resources necessary to maintain it, causing this strategy to be ultimately self-defeating (Garland et al. 2012; Moss et al. 2015). MBIs may help to ameliorate addictive behaviour by offering an effective alternative to thought suppression. Rather than attempting to suppress substance-related cognitions, the emphasis in mindfulness is on changing the relationship with thoughts, learning to stay with and transform cravings and the unpleasant experiences that accompany them (Groves 2014). A pilot RCT employing a MORE intervention for alcohol-dependent inpatients, for example, was found to effect a significant reduction in thought suppression, which was in turn associated with lower levels of alcohol attentional biases (Garland et al. 2010).

The findings of a large, controlled trial have demonstrated that MBRP can effect significant improvements in substance-abuse outcomes (Bowen et al. 2014). Because of its efficacy in improving wellbeing and tackling a variety of emotional difficulties, MBRP is increasingly finding use as an adjunct to support patients on their road to recovery, with some referring to such courses as "mindfulness-based addiction recovery" (MBAR) (Mason-John and Groves 2014).

3. Ontological Addiction Theory (OAT)

Just as early biomedical-based conceptualisations of mental illness eventually evolved to include psychological and sociological dimensions in the subsequent biopsychosocial paradigm, there is growing realisation that a complete account of the causes of human suffering must also include a spiritual dimension.

Metaphysics involves the examination of ontological questions, such as those concerning the nature of reality, existence, and selfhood. A new metaphysical model called *ontological addiction theory* (OAT) has recently been proposed, which advances current approaches to psychopathology by including this important aspect of human existence (Shonin et al. 2013; Shonin et al. 2016; Van Gordon et al. 2018). Based on the assumption that contemporary conceptualisations of mental illness overlook how individuals fundamentally conceptualise themselves and the way that they exist, OAT asserts that individuals are prone to forming implausible beliefs about their existence and that such beliefs can become addictive, resulting in functional impairment and mental illness. Specifically, ontological addiction is defined as *"the unwillingness to relinquish an erroneous and deep-rooted belief in an inherently existing 'self' or 'I' as well as the impaired functionality that arises from such a belief"* (Shonin et al. 2013, p. 64).

There is something of a strange contradiction in Western society regarding the prevailing conceptualisation of selfhood. With humanity's growing understanding of the nature of the physical world, we have reached the realisation that things of the objective world are simply complex structures of particles existing in a state of constant flux. Within this paradigm, there is the commonly held characterisation of the mind or selfhood as an emergent biological software of sorts, which organises our behaviour to safeguard our survival and wellbeing. Within this traditional, predominately materialist worldview, and even at the forefront of modern physics (Van Gordon et al. 2017a), the principle marks of existence of Buddhism appear incontrovertibly true: all things, including ourselves, are subject to change (Pāli: *anicca*) and devoid of an inherently existing self (Pāli: *anattā*). Since phenomena are never fixed in time and space, then all things, including human beings, are of the nature of non-self (*anattā*) and are inherently "empty" because they exist only in a relative sense (Nagarjuna 2005). Yet, though modern psychology understands that selfhood is illusory and a construction of our own psyche, there remains the deeply ingrained habit of viewing the self as a fixed entity with inherent physical and behavioural attributes, and this perspective still dominates many established psychological and psychiatric models (Freud 1961; Maslow 1943; Roger 1959). This is despite the fact that controlled studies have demonstrated significant improvements to wellbeing and wisdom following acquaintance with the idea of a self that is empty of intrinsic existence (Van Gordon et al. 2019).

OAT contends that it is this flawed belief in an inherently existing self that is the main cause of many forms of mental illness. By harbouring mistaken ontological beliefs, individuals reify their sense of selfhood to the extent that they fall into narrow and egotistical response modes (Shonin et al. 2016), pathologically pursuing self-interest and expending disproportionate amounts of energy in furthering self-interest or protecting the self from perceived threats (Van Gordon et al. 2016a). The rewards and punishments associated with such behaviour, furthermore, can exacerbate a person's self-fixation to the extent that it meets the criteria of a clinical addiction (Shonin et al. 2016). Put simply, ontological addiction is when a person becomes self-addicted, placing themselves at the centre of the world, separate from everything around them.

The concept of addiction is largely synonymous with the Buddhist notion of attachment or craving (Pāli: *rāga*). However, the meaning of attachment here is distinct from its use in psychological parlance concerning human relationships and instead refers to the undesirable tendency to cling to transient forms or experiences (Sahdra et al. 2010). As has been discussed, grasping at what brings pleasure and rejecting its opposite creates the cycle of dissatisfaction, disillusionment, and pain that is *samsara*. OAT thus views addiction and its treatment not in terms of understanding and remedying every possible instance or sub-category of behavioural addiction (e.g., drugs, food, gambling, sex, work, etc.) but on tackling the root cause of all addictive impulses. From a Buddhist perspective, this root cause of addiction is of the same nature as the attachment that drives the karmic cycle (i.e., *samsara*) and the preoccupation with what are called mundane concerns. These mundane concerns centre on an individual's preoccupation with the pursuit of pleasure, wealth, fame, possessions, and other things concerning the advancement of the self. That is not to say that Buddhism opposes such concerns per se but only the attachment to such concerns and the dysfunctional ego reification that belies pathological forms of such attachment. In this respect, addiction is viewed as stemming from a kind of spiritual malnutrition; the deluded mind, unaware of its own nature, attempts to concretise the ego-self, blindly chasing material pleasures and rewards that can never bring lasting fulfilment. Release from this cycle of suffering in *samsara* can only be achieved by the extinction of these cravings through transcendence of ego in *nirvana*. Behavioural addiction, then, has its origin in the deeper and more pernicious self-addiction that is the root of all addictions (Shonin et al. 2013).

OAT asserts that without a fixed belief in an independently existing "me" or "I", the conceptual and emotional entanglements that propagate this cycle can no longer gain traction and that treatment strategies should target ontological addiction at its source, undermining self-attachment, deconstructing the ego-self, and dismantling the maladaptive addictive beliefs that have accumulated. This approach is supported by studies showing that lower self-attachment is associated with improved physical and psychological health (Pande and Naidu 1992), enhanced well-being (Sahdra et al. 2010), and reduced psychological distress and chronic pain (Van Gordon et al. 2017b). Furthermore, qualitative studies have shown that acceptance of the self's lack of inherent existence can promote personal, professional, and spiritual development (Shonin and Van Gordon 2015; Van Gordon et al. 2019).

4. The New Wave: Second-Generation Mindfulness-Based Interventions in the Treatment of Addiction

As described earlier, FG-MBIs, with their relatively secularised implementation of mindfulness, have invited concern over the way mindfulness has been removed from its traditional Buddhist roots and the *tisikkhā* (three trainings) principle within which meditation is traditionally taught. Indeed, this apparent denaturisation of mindfulness has raised criticisms over the question of authenticity in these practises, provoking much debate (Grossman 2015; Monteiro et al. 2015; Purser 2019; Purser 2015; Repetti et al. 2016). Some researchers, practitioners, and Buddhist experts believe that mindfulness as it is practised in FG-MBIs has been so altered from its traditional Buddhist conceptualisation that it may even be misleading to refer to the practice as mindfulness (Van Gordon et al. 2019).

SG-MBIs were introduced to place mindfulness back within the *tisikkhā* structure of traditional Buddhist teaching where meditation (right effort, right mindfulness, right meditation) is practised alongside ethics (right speech, right action, and right livelihood) and wisdom (right view, right intention) (Van Gordon et al. 2019). Furthermore, mindfulness has been reframed as an active, enquiring process that is openly spiritual in nature (Van Gordon et al. 2015a). This is because the non-judgemental aspect of Kabat-Zinn's (1994) definition, some believe, does not properly depict the discerning aspect of mindfulness as traditionally practised in Buddhism that prevents the practitioner from becoming morally indifferent (Shonin et al. 2014). SG-MBIs typically follow a similar structure as their predecessors but have been expanded to more fully embody mindfulness as it is practised in a traditional Buddhist setting. For example, the eight-week Meditation Awareness Training (MAT) intervention (Van Gordon et al. 2015a) is openly spiritual in nature, includes ethics as a core aspect of its syllabus, and requires instructors to have several years of supervised practice.

Consistent with the ethics component, MAT integrates meditative techniques that cultivate loving-kindness, compassion, and moral equanimity, while for the wisdom component, insight meditation—such as *vipassanā* or *suññatā* meditation—focuses on cultivating penetrating insight into the nature of selfhood and reality. The rationale for this is that while meditative focus is a prerequisite for attaining the stability of awareness necessary for cultivating deeper insights and ethical and socio-empathic awareness, a fundamental enquiry into the nature of phenomena and reality is also necessary to bring about the spiritual growth required to undermine the powerful self-fixations which have accrued (Chah 2011). In other words, loving-kindness and compassion-based meditation allows the individual to transcend selfhood at an affective/emotional level (e.g., through equanimity, empathy, and compassion), while insight meditations cultivate the deeper awareness associated with non-dual states of being (e.g., insights such as interconnectedness, impermanence, and emptiness of phenomena) (Shonin et al. 2014; Van Gordon et al. 2019).

Within the framework of OAT, Shonin et al. (2016, p. 666) propose a three-phase approach to the treatment of ontological addiction that is held to underlie manifestations of conventional addictions (e.g., drugs, work, sex etc.): "(i) becoming aware of the imputed self, (ii) deconstructing the imputed self, and (iii) reconstructing a dynamic and non-dual self". The first phase is to become aware of the fact that the self is a construction of mind and that there are no credible grounds for believing that there is an inherently existing "I" that operates independently of everything else. This stage therefore focuses upon enhancing self-awareness and laying out the logical foundations for the principles of non-self (or emptiness) which can foster deeper realisation of the inner nature of phenomena. The second phase is to cultivate and practice a variety of spiritual capabilities centring on the aforementioned ethics and wisdom components of Buddhist training. Here, qualities such as compassion, loving-kindness, generosity, and patience are practised alongside insight meditation—such as *vipassanā* or *suññatā* meditation—with the aim of challenging and uprooting the concept of an inherently existent self. As a result, the deep-rooted beliefs that fuel ontological addiction can gradually be eroded as insight into the nature of selfhood evolves and transforms.

It should be stressed, however, that this deconstruction of self is not intended as a deliberate attempt at psychological dissociation or denial of existence but to foster a profound recognition of its constructed, impermanent, and relative nature. Thus, terms such as "non-self" are expedients for shifting focus from awareness-of-self to awareness of the totality of self and other. The final, third phase of this treatment, then, involves reconstructing a self that is dynamic and non-dual in nature. At this stage, though individuals recognise the illusory nature of selfhood, they also understand that they must still operate in an adaptive manner in a world in which they are embodied as distinct entities surviving in a potentially hostile environment. Having recognised the emptiness of inherent existence, however, a true self can be assumed for the purposes of functioning in the world. This reformed self, being based on the insights derived from the first two phases, however, exists as a deeply interconnected entity with a recognition of its ultimate inseparability from the conditions and phenomena around it. By understanding that we, and the situations in which we find ourselves, are inseparable phases of the same whole, it is argued that we can respond more fluidly, spontaneously, and constructively to life's challenges. Being less concerned with self, we are thereby better able to see the big picture, are less prone to narrow self-interest, and less susceptible to the maladaptive cognitive-affective processes in which the ego can become entangled (Shonin et al. 2016).

The importance of this spiritual dimension in addiction theory and treatment is reflected in the widespread adoption of the notion of a higher power within traditional, 12-step programmes for recovery from addiction. Indeed, Groves (2014) has drawn comparisons between these steps, the noble truths of Buddhism regarding the origins and root causes of suffering (attachment or craving), and the role of ethics in recovery from addiction. Consistent with this, Shonin and Van Gordon (2016) list increased spirituality, greater situational and self-awareness, values clarification, and letting go as key mechanisms through which mindfulness can effect positive changes in mental health and addiction recovery.

The formulation of OAT described herein emerged from an analytical review of Buddhist-derived interventions for the treatment of problem gambling (Shonin et al. 2013), and with OAT being so aligned with the concept of addiction—albeit in Buddhist terms—the application of SG-MBIs, such as the MAT intervention to conventional addictions, has been a natural development. MAT intervention studies have since been conducted in respect of (for example) sex addiction (Van Gordon et al. 2016b) and workaholism (Van Gordon et al. 2017c), with the results revealing clinically significant positive changes that were maintained at six-month follow-up. Though these results are encouraging, however, to date there have only been a small number of comparison studies examining whether FG-MBI or SG-MBI approaches are more effective for particular populations (e.g., Bayot et al. 2020; Chen and Jordan 2020).

5. Conclusions and Future Directions

As things stand, it is unclear whether some elements of the MAT intervention (e.g., mindfulness, ethics, or wisdom-based practices) are more useful than others in effecting positive changes in addictive behaviours and whether such advantages may depend upon characteristics of the population under examination. As a result, SG-MBIs might be criticised as being overly reliant on expert opinion regarding best practice in Buddhist-derived interventions. Nonetheless, regardless of the specific types of mindfulness practice to be explored and critically appraised as part of future research (e.g., compassion, loving-kindness, or insight meditation), the growing popularity of MBIs will likely present implications for the training of psychiatrists and other health professionals involved in the treatment of addiction. It is therefore recommended that professionals in this occupation develop a working knowledge of meditational theory and psychospiritual perspectives on addiction aetiology (Van Gordon et al. 2018; Van Gordon et al. 2015a).

There also remain many questions regarding the dose-response relationship, that is, how much treatment is necessary to effect positive clinical outcomes. Related to this, there is also the question of the amount of clinical training required in order to be able to practice effectively in a clinical setting (Garland and Howard 2018) and whether the more stringent training requirements for instructors of some of the SG-MBI interventions are reflected in more positive clinical outcomes than for conventional FG-MBIs.

Finally, most studies of FG-MBIs for addiction have thus far focused mostly on substance misuse, and more studies are needed in respect of behavioural addictions, such as workaholism and sex addiction (Kathirasan 2018). However, the opposite situation seems to currently apply to SG-MBIs, where studies of addiction have tended to focus on behavioural addictions. Thus, future research should return to the question of efficacy of SG-MBIs in the treatment of a variety of addictions—including substance abuse—with the use of more qualitative and longitudinal studies to reveal a clearer picture of the long-term impact of SG-MBIs on relapse prevention.

Author Contributions: Conceptualization—P.B. and W.V.G.; writing—original draft preparation, P.B.; writing—review and editing, P.B. and W.V.G. Both authors have read and agreed to the published version of the manuscript.

Funding: This research received no external funding.

Institutional Review Board Statement: Not applicable.

Informed Consent Statement: Not applicable.

Conflicts of Interest: The authors declare no conflict of interest.

References

Alsubaie, Modi, Rebecca Abbott, Barnaby Dunn, Chris Dickens, Tina Frieda Keil, William Henley, and Willem Kuyken. 2017. Mechanisms of action in mindfulness-based cognitive therapy (MBCT) and mindfulness-based stress reduction (MBSR) in people with physical and/or psychological conditions: A systematic review. *Clinical Psychology Review* 55: 74–91. [CrossRef]

Bayot, Marie, Nicolas Vermeulen, Anne Kever, and Moïra Mikolajczak. 2020. Mindfulness and empathy: Differential effects of explicit and implicit Buddhist Teachings. *Mindfulness* 11: 5–17. [CrossRef]

Bowen, Sarah, Katie Witkiewitz, Seema L. Clifasefi, Joel Grow, Neharika Chawla, Sharon H. Hsu, Haley A. Carroll, Erin Harrop, Susan E. Collins, M. Kathleen Lustyk, and et al. 2014. Relative efficacy of mindfulness-based relapse prevention, standard relapse prevention, and treatment as usual for substance use disorders: A randomized clinical trial. *JAMA Psychiatry* 71: 547–56. [CrossRef] [PubMed]

Brewer, Judson A., Rajita Sinha, Justin A. Chen, Ravenna N. Michalsen, Theresa A. Babuscio, Charla Nich, Aleesha Grier, Keri L. Bergquist, Deidre L. Reis, Marc N. Potenza, and et al. 2009. Mindfulness training and stress reactivity in substance abuse: Results from a randomized, controlled stage I pilot study. *Substance Abuse* 30: 306–17. [CrossRef] [PubMed]

Brown, Kirk Warren, Richard M. Ryan, and J. David Creswell. 2007. Mindfulness: Theoretical Foundations and Evidence for its Salutary Effects. *Psychological Inquiry* 18: 211–37. [CrossRef]

Carroll, Haley A., and M. Kathleen Lustyk. 2018. Mindfulness-Based Relapse Prevention for Substance Use Disorders: Effects on Cardiac Vagal Control and Craving Under Stress. *Mindfulness* 9: 488–99. [CrossRef]

Chah, Ajahn. 2011. *The Collected Teachings of Ajahn Chah*. Tamil Nadu: Aruna.

Chen, Siyin, and Christian H. Jordan. 2020. Incorporating ethics into brief mindfulness practice: Effects on well-being and prosocial behavior. *Mindfulness* 11: 18–19. [CrossRef]

Creswell, J. David. 2017. Mindfulness Interventions. *Annual Review of Psychology* 68: 491–516. [CrossRef]

Elwafi, Hani M., Katie Witkiewitz, Sarah Mallik, Thomas A. Thornhill, and Judson A. Brewer. 2013. Mindfulness training for smoking cessation: Moderation of the relationship between craving and cigarette use. *Drug and Alcohol Dependence* 130: 222–9. [CrossRef]

Fox, Kieran C., Savannah Nijeboer, Matthew L. Dixon, James L. Floman, Melissa Ellamil, Samuel p. Rumak, Peter Sedlmeier, and Kalina Christoff. 2014. Is meditation associated with altered brain structure? A systematic review and meta-analysis of morphometric neuroimaging in meditation practitioners. *Neuroscience & Biobehavioral Reviews* 43: 48–73. [CrossRef]

Freud, Sigmund. 1961. *The Standard Edition of the Complete Psychological Works of Sigmund Freud*. London: Hogarth Press.

Froeliger, Brett, Amanda R. Mathew, Patrick A. McConnell, Cristie Eichberg, Michael E. Saladin, Matthew J. Carpenter, and Eric L. Garland. 2017. Restructuring Reward Mechanisms in Nicotine Addiction: A Pilot fMRI Study of Mindfulness-Oriented Recovery Enhancement for Cigarette Smokers. *Evidence-Based Complementary and Alternative Medicine* 2017: 7018014. [CrossRef]

Garland, Eric L., Anne K. Baker, and Matthew O. Howard. 2017a. Mindfulness-oriented recovery enhancement reduces opioid attentional bias among prescription opioid-treated chronic pain patients. *Journal of the Society for Social Work and Research* 8: 493–509. [CrossRef]

Garland, Eric L., Amelia Roberts-Lewis, Christine D. Tronnier, Rebecca Graves, and Karen Kelley. 2016. Mindfulness-Oriented Recovery Enhancement versus CBT for co-occurring substance dependence, traumatic stress, and psychiatric disorders: Proximal outcomes from a pragmatic randomized trial. *Behaviour Research and Therapy* 77: 7–16. [CrossRef]

Garland, Eric L., Craig J. Bryan, Patrick H. Finan, Elizabeth A. Thomas, Sarah E. Priddy, Michael R. Riquino, and Matthew O. Howard. 2017b. Pain, hedonic regulation, and opioid misuse: Modulation of momentary experience by Mindfulness-Oriented Recovery Enhancement in opioid-treated chronic pain patients. *Drug and Alcohol Dependence* 173: S65–S72. [CrossRef]

Garland, Eric L., Kristin Carter, Katie Ropes, and Matthwe O. Howard. 2012. Thought suppression, impaired regulation of urges, and Addiction-Stroop predict affect-modulated cue-reactivity among alcohol dependent adults. *Biological Psychology* 89: 87–93. [CrossRef] [PubMed]

Garland, Eric L., Susan A. Gaylord, Charlotte A. Boettiger, and Matthew O. Howard. 2010. Mindfulness training modifies cognitive, affective, and physiological mechanisms implicated in alcohol dependence: Results of a randomized controlled pilot trial. *Journal of Psychoactive Drugs* 42: 177–92. [CrossRef] [PubMed]

Garland, Eric L. 2016. Restructuring reward processing with Mindfulness-Oriented Recovery Enhancement: Novel therapeutic mechanisms to remediate hedonic dysregulation in addiction, stress, and pain. *Annals of the New York Academy of Sciences* 1373: 25–37. [CrossRef]

Garland, Eric L., and Matthew O. Howard. 2018. Mindfulness-based treatment of addiction: Current state of the field and envisioning the next wave of research. *Addiction Science & Clinical Practice* 13: 14. [CrossRef]

Goldberg, Simon B., Alison R. Manley, Stevens S. Smith, Jeffery M. Greeson, Evan Russell, Stan Van Uum, Gideon Koren, and James M. Davis. 2014. Hair cortisol as a biomarker of stress in mindfulness training for smokers. *Journal of Alternative and Complementary Medicine* 20: 630–4. [CrossRef]

Grossman, Paul. 2015. Mindfulness: Awareness Informed by an Embodied Ethic. *Mindfulness* 6: 17–22. [CrossRef]

Grossman, Paul, Ludger Niemann, Stefan Schmidt, and Harald Walach. 2004. Mindfulness-based stress reduction and health benefits: A meta-analysis. *Journal of Psychosomatic Research* 57: 35–43. [CrossRef]

Groves, Paramabandhu. 2014. Buddhist Approaches to Addiction Recovery. *Religions* 5: 985–1000. [CrossRef]

Kabat-Zinn, Jon. 1982. An outpatient program in behavioral medicine for chronic pain patients based on the practice of mindfulness meditation: Theoretical considerations and preliminary results. *General Hospital Psychiatry* 4: 33–47. [CrossRef]

Kabat-Zinn, Jon. 1990. *Full Catastrophe Living: Using the Wisdom of Your Body and Mind to Face Stress, Pain, and Illness*. New York: Delacorte Press.

Kabat-Zinn, Jon. 1994. *Wherever You Go, There You Are: Mindfulness Meditation in Everyday Life*. New York: Hyperion.

Kathirasan, K. 2018. The Role of Mindfulness in Treating Addictive Disorders and Rehabilitation. *International Journal of Psychology & Behavior Analysis* 4: 155. [CrossRef]

Ludwig, David S., and Jon Kabat-Zinn. 2008. Mindfulness in medicine. *JAMA* 300: 1350–52. [CrossRef] [PubMed]

Mason-John, Valerie, and Paramabandhu Groves. 2014. *Eight-Step Recovery: Using the Buddha's Teachings to Overcome Addiction*. Cambridge: Windhorse Publications.

Maslow, Abraham Harold. 1943. A Theory of Human Motivation. *Psychological Review* 50: 4. [CrossRef]

Monteiro, Lynette M., R. F. Musten, and Jane Compson. 2015. Traditional and Contemporary Mindfulness: Finding the Middle Path in the Tangle of Concerns. *Mindfulness* 6: 1–13. [CrossRef]

Moss, Antony C., James A. K. Erskine, Ian p. Albery, James R. Allen, and George J. Georgiou. 2015. To suppress, or not to suppress? That is repression: Controlling intrusive thoughts in addictive behaviour. *Addictive Behaviors* 44: 65–70. [CrossRef]

Nagarjuna, Kyabje Kangyur Rinpoche. 2005. *Nagarjuna's Letter to a Friend: With Commentary by Kyabje Kangyur Rinpoche*. New York: Snow Lion Publications.

Pande, Namita, and Radha Krishna Naidu. 1992. Anāsakti and Health: A Study of Non-attachment. *Psychology and Developing Societies* 4: 89–104. [CrossRef]

Purser, Ronald. 2015. Clearing the Muddled Path of Traditional and Contemporary Mindfulness: A Response to Monteiro, Musten, and Compson. *Mindfulness* 6: 23–45. [CrossRef]

Purser, Ronald. 2019. *McMindfulness: How Mindfulness Became the New Capitalist Spirituality*. London: Repeater Books.

Repetti, Rick, Ron Purser, David Forbes, and Adam Burke. 2016. Meditation Matters: Replies to the Anti-McMindfulness Bandwagon! In *Handbook of Mindfulness: Culture, Context and Social Engagement*. Edited by David Forbes and Ronald Purser. Berlin: Springer, pp. 473–94.

Roger, Carl Ransom. 1959. *A Theory of Therapy, Personality, and Interpersonal Relationships: As Developed in the Client-centered Framework*. New York: McGraw-Hill.

Sahdra, Baljinder K., Phillip R. Shaver, and Kirk W. Brown. 2010. A scale to measure nonattachment: A Buddhist complement to Western research on attachment and adaptive functioning. *Journal of Personality Assessment* 92: 116–27. [CrossRef] [PubMed]

Shonin, Edo, William Van Gordon, and Mark D. Griffiths. 2013. Buddhist philosophy for the treatment of problem gambling. *Journal of Behavioral Addictions* 2: 63–71. [CrossRef]

Shonin, Edo, William Van Gordon, and Mark D. Griffiths. 2014. The emerging role of Buddhism in clinical psychology: Toward effective integration. *Psychology of Religion and Spirituality* 6: 123–37. [CrossRef]

Shonin, Edo, William Van Gordon, Nirbhay N. Singh, and Mark D. Griffiths. 2015. Mindfulness of emptiness and the emptiness of mindfulness. In *Buddhist Foundations of Mindfulness*. Edited by Edo Shonin, William Van Gordon and Nirbhay N. Singh. New York: Springer.

Shonin, Edo, and William Van Gordon. 2015. Managers' experiences of meditation awareness training. *Mindfulness* 6: 899–909. [CrossRef]

Shonin, Edo, and William Van Gordon. 2016. The mechanisms of mindfulness in the treatment of mental illness and addiction. *International Journal of Mental Health and Addiction* 14: 844–49. [CrossRef]

Shonin, Edo, William Van Gordon, and Mark D. Griffiths. 2016. Ontological Addiction: Classification, etiology, and treatment. *Mindfulness* 7: 660–71. [CrossRef]

Spears, Claire A., Donald Hedeker, Liang Li, Cai Wu, Natalie K. Anderson, Sean C. Houchins, Christine Vinci, Diana Stewart Hoover, Jennifer Irvin Vidrine, Paul M. Cinciripini, and et al. 2017. Mechanisms underlying mindfulness-based addiction treatment versus cognitive behavioral therapy and usual care for smoking cessation. *Journal of Consulting and Clinical Psychology* 85: 1029–40. [CrossRef] [PubMed]

Valls-Serrano, Carlos, Alfonso Caracuel, and Antonio Verdejo-Garcia. 2016. Goal Management Training and Mindfulness Meditation improve executive functions and transfer to ecological tasks of daily life in polysubstance users enrolled in therapeutic community treatment. *Drug and Alcohol Dependence* 165: 9–14. [CrossRef] [PubMed]

Van Gordon, William, Edo Shonin, and Mark D. Griffiths. 2015a. Towards a second generation of mindfulness-based interventions. *Australian & New Zealand Journal of Psychiatry* 49: 591–92. [CrossRef]

Van Gordon, William, Edo Shonin, Mark D. Griffiths, and N. N. Singh. 2015b. There is only one mindfulness: Why science and Buddhism need to work together. *Mindfulness* 6: 49–56. [CrossRef]

Van Gordon, William, Edo Shonin, and Mark D. Griffiths. 2016a. Meditation awareness training for individuals with fibromyalgia syndrome: An interpretative phenomenological analysis of participants' experiences. *Mindfulness* 7: 409–19. [CrossRef]

Van Gordon, William, Edo Shonin, and Mark D. Griffiths. 2016b. Meditation Awareness Training for the Treatment of Sex Addiction: A Case Study. *Journal of Behavioral Addictions* 5: 363–72. [CrossRef]

Van Gordon, William, Edo Shonin, and Mark D. Griffiths. 2017a. Buddhist emptiness theory: Implications for psychology. *Psychology of Religion and Spirituality* 9: 309–18. [CrossRef]

Van Gordon, William, Edo Shonin, Sofiane Diouri, Javier Garcia-Campayo, Yasuhiro Kotera, and Mark D. Griffiths. 2018. Ontological addiction theory: Attachment to me, mine, and I. *Journal of Behavioral Addictions* 7: 892–96. [CrossRef] [PubMed]

Van Gordon, William, Edo Shonin, Thomas J. Dunn, Javier Garcia-Campayo, and Mark D. Griffiths. 2017b. Meditation awareness training for the treatment of fibromyalgia syndrome: A randomized controlled trial. *British Journal of Health Psychology* 22: 186–206. [CrossRef] [PubMed]

Van Gordon, William, Edo Shonin, Thomas J. Dunn, Javier Garcia-Campayo, M. M. p. Demarzo, and Mark D. Griffiths. 2017c. Meditation awareness training for the treatment of workaholism: A controlled trial. *Journal of Behavioral Addictions* 6: 212–20. [CrossRef]

Van Gordon, William, Edo Shonin, Thomas J. Dunn, Supakyada Sapthiang, Yasuhiro Kotera, Javier Garcia-Campayo, and David Sheffield. 2019. Exploring emptiness and its effects on non-attachment, mystical experiences, and psycho-spiritual wellbeing: A quantitative and qualitative study of advanced meditators. *Explore* 15: 261–72. [CrossRef]

Van Gordon, William, Supakyada Sapthiang, Paul Barrows, and Edo Shonin. 2020. Understanding and practising emptiness. *Mindulness Advance Online Publication*. [CrossRef]

Witkiewitz, Katie, and Sarah Bowen. 2010. Depression, craving, and substance use following a randomized trial of mindfulness-based relapse prevention. *Journal of Consulting and Clinical Psychology* 78: 362–74. [CrossRef] [PubMed]

Witkiewitz, Katie, Sarah Bowen, Haley Douglas, and Sharon H. Hsu. 2013. Mindfulness-based relapse prevention for substance craving. *Addictive Behaviors* 38: 1563–71. [CrossRef]

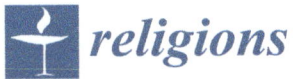

Review

The Significance of 'the Person' in Addiction

Pádraic Mark Hurley

Department of Applied Arts, Waterford Institute of Technology, X91 KOEK Waterford, Ireland; padraic.hurley@wit.ie

Abstract: Van Gordon et al. outline the classification of their Ontological Addiction Theory (OAT), including its aetiology and treatment. In this review article I will from an appreciative perspective question some of its fundamental assumptions by presenting an alternative view on the ontology of 'the person', as distinct from its presently assumed conventional conflation with a contracted separate egoic self. I will propose this view as structurally and ethically significant for the 'embodied' experience of a reconstructed "dynamic and non-dual self", as cultivated in their treatment. Rather than this reconstructed self simply being socially desirable for functional purposes, I will underscore the meaning-generative case for ontological status, in the absence of which, a pervasive 'sense of lack' is evident, with all attendant individual, psychological, social, ecological and ethical implications. This article brings a developmental psychology perspective to bear in appreciating 'personhood' as an emergent, progressively realised and is thus similarly aligned with the intent of OAT in overcoming egoic addictive suffering. This mapping of the territory however populates a blind spot in OAT's diagnosis by affirming unique personhood, a quality of 'integrative presence', meaningfully understood as a psycho-spiritual ontological reality. It offers, as with OAT's stated intent, the merit of avoiding attendant mental health and developmental pitfalls, which can beset what we may discern as an implicit transcendental reductionist assumption operative in OAT, where 'the many' are reduced to 'the One' and there are, it is assumed, no real many. This framing is resonant with the lived experience of healthy 'individuation', a process distinct from the problematic phenomenon of 'individualism', evidenced by the empirical data on post-conventional human development, which potentially provides diagnostic markers for any optimal treatment discernment. It is also attuned to what many recognise as a contemporary Fourth Turning in Buddhism, in its conscious evolutionary recognition of the emergence in non-dual states of a 'unique personal perspective', and/or a relative individuation within the whole. This differentiation has formerly been interpreted through an 'impersonal' lens as an egoic holdover, and potentially inhibits ethical action in the world, as distinct from the ethical import and potential fruits stemming from the ontological affirmation of the person.

Keywords: ego; unique personhood; ontology; epistemology; contemplative traditions; Western Enlightenment; developmental psychology; transcendental reductionism; Fourth Turning in Buddhism

Citation: Hurley, Pádraic Mark. 2021. The Significance of 'the Person' in Addiction. *Religions* 12: 893. https://doi.org/10.3390/rel12100893

Academic Editors: Bernadette Flanagan, Noelia Molina, Christian Zwingmann and Antonio Muñoz-García

Received: 2 September 2021
Accepted: 11 October 2021
Published: 18 October 2021

Publisher's Note: MDPI stays neutral with regard to jurisdictional claims in published maps and institutional affiliations.

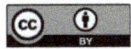

Copyright: © 2021 by the author. Licensee MDPI, Basel, Switzerland. This article is an open access article distributed under the terms and conditions of the Creative Commons Attribution (CC BY) license (https://creativecommons.org/licenses/by/4.0/).

1. Introduction

Van Gordon et al. (2016), in laying out OAT, chart a path from (i) becoming aware of the imputed self, (ii) deconstructing the imputed self, and (iii) reconstructing a dynamic and non-dual self in order to overcome the ontological addiction, described as a "maladaptive condition whereby an individual is addicted to the belief that they inherently exist" (ibid, p. 1). And indeed, overcoming egoic addictive suffering is at the core of contemplative traditions worldwide, whilst subtle significant distinctions remain as to respective 'self-systems'. Set within a conscious evolutionary frame, some of the contemporary mapping of this territory, only relatively recent in its articulation, holds profound implications for our way of being and becoming in the world. Our conceptions of 'reality' and 'illusion', what we value and strive for, our sense of purpose and the very meaning of our lives are all at play. We are therefore exhorted to *choose* our 'view' wisely.

2. Discussion

The evolutionary nature of our cosmos, as we presently understand it, was not within the knowledge sphere of the sages of old. Being conscious of our contemporary 13.8-billion-year story that has shaped and is shaping our human adventure is truly awe inspiring and needs to be integrated within our 'wisdom traditions', if they are to be truly wise. Although science tentatively frames an evolving vast quantitative 'exterior' cosmos, our contemplative traditions *point* us towards a correlative qualitative 'interior', which in post-metaphysical terms (Murray 2019), can be experienced as expansive, spacious, wonder-inducing and transformative for our being, when their insights and practices are applied in our so called ordinary everyday lives. The overlaps identified between the respective contemplative paths of 'east and west' reveal a remarkable common cause during a period in which communications and cross referencing was not supported by the material architecture that we are presently familiar with. It was all communicated through an 'intranet', we might say.

Harvard psychologist and meditation teacher, Brown (1986) for example explored this topic of *universal deep structures* across the source texts of three major traditions, Hinduism, Theravāda and Mahayana Buddhism and derived his conclusions from a precise analysis of the technical language used in the Yogasutras, The Vissudhimagga and The Mahamudra traditions. It is described by Wilber (2006, p. 77) as "an absolutely brilliant and enduring classic in meditative stages". The yoga sutras of Patangali are thought to have been compiled c.a. 400 CE and comprise 196 sutras variously divided into chapters on Samadhi/absorption, Sadhana/practice, Vibhuti-siddhis/powers, and Kaivalya/moksha/liberation. The Vissudhimagga by Buddhaghosa (voice of the Buddha) is a comprehensive distillation, summary and analysis of the Tripitaka, the canons of Buddhist scriptures, Sri Lanka c.a. 430 CE. The 'Mahamudra' comprises a body of quintessential teachings from Tibetan Buddhism, the root text being the *Phyag chen zla ba'd od zer* of Tashi Namgyal or 'Moonbeams of Mahamudra', written in the 16th century.

Significantly, the claim is made by Brown that the distilled deep structures from his rigorous study are *universal* and operate across traditions. He states "[t]he models are sufficiently similar to suggest an *underlying common invariant sequence of stages*, despite vast cultural and linguistic differences as well as different styles of practice" (Wilber 2000a, p. 131, italics in original). They are in effect *trans-lineage*, while their 'surface' features differ, being variously expressed via the matrix of language, culture, social systems, self and biology, etc. Thus contrary to perennialists, who it is claimed fall prey to *the myth of the given* i.e., a lack of epistemic awareness in relation to the structuring of consciousness, where all paths are said to lead to the same enlightened end, Brown argues the evidence suggests "there is only one path but it has several outcomes, there are several kinds of enlightenment, although critically *all free awareness from psychological structure* [ego] *and alleviate suffering*" (Brown 1986, pp. 266–67, my italics) which is pertinent for our topic.

It can be noted also that these cartographies of liberation could analogously draw on Western models (Chirban 1986; Keating 2006, 2008), as found in the 'way of purification', the 'way of illumination' and the 'way of unification' (Underhill 2019), and indeed are included in Wilber's (2000a) integral psychological modelling. In the latter, around a third of one hundred plus comparative charts of human psychological development are contemplative systems, distilled from all the world's major wisdom traditions. Stanich's (2021) recent *Integral Christianity* for example also drinks heartily from the wells of the contemplative dimension of the Christian tradition.

It is noteworthy to highlight the significant post-post-modern or 'integral' nature of this claim, with its supposition of a universal underlying deep structural path. Although at first, this may sound similar to that long critiqued by postmodern scholars, the claim of access to universal deep structures purports to transcend, include and penetrate the postmodern critique of modern (surface) universals and essentialism. Distinct in both *surface* and *depth*, this universal claim may be appreciated within the epistemic and onto-logical assumptions of an *integral participative worldview* (as distinct from a modern and or postmodern worldview), which seeks to integrate knowledge and wisdom across 'east and west' in a timely and timeless manner (Di Perna 2014, n.192).

So if we assume, for the time being, the veracity of this global phenomenon of 'waking up', as testified, recorded and cultivated within our contemplative traditions beyond an exclusive identification with 'ego', which can be understood as a necessary but transitional stage in our development, we enter the contextual birthing canal (epistemic and ontological), wherein 'unique personhood' can emerge. In order to elaborate on this case, I will employ insights from developmental psychology, a significant recent emergent in the scheme of things, in contrast to the millennia of the contemplative traditions just referenced.

3. Adult Developmental Awareness

Suzanne Cook-Greuter (2010) within her seminal publication *Post Autonomous Ego Development*, taking due cognizance of many other adult developmental theories, grounds her own empirical work in the further development of Loevinger and Blasi's (1976) Ego Development Theory (EDT). Her research is widely applied in a myriad of contexts, including in education, business and leadership programmes, with an analysis completed on "more than 9000 tests in more than 200 different academic and business contexts" (McNamara 2013, p. 209). A clear observation from her model is that the goal of Western socialisation for fully functioning adults is what she calls, for relatively transparent reasons, the conscientious/achiever self. Save the requirement of subtle detailed distinctions, mutatis mutandis, this 'structure-stage' of adult development correlates with many other veins of associated research in the field, (Baldwin [1906] 2000; Piaget and Inhelder 1958; Kohlberg 1981; Fowler 1981; Gilligan 1982; Gebser 1985; Kegan 1998, 2009; Commons et al. 1998; Beck and Cowan 2006; Fischer and Bidell 2006; O'Fallon 2012; Torbert 2021). In brief, this *dynamic structure-stage* (as distinct from a common static misperception of 'structure as form') of adult development, can be understood as indicative of the 'scientific rational mind', with all its brilliance and probing capacity, which has led many of us to enjoy 'the goods' of modernity and 'progress'. This structure-stage defines what it is to be an adult from a Western perspective. However, from a developmental psychology perspective, it relies on an unchallenged 'big assumption' of a subject and object distinction. As Cook-Greuter (2013, p. 19) elaborates:

> By most modern Western expectations, fully functional adults see and treat reality as something preexistent and external to themselves made up of permanent, well-defined objects that can be analyzed, investigated, and controlled for our benefit...Most adults ... are not concerned with the basic arbitrariness of defining the objects. They are quite unaware that according to Koplowitz "the process of naming or measuring pulls that which is named out of reality, which itself is not nameable or measurable". They assume that subject and object are distinct, and that by analyzing the parts one can figure out the whole.

One potential takeway from the above is the recognition that our 'everyday reality' is not an ontological given, independent of our perspective. Such a 'naïve' view potentially falls prey to 'the myth of the given'. Rather, the supposition is that we 'enact' reality according to our developmental awareness. Those familiar with integral metatheory may recognize the more complex formulation of a tetra-enaction of reality, according to our AQAL+ shadow constellation (Murray 2015), a distillation of significant vectors, veins and occlusions in human development, with their systemic implications (Bhaskar et al. 2016). This includes at least a recognition of the developmental shaping influence of/on our bio-psycho-socio-cultural conditioning/conditions. Our enacted reality includes not simply our contemplative state-stage development, and what I am referring to as our 'level of being', but significantly also one's structure-stage of consciousness development, or our 'level of becoming'. What merely *subsists* at prior levels *exists* at emerging levels, as they are 'objectified' and become conscious. In short, the nature of such development entails the subject of one stage becoming the object of the subject of the next, and until this developmental transition, we are deemed to be embedded in our views. As Kegan

(2009, p. 52) articulates, "the subject-object relationship, becomes increasingly expansive at successive levels of mental capacity." A positive point to highlight is that empirical evidence from the developmentalists listed above and emerging work from (Murray 2020; Shannon and Frischherz 2020), with considerable nuance, accounting for complexity, simplicity, shadow and without falling prey to simple "growth to goodness" modeling, (Stein 2010), suggests an evolutionary potential towards a desired increased capacity for perspective taking, 'metathinking' and a more 'coherent' experience of reality. What is evident is that contemplative awareness (level of being) needs also to be acutely conscious of developmental perspectives (level of becoming) and their implications for how we view the world and interpret our respective contemplative traditions and their 'original' teachings.

The linkage of change leaders' (or therapists) 'action logics' or developmental levels to organisational transformation and/or with nuance to therapeutic transformation, constitutes a significant 'developmental intuition' within the literature (Forman 2010). According to Torbert's (2021) extensive work in the field, "the change leaders' personal developmental action-logic [when at these later levels, predicted 59% of the variance of the success] is the single most important factor in whether an organisation transforms" (ibid, p. 443). Similarly Brown (2011, p. 1) in "an empirical study of sustainability leaders, who hold post conventional consciousness", documents "how leaders and change agents, with a highly developed meaning making system, design and engage in sustainability initiatives" and lists "access [to] non [post]-rational ways of knowing and [their] use [of] systems, complexity, and integral theories", as a principal finding of his empirical research. Aligned with the above, Scharmer (2018, p. 7), in distilling a core insight from his transformation research, with beautiful simplicity posits, that "the success of an intervention depends on the interior condition of the intervener". While much could be said regarding 'post rational' ways of knowing, it may be optimal for contemplative practices aiming at 'deconstructing ego', to consciously align with developmental perspectival awareness, given its enactive role in cultivating these evidently transformative and effective interventionist capacities. And towards building what O'Fallon (2010) terms "natural therapeutic holding environments" to catalyse 'post-egoic' and personal development.

4. Developmental Implications for Contemplative Paths

Now, within the context of Eastern contemplative-'Enlightenment' teachings, from which Van Gordon et al. (2016) principally draw, a 'traditional' path predominantly assumes an 'impersonal' realisation of identification with 'Source', where 'one' is an expression of this Authentic Self and this Authentic self is One 'Being'. However, the metaphysical and ontological assumptions of traditional paths have been called into question by further developments in modern and postmodern scholarship, originating with Kant's (2008) critiques and the consequent 'turn to the subject' in philosophy i.e., epistemology. The subsequent intersubjective turn along with a compelling revindication and differentiation of ontology, from its prior pervasive conflation with epistemology, i.e., the "epistemic fallacy" (Bhaskar 1975, 2008, 2012), has led many to recognise the subtleties of a "post-metaphysical" perspective in the social sciences, philosophy and spirituality (Habermas and Cronin 2017; Wilber 2006, 2017; Murray 2019), which seeks to articulate and affirm 'truths claims', keenly aware of their fallibilistic and provisional nature, from a humbler perspective. And it is problematic, from an ontological and developmental perspective, to claim as Van Gordon et al. (2016, p. 1) do, that our "imputed self" or ego is a "maladaptive condition whereby an individual is addicted to the belief that they inherently exist".

Much confusion in Western spiritual circles can derive from the pearls and perils of traditional interpretations of Buddhist *no-self* teachings, which when not understood in its appropriate context can have a debilitating impact on attempts to efface the ego, rather than embrace an integrative developmental dynamic (Wilber 2000b, pp. 717–34). On one hand, we can note the adage that we first need to develop a strong healthy ego in order to transcend *and include* 'it' (noting (Van Gordon et al. 2016) *emphasis on transcend* alone), or risk attendant mental health issues (Engler 1986). We paradoxically note that the ego is implicated in the desire to eliminate the ego. Cook-Greuter (2013) cites Chogyam (2002) in *Cutting through Spiritual Materialism* as "perhaps the most cogent analysis of this mechanism," of how the ego is able to usurp ego transcendent moments or states, for its own vain glorification. Thus, while acutely acknowledging pervasive adult 'developmental issues' and the "impaired functionality" that the authors allude to, healthy 'ego development' can evidently be understood, au contraire to Van Gordon et al. as *adaptation* in action at a certain stage or stages in our psycho-spiritual growth (Cook-Greuter 2010). A matured awareness of 'ego states' can duly assist in catalysing ego-transcendence, with regard to integrating the 'individuating' and 'participative' functions of the psyche, which I will discuss further below. An array of contemporary spiritual authors and scholar-practitioners acknowledge, with nuance, that healthy ego development is a prerequisite stage(s), for balanced psycho-spiritual development, participatory enactment and is part of the gradual process of growing 'spiritual individuation', as cited in Ferrer (2017).

Perhaps more pertinently, from an ontological perspective, it is the case that *we always already assume we exist*, as to assume anything other than this involves a significant performative contradiction. This being the case insofar as our very actions reveal tacit assumptions, or a deeper belief, with which we may consciously theoretically disagree but nonetheless, can be excavated through our behaviour. As Bhaskar (2002, p. 70) suggests, "the source of the paradoxical nature of the self is as follows; whatever it is that is said about the self, there is something other than that which is tacitly presupposed", given that as Murray (2019) also reiterates, "all theories are underpinned by, usually tacit, ontological assumptions . . . which are deep, omnipresent and unavoidable". Therefore, if the ego (in the sense of EDT), is a necessary but insufficient stage(s) of our psycho-spiritual development and, as recognised by ego psychology, is 'a construct' (Loy 1999, 2002), what or who is it (without falling prey to transcendental reductionist assumptions), do we *inescapably* assume to 'be real', 'to exist' in ourselves and in each other?

5. Western Enlightenment

Conversely, in the Western Enlightenment tradition, one is alerted to an acute appreciation of the dignities of 'the individual', along with a recognition of the truly evolutionary and dialectical nature of our being and becoming. As Bhaskar (2002, p. 70) comments, "whatever the self is, it is clearly very important in contemporary society, being the bearer of legal, social, religious rights and responsibilities". This carries profound implications and is accompanied by the primary ethical injunction to treat 'each other' as an end in their selves, and to never instrumentalise each other as a means, echoing *the golden practice* or rule. This latter view is exemplified for instance in the societal outlawing of traditional slavery (as distinct from the ongoing systematic nature of 'modern slavery'), and the gradual enfranchisement and inclusion of respective 'out groups' and persons within society over the centuries and decades. This is in stark contrast to the simultaneous egregious dynamics of this enlightenment value of the individual being oppressed and 'one' being seen only as a means, to ideologically gratifying, warring and pervasive consumer ends (International Labour Office and United Nations Children's Fund 2021). In many respects we, at our peril, undervalue our 'personal rights' when failing to acknowledge their historical emergence as a significant recognition of not just a quantitative individual, but a qualitative affirmation and anticipation of our respective integrity of being.

And if *skillful means* connotes working within the context we find ourselves, an application of Buddhist psychology to western clients may do well to bear the bearer in mind, so to speak, while simultaneously recognising that the 'individualism' so valorised in western culture, is a mere shadow, a 'demi-reality' (Bhaskar et al. 2016) of what the western enlightenment's 'original insights' intimated (Taylor 1992). As the ethicist, Neil Levy (2018), maintains:

> With few exceptions, work on moral responsibility in the Anglophone world is resolutely individualist. The individual is not merely the primary unit of analysis and bearer of value; for the most part, individualism is taken for granted to such

an extent that philosophers are no more aware of their individualism than fish are of the water in which they swim.

In brief, the contention is that individualism, as a contemporary social phenomenon in large measure reflects a 'modern self', an ego identity, largely unaware of its own development, which through interdependent construction and shadow dynamics, plays out symptomatically and systemically in our historical moment. The social phenomena of hyper-individualism, narcissism, and relativism are a further intensification of these dynamics in our post-modern culture (Lasch 1979). We can, however, no longer ignore en-masse 'the bads' of modernity such as addiction rates, pollution, climate change, biodiversity loss and child labour for the production of many of our labelled consumer 'goods' and a host of other so called 'wicked problems', indicating symptoms of malaise, that have risen to variable levels of consciousness to characterise our epoch. According to the UN Human Development Report 2020, this age of the Anthropocene "means that we are the first people to live in an age defined by human choice, in which the dominant risk to our survival is ourselves".

And so, aligned with OAT's intent, Edwards (2016, p. 69), while expanding on this implication, remarks:

> Many of these predicaments are self-induced in that we believe in and utilise inadequate political, cultural, religious, scientific and commercial ideologies and their associated identities and practices to deal with these ills and consequently end up reproducing them in new and sometimes even more vicious forms. All this is taking a massive toll on the viability of the planets systems.

Problematic individualism is thus implicated in addiction and no less the Anthropocene. As ironic as it may initially seem, the remedy for individualism and our 'self-induced' predicaments, is a thoroughgoing individuation. Healthy individuation can be understood as an integration of contemplative awareness, where a more conscious union, communion with ones 'ground', 'being' and/or the whole is cultivated, beyond an exclusive identification with the ego, with an acute perspectival awareness, as reflected in the adult developmental literature cited above. It is an invitation for all, by virtue of our 'humanity', akin to that which the integral scholar Stein (2019, p. 274, italics in original) recounts, in that:

> the Judeo-Christian tradition contains a radical enlightenment teaching, with a message about the collective awakening of *everyone everywhere* ... an Absolute Democracy in which each must live so that all will have the ability and dignity to be heard, known and counted. [And pertinently given our topic] ... the core innovation enabling the democratisation of enlightenment ... *is the reclaiming of the personal*".

6. Personal Perspectival Awareness

Thus, the contention emerges that the conflation of the 'personal' with the 'ego' is an unnecessary confusion, and potentially necessitates a catalytic re-orientation in ones 'self-system'. As Stein (ibid, p. 275) further notes, "the universal finds its expression only in and through an infinite variety of uniquely personal forms". This is significant insofar as our present spiritual landscapes are replete with traditional perspectival teachings conflating the personal and egoic, with all attendant risks for abuse and dehumanisation, when 'personal qualities' and an integrity of being are effaced and dissolved (ASI 2021). Notably Ken Wilber (Gafni 2012, p. 398, my italics) has recently awoken to this realisation in that even in non-dual states when:

> you are one with everything that is arising...you still feel a Unique Perspective on how this arises in your experience. [which] would *traditionally be interpreted* as an egoic holdover ... [and] *prevent you from acting in the world on that uniqueness*. And all that really does is gum up action completely.

Wilber (ibid, my italics) thus posits:

> [T]he one true self is realising for the first time that it can manifest and embody in all these different perspectives and *not just force all of them to be reduced to the perspective of the One True Self'* ... there's still just One True Self and it's the same I AMness arising in all these perspectives *that makes them real*.

A subtle recognition of the pitfalls of *transcendental reductionism* is evident here, whereby, as mentioned prior, the many are reduced to the One, and it is assumed, there are 'no real many'. In this awakening process Wilber thus discloses a pithy pointer, insofar as the realisation of *True self + Perspective = Unique Self*. He celebrates this individuation process in that, "[T]his formula ... suddenly lights up all the individuality of the individual organism that had previously gotten wiped out [deconstructed] on the [traditional] way to discovering the One True Self" (ibid).

Gafni (2012) further emphasises the 'personal' nature of this 'unique self' insofar as he distinguishes levels of the personal, and makes the distinction between a conventional appreciation, level 1 personal, a egoic sense of self, and level 2 personal, which transcends a separate sense of self into communion, union with Self, whilst recognising that Self has "a personal face living in you, as you, through you" (ibid, p. xxvi) He describes the Unique Self not as a concept but:

> ... a quality of presence when the ego is set aside, -even temporarily- ... In Christianity this exercises itself as the personal relationship with Jesus Christ that so many sectors of Christendom understand so profoundly-and which is so derided by New Age teachers caught up in the impersonality of so much misunderstood Eastern teaching. In Hinduism the goddesses hold you in radical personal embrace. In classical Judaism the G-o-d loves you and knows your name while in Sufism and Kabbalah she is your most intimate erotic partner. None of this is dogma. It is the first and second person personal realisation that the interior of the face of the kosmos (sic) is the infinity of intimacy. And it is the revelation of the infinite, who yearns to love you personally and uniquely. (Gafni 2012, p. 109)

The supposition here is that this *personal perspectival awareness* was not well understood by traditional contemplative paths, and that it is a relatively recent 'recognition', rigorously researched and articulated, by adult developmental psychology, as referenced above. Personhood thus in the sense employed here, may be tentatively understood as this ontologically assumed, *pre-sense*, that brings *coherence, co-creativity, unity, value and meaning* to our many 'moving parts', in our interaction with our 'environment'. As humans we are compound interdependent beings, as testified by even a meagre appreciation of our present knowledge that 'normal matter', the 0.5% visible portion of our double dark or lambda Λ CDM Universe, is constituent of our very physical bodies, which are ever growing and changing. We are creatures with 'will', 'emotions', 'feelings', 'brain', 'mind', 'memory', 'states', 'intellect', 'multiple intelligences', 'soul', and 'spirit'. All of these to variable degrees in relation to/with/in our surrounding society-systems-environment-nature-cosmos and with other living beings and humans. While we can readily testify to the experience of people (and systems) 'falling apart', 'breaking down', and all the attendant developmentally related physical, emotional, mental, spiritual and social health issues (not least addiction in all its guises), the extent to which we also cohere and unify these parts of our being and becoming is quite extraordinary. Indeed, it might be argued that this objective of cultivating *coherence* is at the very heart of our contemplative and psychological traditions.

Personhood may thus be understood as that unifying and mediating quality that integrates our parts into a meaningful whole, and it is from that pre-sense of 'wholeness' that we can truly and deeply connect and feel connected with others, 'systems' and nature, through a sense of continuity and identity in who we are, while many of our parts can change over time. Indeed, Bhaskar (2012, p. 168) claims that "unless [we] were in [non-dual, unitive] state[s] at least some of the time, you could not do or be anything at all". As he (ibid) points out:

Notice ... in ... your moment of reading, listening, hearing, following me, your moment of communion, not just your ego, ... but your body dropped away ... your cravings, the blind tenacity of your belief in the (exhaustive) physicality of being. And still you were you.

We recognise our family members for who they still are, while so many of the moving parts can and do change. People 'change their minds' regularly about matters and/or grow old as their bodies change. This may of course be extremely challenging as in the case of dementia, where there is a 'loss of self' and other parts of the person, when symptoms like amnesia, agnosia, aphasia and apraxia, etc., are present. However, research in the field, even in the case of advanced dementia, gleans qualitative reports of feeling "still the same" as before its onset, and for ensuring optimal care, strongly advocate that of "utmost importance is that other persons understand that persons with advanced dementia still are persons and support them to feel valuable" (Norberg 2019). Thus, the personal can be understood as relative individuation within the whole and is to be cultivated rather than conflated with the ego, as it implicitly is, in OAT's conventional interpretation.

7. Radical Ontology

John Heron's (1992) theory of personhood, with its extended epistemology, supports the ontological view being proposed here and proposes that core polarities of the psyche toward individuation or participation evolve somewhat predictably within patterned states, as a person matures and learns to balance and harmonise the two modes. He describes the ego as "that experience, [and/or 'state'] where we are out of balance, insofar as we are overidentified with the individuating mode at the expense of the participative". While a lack of space will not facilitate for an in-depth exploration of the implicating causal factors, it is interesting to note *the participative function* and the associated nuanced understanding of 'feeling', as distinct from 'emotion', is described by Heron (ibid, p.16) as:

> the capacity of the psyche to participate in wider unities of being, to become at one with the differential content of a whole field of experience, to indwell what is present through attunement and resonance, and to know its own distinctness, while unified with the differentiated other. This is the domain of empathy, indwelling, participation, presence, resonance and such like.

Heron's (1998, p. xi), model thus critically presupposes:

> ... the human person [as] a distinct spiritual presence in and non-separable from the given cosmos and as such is not to be reduced to, or confused with, an illusory, separate, contracted and egoic self, with which personhood can become temporarily identified.

This echoes Teilhard De Chardin's (1959) profound contention that the artificial separation between humans and cosmos, lies at the root of our contemporary moral confusion. Jorge Ferrer (2017, p. 15) similarly emphasises the "key difference between modern individualism and spiritual individuation is thus the integration of radical relatedness in the later". The practical and ethical significance of such a 'radical ontology' of personhood cannot be overstated, insofar as 'we-space' research (Gunnlaugson and Brabant 2016) also signals how profoundly such an ontology impacts on collaborative success (or lack thereof) in groups, teams, organisations, communities and indeed, given our 'metacrises' (Rowson and Pascal 2021) one might add for, 'nations'. As McCallum et al. (2016) states, with relevance to an ethic of care:

> For us as practitioners, this philosophical view of differentiated and yet unified field of consciousness provides a way of understanding the radically interdependent nature of relationships between parts and whole, individuals and groups, and sub groups within larger and larger collectives ... in the instance of individuals who are recognised with genetic or social "frailties", the degree to which a community understands these individuals not as "other", but as being

integral parts of a larger whole will determine approaches to care, allocation and resources, etc.

The distinction of the 'person', with a core "capacity for feeling" as a spiritual presence and the 'ego', as an alienated part of the psyche "over identified with the individuating mode at the expense of the participative", is understood as an emergent experience within Heron's "states of personhood" (Heron 1992, p. 53). Heron's work strongly correlates with other literature and research within 'the field' (Merry 2020), a selection of which have been cited above. Heron too takes substantive ontological issue with the seeming, hegemonic transcendental reductionism of some traditional eastern teachings, as in the OAT's interpretation, and their implications i.e., positing that "the many are reduced to the one via the concept of illusion: there are no Real many, only the unreal many, illusionary selves that ultimately disappear in the light of the One" (ibid, p. 10). Heron (1998, p. 80, italics in original) critiques this view as "a *repeal* of a conservative creation model," as distinct from cognising the profound import of an evolutionary worldview, for all the contemplative traditions, as exemplified in the momentous, but still relatively unknown 'Fourth Turning' in Buddhism, as we shall observe shortly. Interestingly Aurobindo (2005, p. 482), while echoing the premise in OAT, "[t]he one thing that can be described as an unreal reality is our individual sense of separativeness (sic) and the conception of the finite as a self-existent object in the Infinite,"also critically asserts:

[t]he true Person is not an isolated entity, his individuality is universal; for he individualises the universe: it is at the same time divinely emergent in a spiritual air of transcendental infinity, like a high cloud-surpassing summit; for he individualises the divine Transcendence, (ibid, p. 1008).

Heron (1998, p. 79) is thus concerned that "in elevating the human to the absolute, it ignores the asymmetrical relation between the finite and the infinite" ..and regards it in his model, as "an illusionary state of spiritual inflation". He (ibid, p. 82) thus maintains that "it is important to challenge these claims for the very good reason that they can, for a while at any rate, intimidate and disempower some people from making deep, creative choices about their own spiritual path".

It is also noteworthy is this context that while Van Gordon et al. (2016) qualify a psychopathologising of "belief in god," the assumption from "the Buddhist perspective" that "a belief in a divine and/or ruling being requires that there is a self," is problematic in conception and practice. It is also somewhat ironic in the context of the very aims of OAT, as it is precisely an integrative appreciation of '2nd person concepts of Spirit', or an 'i-thou' 'devotional' practice (central also in Tibetan Buddhism) which potentially recognises higher-deeper, broader, transcendent, immanent and situational levels of thou, "that before which the ego is humbled," (Wilber 2006, p. 160) and which facilitates the cultivation of the 'other' centered favourable character traits, espoused in the OAT approach. As Wilber (2006, ibid) expresses, "[i]n short failing to acknowledge your own Spirit in 2nd-person is a repression of a dimension of your being-in-the world". While we can no doubt acknowledge a pervasive developmental conflation of 'God' with traditional mythic perspectives alone, a developmental orientation which appreciates the '123 of God' (ibid, p. 161), or first person, second person and third person approaches, integrally recognising perspectives and depth, 'East and West' is *more becoming* in a conscious evolutionary age (Corless and Knitter 1990).

Stein (2019, p. 279) likewise notes "the widespread failure to understand this radical truth about the [democratic and personal] nature of enlightenment has kept it from being a legitimate modern belief and aspiration". In a similar vein, De Chardin (1959, p. 283) makes an explicit cultural connection between the discovery of "the sidereal world, so vast" and what he refers to as the *depersonalisation* or *impersonalisation* of modern man, echoing more contemporary insights and remedies from the cosmology of Abrams and Primack (2011) where instead of 'modern humans' feeling lost and insignificant in the vast cosmos, we appreciate our profound integrality with the whole. De Chardin (ibid, p. 285) maintained:

> [F]ar from being mutually exclusive, the Universal and Personal (that is to say 'centred') grow in the same direction and culminate simultaneously in each other. It is therefore a mistake to look for the extension of our being or of the noosphere in the Impersonal.

Fittingly, de Chardin poses the question, "what is the work or works of man if not to establish, in and by each one of us, an absolute original centre in which the Universe reflects itself in a unique and imitable way?" (ibid, p. 287). This characteristic of evolution, he claims, is underscored in any domain, "whether it be the cells of the body, the members of a society or the elements of a spiritual synthesis", (ibid, p. 288) in the principle *union differentiates*. Teilhard thus maintained:

> [T]he peak of ourselves, the acme of our originality, is not our individuality [ego as over identified with the individuating function] but our person; and according to the evolutionary structure of the world, we can only find our person by uniting together...[though] not every kind of union will do ... it is centre to centre that must make contact and *not otherwise* ... [as] the true ego grows in inverse proportion to 'egoism' (ibid, pp. 289, 290).

8. Evolutionary Awareness-A Fourth Turning of Buddhism

The generative implications of our present developing awareness that we live in a vast evolutionary universe is shaping what many are now referring to as the 'Fourth Turning' in Buddhism (Wilber 2014) and somewhat contrary to that which Van Gordon et al. (2016) suggest, regarding interpretations of prior turnings, may well amount to significantly more than another "variation on the same theme" (ibid, p. 4). It may indeed hold significant import for interpretations of "no-self" teachings, the "innermost aspect of consciousness", "transmigration" and "*pashchimadharma* [Sanskrit] or *mappō* [Japanese]" teachings, not discounting their relative insights, within the consciousness of a vast evolving and conrnucopian universe. Indeed each developmental structural stage of 'spiritual intelligence' governs how persons interpret their contemplative/spiritual experience and/or their respective traditions, with a recognition that "the very core of the enlightenment experience will change from stage to stage," (Wilber 2017, p. 9) as we enter anew the hermeneutic circle, moment to moment (Panikkar 1979).

As the reader may recall, in brief, the First major Turning of the Buddhist wheel of dharma refers to the teachings of Siddharta Guatama, represented by Theravāda Buddhism. The Second Turning refers to Nāgārjuna's teaching on 'emptiness', sūnyatā, within the Madhyamika and foundational for the Mahāyāna and Vajrayana schools. The Third Turning focuses its teachings on 'Buddha nature', or *tathāgatagarbha*, embryonic Buddhahood, implying 'enlightenment' is our true and natural state of mind and is represented by the Yogācāra school. This contemporary Fourth Turning of the Buddhist wheel of dharma, (or variously Fifth, if counting tantric/esoteric Buddhism) includes our own era's ongoing discovery of 'evolutionary theory'. It therefore recognizes that the very world of 'form', is itself evolving and if as previously taught, 'emptiness and form' are not two, i.e., nondual, the Fourth Turning in essence recognises that 'emptiness and evolving form', are not two, i.e., nondual. This same complexification of form (for e.g., from strings, quarks, atoms, molecules, to cells, to multicellular organisms, etc.,) is also occuring in humans as attested by the literature referenced, indicated not least by our increasing developmental capacity for perspectival awareness. Thus the supposition is that while tradtional enlightenment remains unchanged in its *Freedom* (Emptiness) aspect, its *Fullness* (Form) has evidently continued to evolve. And as the formula of true self plus perspective indicated, the realised 'true self' is now being expressed in this Fourth Turning through what Wilber refers to as "a post egoic nondual realisation of unique perspective", (Gafni 2012, p. xx) with its attendant ontological, personal and ethical import, as depicted above.

9. Conclusions

Van Gorden et al.'s Ontological Addiction theory presently understood as "the maladaptive condition whereby an individual is addicted to the belief that they inherently exist" risks being enmeshed in a performative contradiction. This is related to an implicit transcendetal reductionsist assumption that is operative in its conception. Any assimilation and an application through skillful means to mental health within a western context will also seek to integrate the insights of the Western Enlightenment and the value of the individual. Critically, this entails a developmental appreciation of the problematic perception of egoic individualism as distinct from the conception of an individuating 'whole person', with ontological import. Thus OAT could positively be supplemented, reconstructed and reconceived as an Ontological Affirmation Theory.

Van Gordon et al. (2016) are correct when they indicate that present mainstream western bio-psycho-social models of medical and scientific opinion are inadequate and operate somewhat broader but shallower in comparison to Buddhist psychology, in their core assumptions of the determinants of psychopathology. This, however, chiefly owes to the lack of a depth ontology in mainstream western models and the incompletion of their own enlightenment project, which critially needs to source its contemplative wellsprings for sustenance, given a present pervasive pyschopathology (in the imparied functional rather than statistical sense) of individualism.

However in contradistinction to Van Gordon et al. (ibid) 'the ego' as perceived through a thoroughgoing developmental lens can be understood as already potentially 'adaptive', insofar as the literature indicates, 'it' evidentially evolves and potentially matures, into a full and flourishing integrative (individuating and participative) personhood. This is aligned with Van Gordon et al.'s (2016) "dynamic and non-dual self", but is critically distinctive, insofar as it affirms and explicitates the radical ontological and ethical implications.

A potential course corrective for OAT, from its implict trancendental reductionism is applicable, if the profound implications of an evolutionary worldview are integrated within the contemplative tradition it draws upon. This is pointedly exemplified and foreshadowed by the momentous Fourth Turning in Buddhism, along with more recent findings in adult developmental psychology, providing possible diagnostic markers in relation to the "therapeutic (and spiritual) discernment [that] is clearly required in order to assess the suitability of a particular individual to receive, and progress through, the various (generic) treatment phases outlined in [their] paper," (ibid, p. 27).

While aligned with Van Gordon et al. (2016) in recognising the core sense of lack that invariably accompanies an egoic sense of self, and its resultant endless cravings for external fullfillment, such as 'addictions' in a myriad of forms, the excavation of inescapable ontological presuppositions, as outlined, reveals who we are, as *persons*, can act as a potential course corrective, to avoid the possible pitfalls of transcendental reductionsim and the oft accompanying egoic inflations and deflations, when the pearls of 'no-self' become perilous. It also underscores a real 'integrity of our being' as we progressively realise the profound evolutionary and participatory insight that 'the whole universe' is, not least evidently in 'the material sense', already in us and we in the whole. Or as Van Gordon et al. (2016, p. 24) somewhat ironically relay it, "[a] person who has realized true self cares for the individual because they care for the whole, and vice versa". Would that they also make explicit the associated ontological presuppositions apt to cultivate and sustain this ethic of care, especially for those who inescapably assume 'themselves' to exist and *be real*.

Funding: This research received no external funding.

Conflicts of Interest: The author declares no conflict of interest.

References

Abrams, Nancy Ellen, and Joel Primack. 2011. *The New Universe and the Human Future: How a Shared Cosmology Could Transform the World*. New Haven: Yale University Press.

ASI. 2021. Code-of-Ethics-for-Individuals. Available online: https://www.spiritual-integrity.org/wp-content/uploads/2021/05/Association-for-Spiritual-Integrity-Code-of-Ethics-for-Individuals-5-16-2021 (accessed on 1 August 2021).
Aurobindo. 2005. *The Life Divine*. Pondicherry: Ashram Press.
Baldwin, James Mark. 2000. *Thoughts and Things: A Study of the Development and Meaning of Thought or Genetic Logic*. London: Elibron Classics, vol. 1. First published 1906.
Beck, Don, and Chris Cowan. 2006. *Spiral Dynamics. Mastering Values Leadership and Change*. Oxford: Blackwell Publishing.
Bhaskar, Roy. 1975. Forms of Realism. *Philosophica* 15: 99–127.
Bhaskar, Roy. 2002. *Reflections on Metareality. Transcendence, Emancipation and Everyday Life*. New York: Routledge.
Bhaskar, Roy. 2008. *A Realist Theory of Science*. New York: Routledge.
Bhaskar, Roy. 2012. *The Philosophy of MetaReality. Creativity, Love, Freedom*. New York: Routledge.
Bhaskar, Roy, Sean Esbjorn Hargens, Nicholas Hedlund, and Martin Hartwig, eds. 2016. *Metatheory for the Twenty-First Century. Critical Realism and Integral Theory in Dialogue*. Oxon: Routledge.
Brown, Daniel P. 1986. The Stages of Meditation in Cross-Cultural Perspective. In *Transformations of Consciousness: Conventional and Contemplative Perspectives on Development*. Edited by Ken Wilber, Jack Engler and Daniel P. Brown. Boston: New Science Library.
Brown, Barrett. 2011. An Empirical Study of Sustainability Leaders Who Hold Post Conventional Consciousness. Available online: http://integralthinkers.com/wp-content/uploads/Brown-2011-empirical-study-of-sustainability-leaders (accessed on 7 July 2021).
Chirban, John. 1986. Developmental Stages in Eastern Orthodox Christianity. In *Transformations of Consciousness: Conventional and Contemplative Perspectives on Development*. Edited by Ken Wilber, Jack Engler and Daniel P. Brown. Boston: New Science Library.
Chogyam, Trungpa. 2002. *Cutting through Spiritual Materialism*. Boston: Shambhala.
Commons, Michael Lamport, Edward James Trudeau, Sharon Anne Stein, Francis Asbury Richards, and Sharon R. Krause. 1998. Hierarchical Complexity of Tasks Shows the Existence of Developmental Stages. *Developmental Review* 18: 237–78. [CrossRef]
Cook-Greuter, Susanne. 2010. Post-Autonomous Ego Development: A Study of Its Nature and Measurement. Available online: https://www.proquest.com/openview/f556d7e8eac2be50b959c2d69a281399/1?pq-origsite=gscholar&cbl=18750&diss=y (accessed on 3 July 2021).
Cook-Greuter, Susanne. 2013. The Nine Stages of Increasing Embrace in Ego Development: A full Spectrum Theory of Vertical Growth and Meaning Making. Available online: www.cook-greuter.com (accessed on 3 July 2021).
Corless, Roger, and Paul Knitter. 1990. *Buddhist Emptiness and Christian Trinity. Essays and Explorations*. New York: Paulist Press.
De Chardin, Teilhard. 1959. *The Phenomenon of Man*. New York: Harper and Row.
Di Perna, Dustin. 2014. Streams of Wisdom. Available online: https://sites.google.com/a/fy.books-now.com/en272/9780989228992-84mentaGEtincma97 (accessed on 3 July 2021).
Edwards, Mark. 2016. Healing the half-world. Ideology and the emancipatory potential of meta-level social science. In *Metatheory for the Twenty-First Century*. Edited by Roy Bhaskar, Sean Esbjorn Hargens, Nicholas Hedlund and Martin Hartwig. Oxon: Routledge.
Engler, Jack. 1986. Therapeutic aims in Psychotherapy and Meditation: Developmental Stages in The Representation of Self. In *Transformations of Consciousness. Conventional and Contemplative Perspectives on Development*. Edited by Ken Wilber, Jack Engler and Daniel P. Brown. Boston: Shambhala.
Ferrer, Jorge N. 2017. *Participation and the Mystery. Transpersonal Essays in Psychology, Education and Religion*. Albany: SUNY Press.
Fischer, Kurt W., and Thomas R. Bidell. 2006. Dynamic Development of Action, Thought, And Emotion. In *Handbook of Child Psychology. Theoretical Models of Human Development*. Edited by William Damon and Richard M Lerner. New York: Wiley, pp. 313–99.
Forman, Mark D. 2010. *A Guide to Integral Psychotherapy, Complexity, Integration and Spirituality in Practice*. New York: SUNY.
Fowler, James. 1981. *Stages of Faith: The Psychology of Human Development and the Quest for Meaning*. New York: Harper Collins.
Gafni, Marc. 2012. *Your Unique Self, The Radical Path to Personal Enlightenment*. Tucson, AZ: Integral Publishers.
Gebser, Jean. 1985. *The Ever-Present Origin*. Athens, Ohio: Ohio University Press.
Gilligan, Carol. 1982. *In a Different Voice: Psychological Theory and Women's Development*. Cambridge, Mass: Harvard University Press.
Gunnlaugson, Olen, and Michael Brabant. 2016. Engaging Collective Emergence, Wisdom and Healing in Groups. In *Cohering the Integral We Space*. US Integral Publishing House.
Habermas, Jürgen, and Ciaran Cronin. 2017. *Postmetaphysical Thinking*. Cambridge: Polity Press.
Heron, John. 1992. *Personhood and Feeling. Psychology in Another Key*. London: Sage Publications Ltd.
Heron, John. 1998. *Sacred Science. Person-Centered Inquiry into Spiritual and the Subtle*. Aukland: Enduymion Press.
International Labour Office and United Nations Children's Fund. 2021. *Child Labour: Global estimates 2020, Trends and the Road Forward*. New York: ILO and UNICEF.
Kant, Immanuel. 2008. *Kant's Critiques: The Critique of Pure Reason, the Critique of Practical Reason, the Critique of Judgement*. Radford: Wilder Publications.
Keating, Thomas. 2006. *Open Mind Open Heart*. New York: Continuum International publishing Group.
Keating, Thomas. 2008. *Spirituality, Contemplation, Transformation.Writings on Centering Prayer*. New York: Lantern Books.
Kegan, Robert. 1998. *In Over Our Heads: The Mental Demands of Modern Life*. Cambridge: Harvard University Press.
Kegan, Robert. 2009. *Immunity to Change. How to Overcome it and Unlock Potential in Yourself and Your Organisation*. Boston: Harvard Business Press.

Kohlberg, Lawrence. 1981. *Essays on Moral Development, Vol. I: The Philosophy of Moral Development*. San Francisco: Harper & Row.
Lasch, Christopher. 1979. *The Culture of Narcissism: American Life in an Age of Diminishing Expectations*. New York: Warner Books.
Levy, Neil. 2018. Socializing Responsibility. In *Social Dimensions of Moral Responsibility*. Edited by Hutchison Katrina, Mackenzie Catriona and Oshana Marina. Oxford: Oxford University Press.
Loevinger, Jane, and Augusto Blasi. 1976. *Ego Development: [Conceptions and Theories]*. San Francisco: Jossey-Bass Publishers.
Loy, David. 1999. *Lack and Transcendence. The Problem of Death and Life in Psychotherapy, Existentialism and Buddhism*. New York: Humanity Books.
Loy, David. 2002. *A Buddhist History of The West*. New York: Suny Press.
McCallum, David, Aliki Nicolaides, and Lyle Yorks. 2016. Exploring the Ego at the Boundary of the I and the We. In *Cohering the Integral We-Space*. Edited by Olen Gunnlaugson and Michael Brabant. US Integral Publishing House.
McNamara, Robert. 2013. *The Elegant Self: A Radical Approach to Personal Evolution for Greater Influence In Life*. Boulder: Performance Integral.
Merry, Peter. 2020. *Leading from the Field*. Minneapolis: Amaranth Press.
Murray, Tom. 2015. Contemplative Dialogue Practices: An Inquiry into Deep Interiority, Shadow Work and Insight. *Integral Leadership Review*. Available online: Integralleadershipreview.com (accessed on 16 July 2021).
Murray, Tom. 2019. Knowing and Unknowing Reality—A Beginner's and Expert's Developmental Guide to Post-Metaphysical Thinking. *Integral Review*. 15. Available online: https://integral-review.org (accessed on 12 July 2021).
Murray, Tom. 2020. Metamodernism, Complexity, Simplicity, and Wisdom. *Dispatches from a Time Between Worlds: Crisis and Emergence in Metamodernity*. Edited by John Rowson and Layman Pascal. Available online: https://www.perspegrity.com/papers.html (accessed on 10 July 2021).
Norberg, Astrid. 2019. *Sense of Self among Persons with Advanced Dementia. Alzheimer's Disease*. Edited by Thomas Wisniewski. Brisbane, AU: Codon Publications. [CrossRef]
O'Fallon, Terri. 2010. The Evolution of the Human Soul: Developmental Practices in Spiritual Guidance. Available online: www.pacificintegral.com (accessed on 3 July 2021).
O'Fallon, Terri. 2012. StAGES: Growing up Is Waking Up. Interpenetrating Quadrants, States and Structures. Available online: www.pacificintegral.com (accessed on 3 July 2021).
Panikkar, Raimon. 1979. *Myth, Faith and Hermeneutics*. New York: Paulist Press.
Piaget, Jean, and Bärbel Inhelder. 1958. *The Growth of Logical Thinking from Childhood to Adolescence*. New York: Basic Books.
Rowson, Jonathan, and Layman Pascal. 2021. *Dispatches From A Time Between Worlds*. La Vergne: Perspectiva.
Scharmer, C. Otto. 2018. *The Essentials of Theory U: Core Principles and Applications*. Oakland: Berrett-Koehler Publishers, Incorporated.
Shannon, Nick, and Bruno Frischherz. 2020. *Metathinking, The Art and Practice of Transformational Thinking*. Cham: Springer.
Stanich, Roland Michael. 2021. *Integral Christianity. The Way of Embodied Love*. Randwick: Bright Alliance.
Stein, Zak. 2010. On the Use of the Term Integral. Available online: www.integralthinkers.com (accessed on 3 July 2021).
Stein, Zak. 2019. Education in a Time between Worlds. Available online: https://sites.google.com/site/gilredupzade3/9780986282676-54clamefGEprobver38 (accessed on 3 July 2021).
Taylor, Charles. 1992. *Sources of the Self. The Making of Modern Identity*. New York: Cambridge University Press.
Torbert, William R. 2021. *Numbskull in The Theatre Of Inquiry: Transforming Self, Friends, Organisations, and Social Science*. Cardiff, CA: Waterside Productions.
Underhill, Evelyn. 2019. *Mysticism. A Study in the Nature and Development of Mans Spiritual Consciousness*. Abingdon: Routledge.
Van Gordon, William, Edo Shonin, Giulia Cavalli, and Mark D Griffiths. 2016. Ontological addiction: Classification, aetiology and treatment. *Mindfulness* 7: 660–71. [CrossRef]
Wilber, Ken. 2000a. *Integral Psychology: Consciousness, Spirit, Psychology, Therapy*. Boston: Shambhala.
Wilber, Ken. 2000b. *Sex Ecology and Spirituality: The Spirit of Evolution*. Boston: Shambhala.
Wilber, Ken. 2006. *Integral Spirituality. A Startling New Role for Religion in the Modern and Postmodern World*. Boston: Shambhala.
Wilber, Ken. 2014. *The Fourth Turning. Imagining the Evolution of Integral Buddhism*. Boston and London: Shambala.
Wilber, Ken. 2017. *The Religion Of Tomorrow*. Boston: Shambhala.

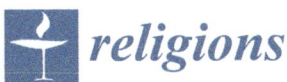

Article

Spiritual Addiction: Searching for Love in a Coldly Indifferent World

Garret B. Wyner

The Chicago School of Professional Psychology, Los Angeles, CA 90017, USA; garretwyner@mac.com

Abstract: I describe "spiritual" addiction as a felt compulsion to seek surrogates in the absence of that spirit of unconditional love underlying core personality change. We awaken to a "real" world akin to a prison in which all sides seem morally compromised, so any choice seems to necessitate sacrificing our conscientious relationship to the truth. Thus, spiritual addiction runs deeper than physical and psychological addictions to include socially accepted "addictions" to all we associate with "success"—including our morality and religion. All that we seek may be grounded in a collectively imbibed prejudice toward truth itself. If so, such a prejudice, underlying spiritual addiction, compromises our will, reason, feelings, actions, and character—including all of our relationships. It underlies the reality of a collective *moral* crisis which, we show, is more deeply a *religious* crisis tempting us to doubt the reality and attainability of that unconditional love that provides a foundation for hope. To overcome the prejudice underlying spiritual addiction, we show how unconditional love can be realized by placing conscientiousness in the foreground of concern as we are guided by the most reliable moral and spiritual witnesses in our history distinct from any religious group claiming to speak in their name.

Keywords: spiritual addiction; faith; truth; hope; reason; religion; love; reality; collective moral crisis

---

Citation: Wyner, Garret B. 2022. Spiritual Addiction: Searching for Love in a Coldly Indifferent World. *Religions* 13: 300. https://doi.org/10.3390/rel13040300

Academic Editors: Bernadette Flanagan and Noelia Molina

Received: 22 August 2021
Accepted: 27 March 2022
Published: 30 March 2022

Publisher's Note: MDPI stays neutral with regard to jurisdictional claims in published maps and institutional affiliations.

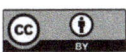

Copyright: © 2022 by the author. Licensee MDPI, Basel, Switzerland. This article is an open access article distributed under the terms and conditions of the Creative Commons Attribution (CC BY) license (https://creativecommons.org/licenses/by/4.0/).

"Most of us achieve only at rare moments a clear realization of the fact that they have never tasted the fulfillment of existence, that their life does not participate in true, fulfilled existence, that, as it were, it passes true existence by. We nevertheless feel the deficiency at every moment, and in some measure strive to find—somewhere—what we are seeking". (Buber 1958, p. 172)

1. Introduction

In this paper, I describe spiritual addiction as a felt compulsion to seek surrogates in the absence of a spirit of unconditional love. This paper will demonstrate how the presence of unconditional love is paramount to core personality change—and how its surrogates, as manifested in various forms of addiction, are rooted in a collective prejudice toward truth itself.

Let us consider the following illustration. The adult daughter of my first psychoanalyst once lovingly referred to him as a "spiritual atheist", which he welcomed. Apparently, there was something about "spirituality" in its contextual connection with his atheism that allowed him to separate it from religion while also enabling him to avoid a wholesale physicalist reduction of the distinctive value of human life. As I took it, he liked to see himself portrayed as a person of character, devoted to the pursuit of truth or, in the language of existentialists, an "atheist of good faith". By contrast, I was once asked by a small group of Christian philosophers what I was working on at that time. I said I was doing independent research on true and false religion in light of the Holocaust and the testimony of a sub-group of Holocaust witnesses, such as Primo Levi, Jean Amery, and others whom I regarded as "atheists of good faith"—even prophetic-type "witnesses"—of an event I believe has cosmic significance for humanity in view of what it reveals about the moral condition of humanity today.[1] They looked confused, perhaps shocked, which quickly morphed into a look of disdain. For "good faith", from their perspective, only applied to religious believers, if not solely to Christians, Protestants, or their particular Protestant denominational sub-group. Of course, my analyst would say the opposite is true: that a theist or "believer of good faith" is an oxymoron.[2] Religious faith seemed to him so manifestly separable from the spirit of a truly good or moral life that only a person governed by blind and/or bad faith could claim otherwise.

How could such a disparity of viewpoints be understood, much less reconciled, if at all? How is it understood and resolved in any case? Consider a couple seeing a therapist in hope of reconciling their marital conflicts. As each partner expresses their point of view, one might think they were from different planets: each side seems fixated on defending themselves by blaming the other. Each uses whatever form and measure of truth or power they can to try to convince themselves, if not their partner and the therapist that they are right and the other is wrong. Reason itself is being used as a cosmic servant, or what Martin Buber called a "thing-like object" or "It" to advance one's own agenda. We have here a form of *faith-in-reason* rather than *faith-in-truth*.

What is the therapist to do? If they are familiar with Aristotle's maxim that in most disputes the truth typically lies somewhere in the middle,[3] they know that the conflict cannot be reconciled insofar as even one of the partners is defensively closed off from empathically seeing and acknowledging truth on the other side. That is, that without a genuinely good faith, or faith-in-truth attitude placed above one's felt need to be right, there can be no reconciliation. Without this, the partners are not "arguing" in the sense of rationally collaborating to see and embrace a more comprehensive truth. To counteract this warfare, the therapist ideally role models such a good faith attitude, i.e., a spirit or character governed by sincerity, empathy, and unconditional love.[4] They provide a safe environment in which the patients are influenced—not compelled—to lay down their defenses and open themselves to see the truths on both sides. Little by little, they begin to trust that truth itself is not against them and that it is only by opening themselves up to increasingly see more clearly a more comprehensive truth that their conflict can be resolved. They may even discover that together they might realize an even higher good then they could alone. Increasingly, they are enabled to not only see but internalize that spirit of unconditional love underlying core personality change.

By unconditional love, I mean something that includes isolated good intentions and actions and good character traits (which Aristotle (1962) called virtues) but also transcends these. I mean a foundation-level state or condition of fidelity toward truth itself, i.e., a way of being. This is not blind or bad faith; nor is it *faith-in-reason* which may invert means and ends as illustrated above. It is *faith-in-truth* itself where the appeal to faith in contrast to—not opposed to—knowledge implies humility or "an absence of a certainty that promotes arrogance".[5] This kind of faith can grow through rational or experiential insight; that is, one evolves from lower to higher forms of faith or trust in truth as one sees that truth more fully as it really is.

Thus, unconditional love implies a supreme love for truth and/or what is truly good; this love supersedes our love for anything else, especially the desire to comply with any individual or group self-centered agendas, e.g., appeals to blood or race, gender, nationality, or even religion and science. Such an appeal is hardly new. Carl Rogers was not the first to appeal to unconditional love as the power for core personality change. Plato refers to love as "the friend of man ... who opens the way to our highest happiness". Freud tells Jung that "psychoanalysis is in essence a cure through love". Viktor Frankl says that "the salvation of man is through love and in love". Additionally, Pitirim Sorokin refers to "the royal road of all-giving creative love" as the only way to create "a mental, moral, or material millennium".[6]

My general aim in this paper is to speak to those sincerely motivated by *this* kind of good faith to consider the possibility that we are collectively suffering from a prejudice toward truth itself that underlies what I am calling *spiritual addiction*. I am claiming that in the process of waking up to what we call the "real" world, this unconditional love appears so pervasively compromised by individual and group self-centered agendas that we are tempted to doubt its reality and/or realizability, which tempts us to embrace surrogates. The practical significance of this cannot be sufficiently underscored: if unconditional love is the power requisite for core personality change (i.e., the fulfilment of human nature), and if such a pervasive conditionality of love motivates spiritual addiction (the compulsion to seek surrogates), then the mere belief that we cannot realize such a good inherently works against that good faith willingness to open our minds and hearts to even see and acknowledge that we are enslaved to our prejudices. We may fail to wake up enough to realize that we are unwitting accomplices in a process leading to our own self-annihilation. Or, to put it in other words, we may not realize that we are sitting on a fence within a vast moral gray area, pretending to be innocent bystanders in fear of taking the reality or our moral freedom and responsibility too seriously on one hand, or not seriously enough on the other. We do not take to heart how this becomes the fertile soil for the creation of previously unimagined forms of evil, such as the 100 million deaths from genocides and democides in the last century alone, along with the literal and imminent destruction of our environment and world. The worst among us feed on our indifference.

1.1. Defining Spirituality

Toward counteracting this consequence, my aim in this paper is to bring into the foreground of our investigation spiritual addiction as a form of *moral* or spiritual lack, which insofar as it is acknowledged moves us, akin to hunger, thirst, pain, or any other lack, to search for what can relieve it.[7] I intend to show that it is the pervasive nature of this morally compromised state that primarily underlies our addictions in general. For what would motivate us to struggle to overcome our addictions if we believe that unconditional love is nothing but a fantasy or illusion and, as such, lacks the requisite power to counteract the escalating forces of destruction we see all around us and within us?

To return to our initial illustration of the conflict between atheists and theists, I intend to show that this collective moral problem is more deeply a religious problem in a way *similar* to the critique of religion by atheists in general,[8] but unlike them, I intend to use the testimony of a sub-set of atheist witnesses of the Holocaust, e.g., Primo Levi and Jean Amery, to show that this collective moral problem is not limited to what we call "religion", but includes atheists and our secular or scientific community as well. Levi's testimony of the absence of any moral difference between atheists and theists in the microcosm of Auschwitz—and the macrocosm of our world today—is not motivated by any scapegoating tactic aimed at blaming the other side to elevate one's own, as if atheists have greater moral power than theists or they alone have the requisite power to counteract our present course toward human self-destruction. Nor are these witnesses claiming that reason in and of itself can provide this power (as Amery (1980) graphically illustrates in the powerlessness of "The Intellectual in Auschwitz"). Rather, their testimony is an indictment of us all, atheists and theists alike. Whatever we call our religious faith and scientific reason, they are just different forms of corruption of the human heart or conscience demonstrating our lack of faith in unconditional love. Stronger still, unlike a great many atheist existentialists, this sub-group of atheist witnesses are not indicting reality or existence itself; nor even any possible super-natural or non-material God at its core. Rather, they are indicting the elevation of individual and group self-centered agendas above true goodness itself. They are referring to our lack of a Buber-like intimately loving, "I & Thou" connection in all our relationships, including our relationship to ourselves. From this vantage point, I claim our collective moral problem is more deeply a religious problem because while the map revealing to humanity the way to realize this love has been transmitted through the mediation of the most reliable religious witnesses in our history, that map has been concealed by spiritually vacuous forms of mainstream religion claiming to speak in its name.

To be clear, I am not claiming there are no real or significant moral distinctions to be drawn between individuals, but that such distinctions are typically drawn within a prejudiced moral gray area. My appeal to Levi as not only an atheist of good faith, but a prophetic-like witness, is especially relevant here. For if he is right about the lack of any difference in *moral* power between atheists and theists, then on what rational grounds can we lay claim to a foundation for hope to counteract the rising dark tide of a moral de-evolution imminently culminating in our self-annihilation? To be sure, some theists may interpret this as a good thing—as an apocalyptic revelation of an end of times scenario—but other theists may view this as a prophetic warning precisely to prevent such a catastrophe. Either way, I suggest that the reality of the challenge itself is becoming increasingly difficult to deny. Levi, at least, is not appealing to a secular or scientific hope in preference to a religious hope, but the lack of an adequate moral foundation for hope on both sides.

The significance of religion, then, enters the foreground of our concern in that it is the *only* historical vehicle in and through or by which such a collective moral education has been revealed. For example, one can easily trace the most therapeutic doctrines in Freudian psychoanalysis to religious history. Thus, the danger of a wholesale rejection of religion lies in throwing away the baby with the bathwater. My appeal to an orientation of good faith subject to an experiential process, by contrast, concedes the atheist's claim that our present forms of religion are morally compromised while nonetheless warning us of the danger of embracing an anti-religion extreme as if we can avoid any faith commitment in some primary value worthy of human trust.

In other words, to resolve this collective moral and religious problem, I distinguish the spirit from the form of religion. By the *form* of religion, I have in mind the tendency of theists to subordinate their faith in truth to faith in themselves or their own doctrines and ritual practices, as though one specific religion (or any) is necessary for the realization of a truly good life. By contrast, the *spirit* of religion refers to faith in truth and true goodness as the one thing needful, so that doctrine and practice are subordinated to that primary value. This spirit, then, is manifested or incarnated in the lives of the most reliable spiritual witnesses in our history (i.e., those marked by the purity of their devotion to the truth and their fullness of insight about reality), though not necessarily in the lives of those claiming to speak in their name.

However, insofar as the contemporary atheist sees no such exceptional moral power in the lives of theists today while theists profess to have that morality they so evidently lack, both remain subject to different kinds of prejudice. They are similar to two antelope so intently engaged in defending themselves and attacking the other that neither sees the lion about to pounce on and devour them both.

In contrast to religious demands for compliance, my aim is to direct our attention to witnesses who do not ask us to exercise blind faith in them but invite us to look and see for ourselves what is truly worthy of our deepest trust. Such a spiritual religion of the heart calls us toward potentially endless creative development on the stable foundation of truth. It has power not only to breathe new life into what is of genuine value in any form of religion we may identify with, but also to encourage us to create new forms by the revelation of a transcultural religion of the heart consistent with Augustine's maxim, "love and do as you please". That is, place your faith in truth and true goodness and you will fulfill the spirit of any genuine moral law.

1.2. Structure of the Paper or Steps to Realize This Aim

I will first present the case of a patient, Brandon, who, as with Levi, has sufficiently awakened to the "real" world[9] that his awareness of our present condition is undermining his hope for humanity and himself. This awareness of our contingent condition and belief about our prospects for hope underly his felt unwillingness and/or inability to pursue socially accepted goals. My aim is to use this case to bring into the foreground of our investigation both the character of this spiritual emptiness and what can implicitly fill it. We shall especially narrow in on Brandon's claim that despite this increasing awareness of the real world, there is also a growing experiential awareness of the reality of unconditional love, which has the power to counteract the aforementioned rising dark tide. It is this, he claims, that has kept him alive over the past two years. This faith in true goodness, then, presents itself to him as an alternative to both a naïve and illusory false optimism on one hand, and a pessimistic, if not wholly nihilistic, insistence on the unavoidability of human selfishness on the other.

With this case before us, we will then briefly ask ourselves whether, or to what extent, our current addiction literature (along with our broader educational context) speaks to this problem. To this end, we will primarily look at Lance Dodes' theory of psychological addiction as underlying all addiction. My intention here is not to provide a meta-analysis or critique of all prevailing theories of addiction, nor even to examine a theory of addiction that is the most recent or widely accepted. Rather, I am merely using Dodes' theory as a kind of rhetorical device to bring into the foreground of our investigation the possibility of a deeper spiritual addiction underlying addiction's physical, psychological, moral, and social symptoms. My hope is that such an example may be sufficient to illustrate the general avoidance within current theories of precisely the foundation-level moral and spiritual problem at issue here.

Toward providing a solution, I narrow in on this deeper moral and spiritual problem implicit in Dodes' account. I highlight the way all prejudice works by aligning itself with what is, or purports to be, the highest revelation of truth and value in our history. That is, the only way the power of truth can be avoided, manipulated, or controlled is by appearing, akin to a shapeshifter, to be the very thing one is not. Thus, we see why every original religious (or scientific) form of revelation actually manifesting the spirit of truth is invariably followed by a chameleon-like imitation without it.

We are then prepared to see why the most subtle barrier in our way to such a truly good or spiritual life is what I call "good parent (teacher, therapist, leader) syndrome". That is, the tendency of those in the highest positions of authority to compare themselves *within* a morally compromised norm rather than raising the moral bar by comparing themselves with the very best moral or spiritual examples in our history. I suggest that what is most needed here is not merely our acknowledgement of this prejudice in the highest places of authority, but the understanding of the likely cost of this acknowledgement, viz., the possible loss of one's following, along with the likelihood of others using this acknowledgement to elevate their own lust for power. However, I also point out that this is precisely the cost we must be willing to pay if we are to serve a truth and goodness greater than ourselves.

2. Case Presentation
2.1. Brandon

Brandon[10] is a 35-year-old single heterosexual male, out of work for the past 2 years,[11] and on the verge of becoming homeless. He refers to his general condition over this period as being profoundly depressed and in an almost constant state of anxiety that intrudes into his sleep and most of his waking hours.[12] Although not actively suicidal, in his darkest hours, he has wondered if it might be better if he was dead rather than suffer this "endless pain". In such moments, he sees no light at the end of the tunnel, as if life were an unbearable burden which he must bear, if only to spare his mother and a few close others from blaming themselves for his death.

2.2. A Typical Day

Brandon typically wakes from a sleepless night to an onslaught of anxious thoughts and feelings that threaten to overwhelm him. He consistently arrives at his 7 a.m. daily psychotherapy sessions 20 min late, wearing dirty clothes, un-showered, and disheveled with unkempt hair and beard. He complains of the squalor in the temporarily free apartment in which he lives: clothes, take-out food containers, cigarette butts,[13] and empty beer and liquor bottles strewn across his dirty bedroom floor and the corners of his bed. He condemns himself for his felt *unwillingness and/or inability* to clean this mess up. He lacks the motivation to even buy food more than once a day. He insists he cannot muster the strength to look for a job.

When asked, he can predict beforehand what is likely to occur each day. After therapy, he will drive to a local liquor store to buy whatever number of whiskey shots he feels in that moment he will need to make it through the day. He will drink 1–2 shots in the liquor store parking lot in hope this will provide enough motivation to buy something to eat before returning home to play online multiplayer video games for most of the day, interspersed with drinking alcohol and smoking cigarettes and cannabis.

2.3. Therapy and an Existential Crisis

Most surprising to his parents, relatives, and friends is that Brandon has been in therapy for the past 10+ years, along with periodic psychiatric evaluations and treatment with psychotropic medications. When asked why he does not find another therapist, he insists that without this therapist he would probably be dead. To be clear, for most of this 10-year period he was not in the same condition he is in now. Prior to these past 2 years, he only went to therapy once per week, and by outside behavioral appearances, he was very successful—working as a producer with a six-figure salary, living in a nice apartment, with a large and supportive social network of friends. However, his increasing experience of the "real" world—especially in the form of a toxic work environment, culminated 2 years ago in an existential crisis, at which time the floor his life was standing upon seemed to give way. His increased reliance on the addictions mentioned above were inadequate to enable him to cope with his anxiety, which culminated in him quitting his job.

2.4. Moments of Hope

Brandon's experiences over the past 2 years have not been entirely dark. In certain moments he has felt hope in the dawning of a new day, or less anxious after meditating with his therapist for 5–10 min at the start of his sessions. He has especially felt calmer after taking a walk with his therapist along the LA River. Above all, he has experienced bursts of optimistic energy when his therapist has been able to provide a mirror for him to see his real strengths and prospects for hope. Thus, despite his seeming lack of outward progress from the vantage point of socio-cultural values such as having a good job and other signs of "normal" functional behavior, he senses and, at times, sees a form and measure of real inward growth. When he does, he finds himself more able to vividly recall, and be nourished by, not only seemingly isolated or random glimpses of light at the end of his dark tunnel, but a more tangible sense that his struggle—even over the past 2 years—might actually be symptomatic of a deeper, ongoing form of progress. He can imagine that his suffering is rooted less in any deficiency limited to or originating in him than in a deficit he had imbibed from his infancy from a broader social context, and that his addictions are symptomatic of a deeper and more pervasive spiritual lack or deficiency. He can sense that the profound emptiness and pain he feels revolves around a form of collective cold-indifference, rather than any alleged happenstance, and he can understand that his pain might even be of value in moving him to look to see more clearly and acknowledge more deeply a human-caused moral complicity—this acknowledgement being the only thing that could relieve his suffering.

2.5. A Closer Look at Brandon's Addictive Behavior

Although in the past 2 years Brandon has been able to do without alcohol, other addictive substances, and even video games for several months at a time, over the past 6 months or more, he has averaged 8–10 drinks a day. He knows that whatever amount of alcohol he buys he will drink; that the more he drinks, the more depressed he will become; and that the more depressed and anxious he feels, the more he will drink. It seems clear to him that his depression, rather than his alcohol consumption, lies at the root of his problem. Alcohol is not the driving force underlying his addiction. It is precisely because of this that he does not know how much liquor he will buy until he actually arrives at the liquor store and sees how he psychologically feels. This decision has essentially nothing to do with physical symptoms of tolerance or withdrawal. Reason and willpower in the moment of acute anxiety and despair seem to play virtually no role in his "decision" to drink. He does not seem able to even re-direct his attention to less anxiety producing thoughts that might move him in a direction opposed to the thoughts and feelings driving his addictive behavior. In short, Brandon feels virtually powerless to do anything constructive, as if the only thing he is able to do is embrace or succumb to the seduction of those addictive behaviors that momentarily shift his attention away from his emptiness and pain. He does this despite knowing that these actions will invariably leave him feeling worse at the end of the day and, as the days and months add up, even more hopeless by reinforcing his conviction that he cannot change.

2.6. A Concrete Example of Brandon's Powerlessness

One Monday, Brandon came to therapy feeling unusually confident in his ability to buy only four shots of alcohol that day, in part because he had only three and a half shots on Sunday, two shots on Saturday, and one shot on Friday. He was especially motivated because of plans to visit his family on the East Coast in a few days. He wanted to arrive sober, clean-shaven, and wearing clean clothes. However, despite this relative progress, he felt so paralyzed by anxiety that he could not even clean his clothes at the laundromat and considered having the cleaners wash them for him. However, he felt ashamed at the thought of not being able to clean them himself. His therapist asked, "How would you feel at the end of the day if you succeeded in drinking only three shots (instead of four), ate a healthy breakfast, and had clean clothes even if washed by the cleaners"? Brandon said he would feel pretty good. So, after leaving therapy, he went to the liquor store and purchased three shots, drinking only one before going out for breakfast.

While eating, however, he began to dissociate, as if he was being assaulted by two different and opposed spiritual (non-audible personal) voices. On one hand, there was the "usual" voice of his therapist, attuned to his experience and striving to collaborate with Brandon's truest and best sense of himself. On the other hand, he imagined his parents and relatives, friends and broader social world shaking their heads at him for being a failure or loser without a job and a weakling for being unable to control his own behavior. Worse, in this moment he imagined his therapist judging him in the same way, as if—despite what his therapist might have said to the contrary—he sensed his therapist was frustrated with him and in that frustration judging him for stubbornly refusing to play a responsible role in his own recovery. He believed his therapist, similarly to his family and everyone else, did not understand what he was experiencing. Thus, instead of helping him, they were actually collaborating in his suffering, even if unintentionally. This made him feel unbearably alone. He felt condemned in their eyes, as if the primary causal root of his addictions was some moral deficit in him for which he should feel guilty and ashamed. It was in that critical moment (Dodes 2002, p. 54) that Brandon felt driven to not only drink his remaining two shots, but to rush to a liquor store to buy a fifth of whiskey. He then sat in his car for 2 h, drinking about two more shots from that bottle,[14] feeling overwhelmed with guilt, shame, and sorrow as he tearfully and unsuccessfully tried to find the strength of will to wash his own clothes rather than suffer the ignominy of depending upon a cleaner to do it for him.

2.7. Therapeutic Misattunement and Confession

Brandon did not go to the cleaners. However, he did feel safe enough the next morning to tell his therapist what he had experienced the previous day. He said he sensed, on a gut level, his therapist's frustration with his lack of "sufficient" outward or behavioral progress. He felt that his therapist had shifted from remaining empathically attuned to Brandon's experience to being more concerned with Brandon's outward behavior, regardless of his therapist's underlying motives.

As Brandon talked, his therapist reflected on similar experiences of his own and how such a lack of attunement and understanding from those he had most relied upon had negatively impacted him in the same way it did Brandon. This moved him to confirm or validate Brandon's intuitive experience. He did not defensively attribute it to Brandon's "subjective perspective" while inwardly holding an opposing perspective. Rather, he openly acknowledged his feelings of frustration and his felt need for validation as a "good-enough" therapist (Winnicott 1965), as they collaboratively explored their shared sense of broader social forces influencing us all to "fit in" to group self-centered agendas at the cost of sacrificing allegiance to one's own conscience, i.e., what Brandchaft et al. (2010) would call "systems of pathological accommodation".

2.8. Toward a Cure

In that moment of authentic, empathic connection, or what Buber (1970) called a dialogical I and Thou understanding, Brandon no longer felt unbearably alone as he did the day before. He said that the previous day's experience of abandonment by his therapist felt worlds apart from the spirit he now sensed emanating from his therapist, as if he were a truly ally, struggling as best he could to understand Brandon's inner world. His therapist was once again standing with him not only as a fellow traveler struggling to climb the same mountain, but also as a guide with a bit more experience to help Brandon see a way out of his present disorientation and darkness. In other words, his therapist seemed able to hold a true hope for him, which Brandon could not yet see for himself, but could nevertheless rely upon until he could see it for himself.[15] His therapist's awareness of this objective truth about Brandon's condition also brought with it a kind of moral power[16] that could and did enliven Brandon's will to care for himself. This power[17] seemed greater than the therapist and Brandon themselves, yet it was experienced by them both in a way that reassured Brandon that there really was a way out of his present darkness.

This is what seemed lacking in that moment when Brandon found himself in despair in his car. It seemed as if his therapist, in his own frustration, was trying to influence Brandon to rely upon his <u>own</u> will separate from his own experiential sense of such a true hope and that sense of hope he previously saw in the eyes of his therapist. In that moment of frustration, his therapist placed himself between Brandon and that revelation of hope instead of helping Brandon see it more clearly and fully for himself. In that moment, therefore, his therapist lost sight of the vital instrumental role he played in tangibly collaborating with that spirit of truth and love on Brandon's behalf. In short, in that moment, his therapist had, in fact, abandoned Brandon to his own resources rather than continuing to empathically suffer with him to help him see and feel that truth for himself.

2.9. A Call for a Collective Confession

What especially hit home for Brandon's therapist was not merely the realization of his own empathic misattunement, but the realization of his own need for a far more intimate and continuous experiential connection with that spirit of truth and love that could alone make tangibly present the meaning, purpose, and primary value of human life. This is not an appeal to a spiritual life separated from our physically embodied life. Nor is it an appeal to a spirit that only speaks to theists. Rather, it is an appeal to a spirit of truth and love speaking in and to and through each and every one of us, which can only be actualized and internalized within us when we are willing to invite it in. For it cannot compel us without violating who or what we are. This is what Brandon most needed in that moment when he sat sobbing in his car, desperately trying to hear that loving voice within himself, but he could not because it was obstructed—not only by a coldly indifferent world, but by the one person he had come to trust more than anyone else.

2.10. Toward Further Elucidating the Meaning of Spiritual Addiction and Why It Matters

I contend that Brandon's case illustrates no mere subjective psychological problem limited to him or within him. Despite real and significant subjective differences in our experiences, there is a sense in which we may all suffer from such a spiritual emptiness or addiction not grounded in our neurobiology, nor the more specific deficits of our individual parental and cultural upbringing. I am not appealing to an Alcoholics Anonymous (AA)-type moral, religious, or even spiritual diagnosis of this problem and solution—at least not as this is commonly understood.[18] On the contrary, I contend that the primary barrier to a truly healthy spiritual life is an implicit, if not explicit, assumption by both theists and atheists today that a truly conscientious or altruistic life is impossible to realize, if not pathological (Oakley et al. 2012).[19]

In more religious terms, I am referring, to take just one example, to Gandhi's criticism of a pervasive tendency he observed among Christians of his day to lay claim to privileged spiritual status while also defending a religious doctrine of salvation in sin rather than a doctrine of salvation from sin that can speak to the moral struggle of atheists and theists of good faith alike (Gandhi 1993). Salvation from sin might be compared to fidelity in a truly healthy developing marriage, which requires an increasingly strong commitment and eschews any alleged necessity of being unfaithful at all, much less repeatedly or habitually. The idea of salvation from sin can speak to the moral struggle of atheists and theists of good faith alike. The collective moral indictment, of course, does not deny real and significant moral differences between us as atheists and theists. It only points to a problem which, although suffered by us all, is all the more suffered by conscientious atheists and theists, which places them in a different camp from the unconscientious on both sides.

3. Review of the Addiction Literature

Demonstrating that there is a general moral and religious bias in the addiction literature, along with an account of its causes, would require an investigation beyond the limits of this paper. Specifically, it would require an examination of the ontological, epistemological, and ethical commitments or assumptions of current research as grounded in Hume's empiricism, Kant's failed attempt to overcome Hume's epistemological skepticism, and current post-modern subjective interpretations of Husserl's phenomenology.[20] Since I cannot do this, it must suffice for me to posit that the current naturalistic or physicalist emphasis for understanding addiction is an extreme reaction to a prejudiced religious cultural context, a reaction which has, over the past 100 years or more, increasingly broadened to include psychological and broader environmental influences. This corresponds with major psychotherapeutic shifts in orientation and emphasis beginning with classical behaviorism (physical), psychoanalysis (psychological), humanistic-existentialism (free will and moral responsibility), multi-culturalism (broader social influences), and transpersonalism (self-transcendent good). Despite their initial emphases, as each of these orientations have evolved, they have adopted a more integrated and interdisciplinary orientation. My use of Lance Dodes' psychological approach to addiction, therefore, may be viewed as a rhetorical device to bring the moral/spiritual aspect of addiction into the foreground of investigation while fully conceding the appearance of me simplistically dismissing the real and significant contributions of this collaborative struggle to make sense of and resolve our most foundation-level human problems.

3.1. Physical Addiction

Clearly, Brandon has an unhealthy relationship with alcohol manifested in symptoms of physical withdrawal and tolerance (Dodes 2002, p. 70). However, he has also been able to overcome this physical dependence and be alcohol-free for many months at a time. The same holds true of his addictions to other substances, e.g., nicotine and benzodiazepines. This confuses him: if he sometimes feels a non-compulsory *desire* for social drinking without any felt *necessity* to drink, while at other times he feels a form of *compulsion* to drink despite a *desire* not to drink, why should he believe alcoholism is a neurobiological *disease*, necessitating life-long abstinence?[21] Why should he have to abstain from alcohol but not substances such as benzodiazepines, etc.? More importantly, if he can lower his anxiety, as well as lessen his feelings of depression, by re-directing his attention by means of meditation or other mindfulness practices, then why believe these symptoms are primarily, if at all, rooted in his biology?[22] He wants to know what this power is, and how to gain access to it, so that it might free him from his enslavement to this, that, or any addiction. Brandon's earlier described experience, along with his own familiarity with drug addiction studies such as the famous Rat Park experiments,[23] are consistent with Dodes' claim that there is virtually no scientific evidence for any genetic or neurochemical basis for any addictions, regardless of results from twin studies, adoption studies, or direct gene studies, along with similar arguments against addiction as being rooted in one's brain chemistry (ibid., p. 98ff).

3.2. Current Approaches to Addiction

More current approaches to addiction as physical claim to be integrated by including environmental considerations. Yet, insofar as "environment" is used in such approaches as a catch-all term to include anything other than what a researcher regards as most acceptably physical, such approaches may not imply any shift of ground. As Peele and Alexander (1998) put it, "this new theoretical synthesis is less than meets the eye: It mainly recycles discredited notions while including piecemeal modifications that make the theories marginally more realistic in their descriptions of addictive behavior". For example, the authors of a 2021 journal article (Heilig et al. 2021) acknowledge widespread scientific criticism of substance addiction as a brain disease, but nonetheless assert "that the foundational premise that addiction has a neurobiological basis is fundamentally sound". They point out that the brain disease model was originally presented as an "effective response to prevailing nonscientific, moralizing, and stigmatizing attitudes to addiction", which treated addiction as simply "the result of a person's moral failing or weakness of character, rather than a 'real' disease".[24] They concede that "any useful conceptualization of addiction requires an understanding both of the brains involved, and of environmental factors that interact with those brains". They state that the disease model "in no way negates the role of psychological, social and economic processes as both causes and consequences of substance use".[25]

In short, such a token concession to environmental causes may be interpreted to support the authors' fundamental materialistic prejudice: "If not from the brain, from where do the healthy and unhealthy choices people make originate"? Or, as powerfully articulated by Francis Crick, "You, your joys and your sorrows, your memories and your ambitions, your sense of personal identity and free will are in fact no more than the behavior of a vast assembly of nerve cells and their associated molecules". This is hardly the humility that the atheist "Four Horsemen" (Hitchens et al. 2019) lay claim to as the mark of scientific investigation. As Sam Harris puts it, "Scientists in my experience are the first people to say they don't know. If you get scientists to start talking outside their area of specialization, they immediately . . . say things like, 'I'm sure there's someone in the room who knows more about this than I do' (ibid., p. 52)". Or, as Richard Dawkins puts it, "Science may or may not . . . solve these Deep Problems. And if science . . . can't answer them, nothing can. Certainly not theology (ibid., p. 21)". To me, at least, such claims are hardy exceptions to a rule. They purport to go far beyond any mere criticism of current moralizing views of addiction. On the contrary, they express a widespread and rationally unsupported naturalistic and deterministic bias rejecting the indeterministic causal role of human moral freedom and the knowledge of objective moral values. As such, it appears to me as a strawman argument used to simply dismiss an entire cumulative history of human experiential moral wisdom as unworthy of serious rational inquiry.

3.3. Psychological Addiction

With respect to Brandon's addiction to video games, which obviously does not involve withdrawal and tolerance, such a disease model of addiction seems unable to account for the specific character of the compulsion involved. According to Dodes' alternative account: "An addiction, then, is truly present only when there is a psychological drive to perform the addictive behavior—that is, only when there is a psychological addiction" (ibid., p. 74), regardless of whether the addiction also involves substances capable of causing symptoms of withdrawal and tolerance. In keeping with Dodes' account, Brandon is aware of an inner psychical conflict between his desire for healthy functioning[26] and his desire for the object of his addictive behavior. Although in some moments the object of his addictive behavior powerfully moves him to embrace it above his health, at other times his concern for his health exercises a more powerful constraint such that he is both more willing and able to act in a healthier way. In the moments when he believes/feels most socially invalidated and/or overwhelmingly anxious, trapped, or out of control, he feels a more powerful need to embrace the addictive object to momentarily restore a sense of control. In other moments, by contrast, when he believes, sees, and feels a sense of worth and/or hope for positive change, the aforementioned sense of powerlessness is diminished.

3.4. AA Model of Spirituality and Addiction through the Lens of Lance Dodes

Given my primary concern with spiritual addiction, let us now turn to Dodes'[27] critique of AA in view of what seems to be his implicit rejection of any type of moral, spiritual, and especially religious basis for addiction. This seems especially needful given that AA is the most widespread, if not the only, kind of treatment available to those suffering from addiction. It is not surprising, therefore, that most of the myths about addiction Dodes describes are implicitly if not explicitly ascribed to AA. As mentioned, Brandon's own experience resonates with a cause of addiction deeper than the biological or physical, but as an atheist/agnostic, he is also extremely skeptical of religious ideations that presume an absolute moral authority he believes they lack. Thus, he is inclined to agree with Dodes' critique of AA-type religious explanations of addiction and their associated moralizing accounts.[28]

Dodes claims that according to AA, an "addict"[29] such as Brandon must hit rock bottom (ibid., p. 93), which Dodes interprets as AA saying that Brandon is to regard his slips or setbacks as "failures" within a process that must necessarily culminate in a "near total collapse" before he can realize the disease at the root of his addiction(s). If Dodes' interpretation is correct, then according to AA, this collapse would lead Brandon to the realization of the necessity of surrendering his will to a higher power (ibid., p. 95ff). However, given Brandon's ability to control his addictions for periods without such a total collapse in addition to his atheistic orientation, how could he conscientiously identify with these claims despite his felt need for some kind of tangible social support?

With regard to surrendering his will to a higher power in particular, if this is intended by AA (as per Dodes) to mean giving up any form and measure of agency to another—even to a "god"—how is such a wholly dependent relationship supposed to enable the addict to play even a collaborative role in one's own recovery? Brandon already feels pressure by both religious and secular groups to blindly conform to their respective forms of prejudice; how much more, therefore, is such an absolute demand by AA likely to compound this problem? This lies at the heart of his problem, viz., not merely the moral conflict he senses between his willingness and ability to act in his own best-interest, but the influence of a broader social context demanding blind conformity to group agendas above his own conscience. On one hand, he senses that there is some active and collaborative role he can and should play; on the other, he feels the need for a self-validating collaborative relationship with others, such as his therapist, in the healing process.

Another myth that Dodes attributes to AA is the necessity of counting one's days of sobriety (ibid., p. 96ff). Dodes states that "restarting from zero is the dark side of this tradition" and that "it is both punitive and unrealistic (ibid., p. 96)". That is, he interprets AA to be treating such slips as "failures" or as "backsliding" into the same condition one was in before. If so, then it would seem not only inaccurate and punitive, but even more likely to feed the self-condemnation that already seems to be driving Brandon's addiction. By contrast, Brandon would definitely concur with Dodes that his slips do not imply that he has failed to make any real and significant progress toward overcoming his addiction, and that the temptation to believe the contrary might actually blind him to see the real progress he has made and is making.

Brandon's progressive awareness is also especially relevant for Dodes' interpretation of AA's claim that the addict has a problem with knowing reality. As Dodes points out, there seems to be no evidence that those suffering from addictions have more of a problem with knowing reality than the non-addicted. Not only do studies show the opposite is true,[30] but the more Brandon has awakened to see the real world, the more he seems to find his overwhelming anxiety and despair reasonable. In other words, he is suffering from a form of existential anxiety and despair grounded in a collective lack of meaning, purpose and value for human life generally as well as his own life in particular, which is fueling his addictions.

3.5. Further Reflections on Dodes' Myths

While in some ways, Dodes' "debunking" of AA myths supports our understanding of addiction through Brandon's eyes, in other ways it misses some important alternative explanations. It dismisses the spiritual as a monolith rather than considering AA's interpretation as only one possibility. Looking closer at Dodes' assessments, we can see where a spiritual interpretation might actually be helpful in the understanding of addiction and further our pursuit of the idea of a spiritual addiction underlying addiction as a whole.

First, with respect to Dodes' rejection of one needing to surrender to a higher power: does this not equally, if not all the more so, apply to any so-called secular or scientific theories claiming authority for the correct understanding of addiction and its treatment? Is Dodes, for example, not asking his patients to willingly surrender their self-reliance to him (a higher power) to gain sufficient access to that knowledge requisite for change that he has privileged access to? On the other hand, let us assume that the most reliable religious witnesses in our history[31] acknowledge the necessity of some form of self-surrender to a higher power. This surrender may refer only to a willing surrender to what one increasingly sees to be of the highest value for one's life, along with surrendering previously held prejudices obstructing one's way to that good. This kind of surrender implies no rejection of the self or one's will or freedom. On the contrary, by opening the door to the highest vision of reality we are capable of, it expands our freedom and creative potential indefinitely. It might be compared to a willing commitment to a partner within a collaborative relationship that not only nourishes each partner individually, but also enables them together to create a value greater than each could realize alone. Thus, Dodes' interpretation of that self-surrender to a higher power that reduces a person to a slave in relation to a tyrant is not representative of the viewpoint of the most reliable religious witnesses in our history. As John Wesley put it, "You cannot force the conscience of anyone. You cannot compel another to see as you see. You ought not to attempt it. Reason and persuasion are the only weapons you ought to use".

I should add that the relationship between free will and the grace (love or goodness) of any form of higher power (e.g., the love of a parent, therapist, medical doctor, or even a good God) is one of the most if not the most complex and controversial problems in our moral and religious history. Within Christianity, for example, one finds apologists on both extreme ends. Nor can any of us avoid taking our own stand in a way that invariably manifests itself in all our relationships, including psychotherapy. This may help us to appreciate Brandon's struggle over the extent to which the lack of power he feels over his addictions is rooted in his own will and/or an inability influenced by imbibed prejudices and ongoing social demands to pathologically accommodate to this or that group's agenda. It is more than likely, therefore, not only for atheists biased toward religion, but also for theists biased toward atheism, to embrace one extreme or the other in a way that misinterprets their true relationship.

As for Dodes' interpretation of AA's dark side in insisting on the necessity of counting one's days of sobriety, Dodes is not, presumably, claiming that slips are necessary, much less inherently good. On the contrary, one might reasonably believe that it is precisely because repeated slips tend to reinforce addictive habits that this might motivate greater vigilance in the effort to form healthy habits. However, as difficult as it is to overcome unhealthy habits in the formation of healthy ones, it may be as difficult, if not more difficult, to maintain the reformed habit. The longer one is able to do so—and this almost universally by means of positive reinforcement from one's social surroundings—the greater the power to maintain or retain that progress. Thus, the demonstrable ability to remain sober for a long period of time (by means of a potentially validating social context such as an AA group) may actually work to: (a) empirically confirm the addict's conviction that he can overcome his addiction indefinitely; and (b) further motivate greater vigilance (in relying upon such a cohesive social support network) to overcome even the most subtle temptations towards strengthening his resilience. In short, in opposition to Dodes, AA's counting one's days of sobriety need not imply that one has made no progress or has fallen back to where one was at the start. I believe the relevance of this for a spiritual cause of addiction revolves around the appeal to such a life-long social context. In view of our distinction between the spirit and form of a religion (or any group), we would do well to ask whether one's identification with any AA group promotes just another form of prejudicial group mind or, alternatively, works to increasingly nourish one's relationship with that spirit of truth and goodness that liberates us to be our true selves whether in or outside the group.

Finally, as for Dodes' interpretation of AA that the addict may know reality even more than the non-addict—while at odds with AA's specific spiritual beliefs—does not imply that both the addict and so-called non-addict are free of a more deeply shared prejudice toward reality itself. Indeed, this is the testimony of the most reliable religious witnesses in our history. They include but do not reduce reality to physical reality. They appeal to a far broader reality, along with a far broader empirical or experiential awareness of it than the narrow empiricism of our day. For present purposes, the latter, in contrast to the former, treat our ability to experientially know moral, spiritual, and religious values as no less confirmable as our knowledge of anything else.[32] As in Plato's "Allegory of the Cave", those who have gone so far as to discover that they are being deceived by blind leaders of the blind (theistic or atheistic) are still far from seeing reality outside the cave. Thus, behind the veil of darkness and despair that we increasingly discover characterizing our so-called "real" world is the possibility of a reality of truth and love, wonder and beauty that extends far beyond our ability to imagine, much less see, relative to our present condition in the cave. It is not that we all cannot see it and realize it, but that we cannot see it insofar as we continue to believe there is nothing to be seen. This is why these witnesses, as opposed to atheists and theists demanding blind faith in them, call each and every one of us to open our eyes to undertake the requisite experiential process to see the truth for ourselves.

Is this not consistent with what good therapists attempt to do with their patients? Do such therapists not travail with and for their patients, to help them see that their despair for themselves and humanity is rooted in our collective unwillingness and/or inability to see and adequately mirror the true worth of our children? Insofar as the therapist can do this, the patient is enabled to see through the veil of that overarching prejudice to find the freedom to love.

4. Analysis and Solution

Having looked at some of the characteristics of spiritual addiction in Brandon's case and having briefly examined Dodes' account of psychological addiction, I now want to bring into the foreground Dodes' implicit acknowledgement of the primacy of moral values in the problem of addiction. In so doing, I intend to expound my own view of addiction as a reaction to a form of moral or spiritual bankruptcy.

Moral vs. Social Power and Weakness

Dodes repeatedly refers to the way in which addicts such as Brandon tend to be incredibly cruel in blaming themselves for being unable and/or unwilling to overcome their addictions (ibid., p. 12). They believe they should feel guilty and ashamed. These beliefs may be so convincing that the addict feels almost driven to suicide to relieve this constant emptiness and pain (ibid., p. 13). Dodes rightly claims that the moral beliefs driving this suffering are both false and the cause of the addict's suffering, and he attributes them to a prejudicial social context. But why does the addict believe these claims? How does Dodes know that these beliefs are false? How can a patient, such as Brandon, be helped to distinguish these false, socially imbibed prejudices from true values within a process of coming to know them as the apparent means to overcome any form of addiction?

First, insofar as we are willing and able to empathically sit with Brandon sobbing in his car, we may feel less inclined to blindly assume that he is willingly deceiving himself and/or others. He certainly seems to be deeply suffering from forces he does not understand and thus has no immediate control over. We may also find ourselves more willing and able to empathize with him insofar as we too feel the weight of the demands for blind conformity to group prejudices. Additionally, if we can recognize these things, we may also begin to appreciate, with Brandon's therapist, the possibility of a role we may all be playing in Brandon's suffering as long as we avoid putting such prejudices to the test of our own evolving experience of the truth. Is this, or something similar to this, not what Dodes is directing our attention to with respect to false yet pervasively accepted moral and religious judgments of the addict?

Dodes is right: the fact that a person suffering from an addiction, such as Brandon, may believe and feel he is primarily or solely responsible for his addiction does not imply that that belief is true (or true in the specific sense that he believes). As Dodes puts it, "we live in a culture that frequently treats people with addictions as if their problem was caused by a moral deficiency . . . even though this is not true (ibid., p. 79)". Notwithstanding these culturally imbibed moral beliefs, myths, or prejudices and their correlative feelings, the person suffering from an addiction is not, according to Dodes, morally culpable, stupid, or even morally weak. However, "since no one has helped them find a reasonable explanation for their addiction, it is easy for them to assume it's due to moral weakness or stupidity as if these were the only logical explanations" (ibid., p. 12). In support of his contention that the problem of the one suffering from an addiction is not due to his unwillingness to act rightly, as opposed to some form of innocent ignorance and correlative powerlessness or inability, he appeals to one case after another in which those suffering from an addiction believe and feel, similarly to Brandon, that they "can't stop" (ibid.), that in the case of addictions we are confronted with a form of subjective inability as opposed to any mere unwillingness to change.

Dodes then claims (ibid., p. 14) that what is driving or causing any addiction is something psychological <u>within</u> the individual. What precisely does he mean by this? A reasonable interpretation is that Brandon has been psychologically indoctrinated by outside social forces to believe (falsely) certain cultural moral myths or prejudices which, insofar as he continues to believe them, he lacks the requisite power to counteract them. Yet, as previously mentioned, Dodes seems to sweepingly reject any form of moral, spiritual, or non-physical cause other than what he calls "psychological", which itself begins to seem suspect given his appeal to drives. At least it suggests an appeal to Freud's biologically instinctive drives—a word that fails to distinguish influencing or constraining causes applicable to human freedom from physically determining forms of causation applicable to creatures that lack this freedom. Dodes describes a patient who believes he is inherently a failure, and thus feels like a failure, and is thus moved to act like a failure, which, in turn, seems to confirm the patient's original false belief. As the patient puts it, "Once a failure, always a failure" (ibid., p. 46). We do well to look at the lawful sequence between belief, feeling, action and confirmation.

Dodes seems to conclude from such cases that the uncontrollable drive underlying addiction is not rooted in awareness but in unconscious feelings. But again, what does he mean by this? Feelings are not vacuous or directionless. One is not merely anxious or depressed, but anxious and depressed about something. Additionally, this is not contradicted by the fact that the something in question may not be unconscious in the sense of not being immediately in the forefront of one's awareness. Indeed, what else do psychotherapists do but help the patient to see increasingly more clearly for themselves what things are influencing or motivating those feelings? An appeal to moral feelings, such as feeling guilty, ashamed, or worthless, is inseparable from moral beliefs and the objective moral values of those beliefs and, as such, they are not literally unconscious.[33] In short, what is motivating the addiction is not mere subjective feelings or instinctual drives, but precisely false or conflicting beliefs about moral values or moral reality.

To apply this to Brandon's case, such an acknowledgement of his and our capacity to know such values implies no imposition by the therapist on the patient of any set of moral beliefs, religious or anti-religious. This is consistent with helping a patient to distinguish what is true and false with respect to any kind of object. It appeals to the patient's own ability to see and distinguish for themselves what truly is and is not in their own best interest. In other words, given such a treatment goal, the patient's will certainly plays a necessary role in recovery, at the very least in the form of the willingness to acknowledge that there is a problem to be resolved and to collaborate with the therapist and/or others in discovering what that problem is. In this case, this certainly involves putting the patients' imbibed moral prejudices to the test of their own evolving experience.[34] For example, a patient has been told by his parents that he is a "bad child" and treated as such throughout his childhood. Of course, there are many "bad" actions that the parents can point to in seeming justification of their claim. But what originally motivated those actions? As this is explored in detail and in depth, the child may come to realize that he believed he was worthless because his parents treated him that way, even to the point of making him the family scapegoat so the parents could avoid addressing their own shortcomings. As the child comes to see with increasing clarity this theme repeating itself in one case after another, this brings with it increasing power over his previously held "vague" and false beliefs about it. As Plato-Socrates, and the entire Western tradition of philosophy, have claimed, "knowledge (of the right kind) is power". They are referring to experiential knowledge as opposed to mere abstract knowledge.[35]

If all this is true, then the problem of addiction is a problem of moral weakness after all, which is not changed by the fact that it is not limited to, nor even necessarily originating in, the person suffering from an addiction, but is primarily or initially rooted in a prejudiced social environment working against the development of that experiential moral insight that increasingly brings with it the power to overcome any addiction. What the patient needs, therefore, is a genuinely empathic, caring, and insightful therapist (and/or other) willing and able to provide a safe, non-morally judgmental environment within which the patient can learn to distinguish true from false moral judgments, knowledge which brings with it the power to will and act in accordance with it.[36] However, insofar as I am right about such a pervasive morally prejudicial context, we may also appreciate how difficult it may be for a patient or any of us to access this moral reality and its power.

The problem of moral weakness, therefore, is not properly accounted for by appealing to what the person suffering from an addiction is willing or able to do in the present moment, as if Brandon was supposed to simply "lift himself up by the boot-straps" and stop drinking. Nor is the problem of moral weakness limited to those we call addicts alone. It has to do with a pervasive lack of moral awareness and its correlative form of power that would, if it were sufficiently present, empower us to realize the best versions of ourselves. The root cause of our addictions as unhealthy displacements, therefore, is not limited to this or that person's "psychology", inner subjective world or "psychic reality". Nor is it limited to any shared characteristics of "addicts" alone in contrast to "non-addicts" by virtue of any posited "addictive psychological predisposition", as Dodes seems to suggest. Rather, it lies in the way we initially imbibe a form of collective moral prejudice that powerfully influences us to place our individual and group self-centered agendas above our conscientious fidelity to the truth.

5. Social Influences or Causes
5.1. Parental Asymmetrical Role

Toward a better understanding of the origin of this prejudice[37] and the way to overcome it, let us take it for granted that our parents play the most powerful role in the initial formation of their children's character—for better or worse. In the best sense, "good-enough" parents both embody and outwardly manifest a kind and degree of love or goodness that even an infant can viscerally sense is trustworthy. The child feels uniquely loved, not only because he is inherently loveable and thus should be loved, but because the child is loved. This intangible spirit of love is tangibly incarnated in the life of these loving parents and increasingly internalized by the child as both a specific and generic kind of "voice", or inwardly felt presence, that initially defines the child's core sense of self and self-worth.[38] Additionally, insofar as the child's connection to this voice is maintained and strengthened by the social context in which the child lives, it all the more deeply and powerfully roots itself to define the quality of the child's will, mind, feelings, actions, habits, character, and life as a whole, as it extends outwardly to positively influence everyone and everything he comes in contact with.

However, where is such an unconditional love to be found outside of movies or the story books we read to our children? Sooner or later, at least, we come to realize that most parents tend to fall short of being "good enough" in this sense. But what precisely does this mean? Instead of the child awakening to find such an internalized purely good inner voice grounding his life, he[39] finds an opposing harsh or critical voice enmeshed with it. In some cases, this self-invalidating inner voice may have so much presence and power in and over him that he feels possessed by or enslaved to it. Despite all his attempts to vanquish it by reason[40] or mere force of will on the one hand, or by concealing it from himself on the other, to minimize the suffering it causes him, it may seem to be an alien presence so fully in control of him that he feels powerless to free himself from it.

Note that the presence of both positive and negative inner voices within the child is entirely consistent with a parent providing for their child's so-called "basic needs". For it is precisely here where we may appreciate humanistic-existential psychology's emphasis on a uniquely human moral or spiritual need that is necessarily manifested in the intentional act of providing for any and all of our children's needs.[41] In other words, love is not a spiritual luxury or addendum to human life, but rather its presence or absence essentially defines the character of all that we think and do. To put it in still another way, as with breathing polluted air, this critical, judgmental, invalidating inner voice should not be present within us at all.

What, then, if the child awakens to a broader social real world only to find the same conditioned, compromised, or polluted love everywhere?[42] In Brandon's words, "this infection is present in every one of us in varying degrees, and largely undermines the pursuit of the voice of truth and goodness. Which is why it is more important than ever for therapists (and all other authority figures) to reflect on their own myriad potential 'infections,' predispositions, or prejudices". In this way, he's certainly right. How else can this moral infection be eliminated and the conscience restored to a state of purity? Without this, we are all the more tempted to believe that this pervasive selfish cold-indifference infecting the love we all profess defines the very essence or nature of what it means to be human, if not also the character of reality itself.[43] The root problem here, therefore, does not revolve around an opposition between religious "faith" on one hand and atheistic "reason" on the other, but around the temptation to place our faith and reason in serving one side or the other above our fidelity to the truth.

In short, given the child's relative lack of experience, how he initially viscerally feels and subsequently conceives of himself and reality depends almost entirely on the beliefs or conceptions—not yet veridical perceptions—he initially imbibes on his parents' knees. But as his experience broadens, he is increasingly able to see for himself whether or to what extent the beliefs or prejudices he has imbibed are consistent with his growing awareness. If the two are at odds, and if his parents and the groups he most identifies with demand he choose their side above his own conscience, he suffers a form of existential anxiety, moral suffering or spiritual trauma, i.e., a conflict at the very core of his being.[44] Note that the dilemma arises not solely or primarily because of the parents' or in-group's prejudices, but because of their complicit refusal to acknowledge these prejudices, which influences the child to either assume that what is missing must be his fault or, at least, to avoid as taboo looking too closely at precisely what is missing. If the child is punished for daring to express his own voice as in the old saying, "children are to be seen and not heard", he is increasingly less likely to speak up again. He viscerally senses he must comply, "brown-nose", or embrace a "false self" or form of "imposter syndrome" to survive in such a world.

What is the child to do in such a social context or world? How can we resolve this dilemma of sitting on a moral fence in which either extreme of being too good or too evil seems too costly? As illustrated in Brandon's own comment above, what is needed is for us to acknowledge that there is a problem regardless of whether or to what extent it is understood. This would then motivate us to look more closely at the nature of that problem, lack, or need so that, as with hunger or thirst, we would be moved to search for the kind of thing that can alone meet that need. We would be moved, therefore, to search for a safe enough non-judgmental social environment in which we can express our own voice, i.e., what we actually think or believe and feel. Within such an environment, akin to standing with another on a mountain trail, we may then undertake an experiential developmental process—a road less travelled, leading toward an ever more comprehensive vision of the truth as worthy of our deepest trust. Indeed, every culture in our history refers to such a process by means of familiar metaphors such as climbing a mountain, swimming toward a beacon of light, or the search for the way out of Plato's Cave. Such a process effectively reverses or counteracts the opposing process of our initially prejudiced moral education. This is the core issue I am claiming underlies spiritual addiction, viz., that we are generally attempting to sit on a fence, holding onto opposing fundamental primary values, as if this could be done without real and indelible moral consequences.

We may now better appreciate Brandon's moral progress despite his symptoms. Despite the appearance of failure in view of behavioral symptoms that include feelings of despair, suicidal ideology, and functional paralysis, he states, "my present concern is how to move forward in life given my growing realization that the prejudices I've imbibed do not align with my current values. It's not that I don't have more prejudices to overcome. I am aware that I am sitting on the fence of indecision, which is increasingly moving me to take to heart my own measure of responsibility. As Walden put it, 'As if you could kill time without injuring eternity.'" He is increasingly realizing, I believe, that there are moral laws, no less than physical and psychological laws, involving real and unavoidable, immediate and indelible moral or spiritual consequences of every moral intention and action, including our attempts to sit on the fence of indecision as alleged "innocent bystanders" (Merton 1966). Similarly to choosing to remain in a toxic marriage, the choice to sit on this fence works to increasingly enslave our will or heart, along with our mind or reason, feelings and actions to that toxic spirit, until we become unwitting accomplices in our own spiritual, psychological, and physical self-annihilation. We are in desperate need of genuine moral guidance.

But where do we find this guidance? To answer this question, perhaps we might consider "when" as opposed to "where". For if the great obstacle in our way of realizing a truly and fully altruistic life revolves around such a relatively prejudicial and complicit form of ignorance, it may no longer be surprising that the primary means by which this ignorance is maintained is by the use of false comparisons, such as the identification of "normal" with "healthy". Within such an unhealthy norm, we tend to compare ourselves with others within the same morally or spiritually diseased condition, which not only blinds us to the reality and danger of such a soul-destroying disease, but in so doing makes us increasingly insensitive to that healthy moral pain of true guilt moving us to search for a viable cure. What we need, therefore, is not to deny, run from, or medicate-away this pain, but to heed what it has to teach us. Instead of comparing ourselves to the worst, or seeming worst, among us to make us feel better by elevating an impoverished self-image, we need to lift rather than lower the moral bar by looking for guidance from the spiritually healthiest or most unconditionally loving in our collective history instead of limiting ourselves to those within our immediate empirical social surround.

5.2. Simplicity of the Law of Moral/Spiritual Personality Change

We have looked at the way a child raised in the healthiest environment would imbibe that spirit of unconditional love and be initially formed in its likeness, just as a child raised in the most malignantly narcissistic environment would imbibe that spirit. Both extreme possibilities, along with the vast moral gray area in between, would all be instances of a single "law of love": that who or what we most love or entrust ourselves to, we become similar to.[45] Despite this initial influence, however, we observed that by virtue of our moral freedom, we can change in any direction. A child raised by the very best of parents can choose to continue on that path or act contrary to that initial influence.[46] By virtue of the same law, even if one's parents and broader social context fall far short of such loving care, insofar as the child is willing and able to search for healthier role models—even in our collective past—that capacity can be nourished. Thus, we observed the potentially life-changing impact on the young[47] of genuinely good teachers, therapists, and leaders, as well as good friends, partners, and groups, whether past or present. Indeed, such a genuinely healthy social support network is rightly considered the cornerstone of psychotherapeutic cure across theory and technique (Sorokin 1954, p. 61ff). But why can we not build such a truly tangible social support network on the foundation of a moral education of humanity itself evolving over time?

5.3. On the Complexity of Personality Change: The Role of Religion

Let us consider Gandhi's criticism of Christian missionaries in India as a relatively recent case to help us distinguish true from false forms of not only moral but more deeply religious claims about reality. Gandhi and others at that time describe how "Christianity" became a stench rather than a rose-like aroma for desperate Hindu and Muslim Indians who felt forced to convert to Christianity in exchange for food and medical care from Christian missionaries (Gandhi 1993, p. 45).[48] But given Gandhi's belief in the equality of all (major) religions, what may seem paradoxical is Gandhi's profound heartfelt connection to the Jesus of the Gospels while remaining a life-long Hindu. Along with Martin Buber's identification with Jesus as his big brother in a common Jewish faith, or the affection for Jesus expressed by the Buddhist master Thich Nhat Hanh in his *Jesus and Buddha as Brothers* (Nhat Hanh 1999), such examples may help us to distinguish our willing faith in the spirit of religion as incarnated in the tangible lives of its most reliable witnesses in our history from religious group self-centered agendas demanding blind faith in their doctrinal claims and ritualistic practices. Specifically, the Christ-like moral character of C. F. Andrews and Gandhi inspired Indian Hindus and Muslims of good faith to follow their moral example without any felt need to convert to any religious group. Properly understood, a Jew such as Martin Buber, a Buddhist such as Thich Nhat Hanh, a Hindu such as M. Gandhi, and an atheist such as Primo Levi might be far more "Christian" in sharing Christ's spirit than the vast majority of professed Christians. In this we may sense the possibility of a transcultural religion of the heart. We will return to this point shortly.

This example may also help us to appreciate Levi's testimony of a process of moral de-evolution opposed to religious claims of a *moral evolution*, or a process of revelation and providential redemption, of humanity. In precisely the same way as deceit, albeit not necessary, is inseparably dependent upon the truth it rejects, so too such a moral de-evolution may be inseparably dependent on a collective moral evolution. In other words, this morally devolving process may not be rooted in this or that particular religious tradition, but in a form of generic religious prejudice that atheists as outsiders may be all the more capable of recognizing.[49] However, this implies nothing about the character of the most reliable religious witnesses in our history, e.g., an Abraham or Moses, Socrates, Buddha, or Jesus whom we might well imagine getting along fabulously not only with one another, but with atheists such as Levi and Amery, in a way that the majority of their professed followers could not. In short, regardless of our identification as atheists or theists, we may be unable to see the wheat because of the weeds.

Such a generic form of religious prejudice may not only erect the greatest barrier to seeing what the most reliable spiritual witnesses in our history share, but also blind us to the tangible reality of this collective moral evolution or progressive revelation and process of human redemption underlying a true sense of hope. We may understand why this collective moral problem is a religious problem in view of the role religion has historically played in transmitting or obstructing the revelation of moral truth. It strikes at the very heart of our deepest moral commitments. Therein lies its power. For, in reaction to this pervasive religious dogmatism or prejudice, our contemporary naturalistic or anti-supernatural attitude may be throwing the baby away with the bathwater. In short, I am claiming that spiritual addiction is not only a response to a collective moral problem, but more deeply a religious problem, because of the way spiritually emptied forms of religion conceal the testimony of its most reliable witnesses. They do not support moral character as the one and only mark of a genuine spiritual life for atheists and theists alike. But how can such religious prejudice be overcome insofar as professed believers are unwilling to humbly acknowledge their infidelity to their own teachers and teachings? How can it be overcome unless we are willing to seek the spirit of truth and unconditional love above any form of religious, anti-religious, or group identification?

5.4. Good Parent Syndrome

More subtle even than this conflict between the "spirit" and the "form" within religion is the way the same problem of systems of pathological accommodation may infect any new form of revealed truth. Thus, the spirit of science becomes conflated with just a new formalism. Science becomes the new religion and scientists the new priests or apologists for the new faith now claiming absolute authority to know the truth. In other words, despite the collective nature of a problem including all of us, it especially revolves around those in the highest positions of power responsible for our education today. Indeed, the relatively good qualities of our parents, teachers, and leaders within such a vast polluted moral gray area all the more tempts us in our need for guidance to close our eyes to their real shortcomings as if to dare compare them to a higher moral standard was akin to an act of betrayal.

To repeat: I am not claiming that there are no real and significant moral distinctions to be drawn within the normal condition of our world. But how can we clearly draw such distinctions insofar as we continue to choose to remain in the haze of the norm of this vast moral gray area in which we now live? How can we see that fullness of light that alone reveals the way to a true hope if we refuse to allow that same light expose the barriers to that way? If we, together with Levi, have dared to awaken so far as to see that there is no specifically moral difference in the lives of modern-day professed atheists and theists,[50] then it may not be surprising that we would all be tempted to lose faith and hope in any true providential revelation, calling out to and within each and all of us to collaborate with it for the sake of the redemption of us all.

From this perspective, the suicides of the most reliable atheist witnesses of the Holocaust, such as Primo Levi (1986), Jean Amery (1980), and Paul Celan, may appear less, if at all, as an intrapsychic problem with them (as if their testimony about humanity was warped by the extremity of their traumatic experiences) than a problem with our unwillingness to embrace their good faith. I will return to this point in a moment. However, for now, I must point out that even in the case of these witnesses we must distinguish what they see, and thus bear witness to, from what they are merely tempted to believe. They see and bear witness to our continued collective complicity in denial and the present and impending consequences of that denial. They are merely tempted to believe that this denial signifies that we are past the tipping point for hope.

Yet, unlike the atheist Four Horsemen, even they concede that this is not an indictment of reality, truth, or true goodness—nor even an indictment of any possible God or "spiritual higher power" at its core whom they do not see and thus cannot bear witness to. It is an indictment of us all, including themselves. However, it is even more an indictment of what is called religion today, for they see no such morally healthy "social support network" in the lives of contemporary believers or non-believers. The one and only mark of any true religion of the heart is that support network: the incarnation of unconditional love in our lives. In "Christian" terms, they have not rejected any "living gospel" that they have allegedly "heard" because it is practically nowhere to be seen or found. Indeed, as paradoxical as it may sound, the good faith of these atheist witnesses may be all the more manifest in their suicide, i.e., a form of despair arising from their unwillingness to live in a world in moral denial, actively working to quench the spirit of love in their and our hearts.

The practical implications are radical: on the one hand, the existence of a single such atheist witness, having the moral character and insight of a Primo Levi, powerfully indicts the character of the "faith" of the majority of believers today. For would such a witness not embrace a life devoted to truth and unconditional love if he truly saw it tangibly manifested in even a single case? On the other hand, if there is such a hope for humanity and if that hope is most fully revealed in the lives and testimony of the most unconditionally loving and reliable religious witnesses in our history, then how can we enter into such a life unless all of us—professed believers especially—humbly acknowledge that they and we have been tried and found wanting?

What I am calling "good parent syndrome", therefore, is not only rooted in the need for such a collective confession. It is not specific to parents, but more broadly refers to anyone in the highest positions of authority or power,[51] having the responsibility to educate or guide the rest of us. This is where confession is most needed; if they profess to have a form of integrity and power they lack, they tempt those they are called to serve to doubt the reality and realizability of the real thing. That is, they tempt their followers to doubt not only them, but all authority, including the authority of the spirit of truth itself manifested in the lives of its most reliable witnesses in our history. This was the lesson that Brandon's therapist took to heart from his own failure.

Let us apply Brandon's question to each and all of us, "To what extent is my problem a problem of will or ability? Is it a problem with my unwillingness to do what I know to be right? Or is it a problem with my inability to live the kind of life I know I should because of some form and measure of real ignorance? Is it primarily a problem with me or, rather, with my dependence on this or that group within a prison-like world demanding blind compliance to its will? What I am now willing and able to do about it"?

As I have tried to elucidate, this problem revolves around our will in relation to our awareness of a reality greater than ourselves. It involves our willingness to engage in an experiential process, such as climbing a mountain, of moving from (lower) forms of faith to (higher) forms of faith by (means of increasing) rational insight. If we, as with Levi and Amery, believe that there is no true hope, we cannot but act upon that belief and, in so doing, feed that despair in a way that enables it to evolve into ever more subtle and malignant forms infecting everything we will, think, feel and do on a level deeper than we can consciously or immediately control. We cannot simply will into being faith and hope in a supreme value that we secretly doubt or mistrust. This brings us back to another question we applied to Brandon at the start: what does "holding the hope" for a patient mean other than an actual ability to see a real hope for the patient which the patient cannot yet see or fully grasp for himself? As long as the patient cannot see (in contrast to being unwilling to see) any such faith and hope as he looks into the eyes of his therapist, he may be further tempted to believe that there is no such hope, which undermines his motive to even examine whether that belief is true.

In this sense, the main barrier to healing our collective spiritual addiction—both on an individual and collective scale—is not the worst individuals and groups among us, but the best. Relative to an unhealthy or morally compromised norm, the best among us may well be far more aware than most of us, but relative to a morally healthy norm, they may literally be worlds apart. As with the "priests" in every age who attempt to usurp the true ministry of the spirit, our present-day priests (parents, teachers, therapists, group leaders, or scientists) may rightly fear the consequences of acknowledging their true condition. They might lose their following, and others might use that confession to promote themselves. But perhaps that is the price we must pay, or the cross we must bear, for any of us to presume to take on that power and its responsibility. Additionally, insofar as we dare to do so, it might even inspire others to do the same. It might even go so far as to motivate an historically unprecedented collective confession or cry from the heart, in spirit and in truth, that can avert the gravest danger we have ever faced.

6. Conclusions

In this paper, I have described spiritual addiction as a felt compulsion to seek surrogates in the absence of that spirit of unconditional love underlying core personality change. I described our awakening to the real world as akin to a prison in which all sides seem morally compromised, so any choice seems to necessitate the sacrifice of our conscientious relationship with the truth. Thus, I argued, spiritual addiction underlies not only physical and psychological addictions but also socially accepted "addictions" to all that we associate with success. It strikes at the heart of our most cherished value priorities including what we call morality and religion. All that we seek may be grounded in collectively imbibed prejudice toward truth itself compromising our very selves and all our relationships to one another.

I used the case of Brandon to illustrate that at the root of this problem is not merely the fact of such an imbibed prejudice but our collective unwillingness to acknowledge it, and the seriousness of the consequences of that denial. I argued that as long as we continue in this denial, this will only allow the disease to continue on its deadly course. I claimed that the relative lack of individuals and groups in our world today living a truly conscientious, altruistic unconditionally loving kind of life tempts us to doubt the reality and/or realizability of such a life. Stronger still, we are tempted to project this problem with humanity onto reality itself as if this spirit of selfish, cold indifference is rooted in the essence of being human, woven into the very fabric of reality itself, as well as any possible "god" it its core. This, I claimed, lies at the root of our spiritual addiction. Similarly to Brandon, we are all suffering from a form of existential anxiety in fear that there are no true grounds for hope. Additionally, insofar as we merely believe it, we feel it, along with our felt powerlessness to overcome it, which moves us to seek relief by embracing one surrogate or another. We feel angry at forces within us and outside us that we do not understand. We feel hopeless, as if we are unable to truly and substantially change.

Toward finding a way out of this prison, I claimed that insofar as we are willing to acknowledge our desperate condition, the same light that exposes this condition also powerfully moves us to search for a way to overcome it. Denial and despair are not our only options. As we open our eyes akin to children with a beginner's mind, we enter into a step-by-step experiential process that can enable us to see with increasing clarity that none of us can avoid a faith commitment, along with the lawful consequences of that choice. We must and invariably will choose who or what we will most trust and, depending on the kind of spirit we choose to embrace, will determine what we will become. In this sense, not only can no one avoid a faith commitment, but no one can avoid faith in some kind of "god" or primary value. The only practical question is what type of "god" we will place our faith in—a god defined by truth and unconditional love or a displacement, surrogate, or idol.

This, I claimed, is the problem underlying Brandon's many addictions. Although he suffered from depression and anxiety even as a child, it did not come to a head until he had within his reach those primary values our society holds before us as practically the necessary and sufficient conditions for a "good life". In Brandon's case, it took the form of him becoming the youngest producer in the history of his company and having the realistic prospect of making more than enough money to provide not only for all his so-called basic needs, but all his material desires as well. Yet, for the sake of this worldly success, he would have to subjugate himself even more than he already had to a toxic work environment. He felt dependent on that job, as he once did his parents, as if it were the one and only means to "live the dream" or realize his hope of creating something of value with his life. Yet, the spiritual toxicity of that environment little-by-little, day in and day out, chipped away at that dream in a way he could foresee would finally result in the loss of his true sense of self and self-worth.

But that is not all, nor is it the worst of it. What he had discovered in his workplace, he was also discovering in every other form of relationship in his life. No longer was the problem merely the shortcomings of his parents or his present work environment, but a toxicity infecting the marriages and families, friendships, communities, and workplaces he saw all around him. Everywhere he looked he saw what the poet, Jones Very, called "The Dead"—one and the same tyrannical spirit demanding we choose a side within a prison-like world in which all sides are compromised. He felt he could find no individuals, much less a spiritual community of individuals, that might constitute for him a truly safe and unconditionally loving relational home (Stolorow 2011). He thought that he and we were all locked within a so-called "real" world governed by immoral and thus irrational forces, where the only law is the blind lust for power to be on top. By means of Brandon's case, we considered the practical implications of such a collectively unmet spiritual need and why the moral weakness or powerlessness at issue runs far deeper than one's individual willpower.

We then journeyed beyond this sketch of such a collective spiritual addiction by painting in broad strokes the way to overcome it. We realized there are necessary implications for change grounded in our willingness to acknowledge rather than deny this addiction. We can see that the relative lack of individuals and groups today capable of bearing witness to such an unconditionally loving life does not imply, nor is it experientially a fact, that there are no such examples permeating our collective history up to the present day. Thus, in precisely the same way that we can and do find tangible role models for any other goal-oriented behavior by means of their words in books or even a podcast, the same applies to moral and spiritual guidance. Given the unprecedented growth of our technology, we have all been brought together as we never have or could before. We now have tangible access to the most reliable spiritual witnesses in every culture in our history. If we choose to undertake such a spiritual journey, guided by such witnesses, we will increasingly be enabled to not only overcome our prejudices, but in so doing increasingly internalize the same kind of intimate connection they had with that voice or spirit of truth and love. Importantly, however, despite the real instrumental or mediatorial value of these historical witnesses, their job description is not to have us place our faith blindly in them—nor even in any one of them as the very best—but to help us see for ourselves that the same spirit of truth and love that was so fully incarnated in and through them is right now striving to reveal itself in and to and through us all. Even that spirit's exposure or indictment of our present condition is not motivated by wrath but by love. Additionally, because it is love, it cannot compel us without violating who and what we are. Such a love can only entreat us to avoid the necessary consequences of our own bad faith by calling us to lay aside our differences as atheists and theists, Jews and Christians, in a collaborative search for that light and power of love that can transform us all.

To apply this more directly to Brandon's case, let us recall his conflict with his therapist. We may now appreciate the sense in which the problem there was not merely his therapist's momentary lack of empathic attunement. Nor was it resolved by his therapist's willingness to merely acknowledge it. Rather, it forced his therapist to acknowledge the compromised condition of his own heart and the extent to which he was and is responsible to do all he can on his part to retain his moment-by-moment connection to that spirit of truth and unconditional love that is life. How else was he to truly "hold the hope" for Brandon, his patient?

He realized that there is no psychological "treatment" that can heal our spiritual addiction. We are not thing-like objects to be "fixed" through any such impersonal means. As a hundred years of psychological efficacy research has come to realize,[52] we cannot separate any technique (including religious ritualistic practices or universal spiritual disciplines) from the intention or motive of those using it, nor, therefore, from that intimacy of interpersonal connection in which alone lies the "one thing necessary" for any genuine cure. The treatment "tool" is you and me. It does not require that we become "great" thinkers or philosophers, medical doctors or psychologists, scientists or priests. Indeed, if this drive for greatness is our primary motivation, it only feeds that hubris that distances us from that genuine humility which is the necessary condition for our access to a love greater than ourselves. This goodness is what Brandon said has kept him alive despite his darkest moments of despair. He believes in the reality and power of love. He has seen it, felt its presence, heard its call. Even now it is calling out to him and us despite our suffering, as if that suffering was uniting us to wounded others and them to us in the realization that none of us can undertake this journey alone. Perhaps we are all children; all climbing a mountain that at its peak may only reveal one new horizon after another beyond our ability to fathom.

> "I will remind you of an innocent and ancient story, of a king and his new clothes . . . Tailors deceived a king, telling them they would weave him a wonderful suit which would be invisible to any but good men . . . In the end the naked king paraded out into the street where all the people were gathered to admire his suit of clothes, and all did admire it until a child dared to point out that the king was naked . . . Have you and I forgotten that our vocation, as innocent bystanders—and the very condition of our terrible innocence—is to do what the child did, and keep on saying the king is naked, at the cost of being condemned criminals? Remember . . . if the child had not been there, they would all have been madmen, or criminals. It was the child's cry that saved them." (Merton 1966)

Funding: This research received no external funding.

Institutional Review Board Statement: Not applicable.

Informed Consent Statement: Written informed consent has been obtained from the patient(s) to publish this paper.

Data Availability Statement: Not applicable.

Conflicts of Interest: The author declares no conflict of interest.

Notes

[1] I define "witness" as one marked by both their authenticity or conscientious devotion to the truth and their relative fullness of experiential insight.

[2] It is worth pointing out that despite the popular appeal to "faith vs. reason", no one can avoid faith commitments, as without them our beliefs could not be subjected to a process of experiential verification and thus serve as true premises in sound arguments leading to an advance in our discovery of truth. This is different from blind and/or bad faith, implying either unexamined prejudices and/or an unwillingness to subject our prejudices to rational verification.

[3] This should not be taken to mean an exact 50/50 split, but anywhere in between the two sides. However, I am not suggesting that there are no cases of perpetrators and innocent victims.

[4] The humanist psychologist Rogers (1961) presents these qualities as the mark not only of the ideal psychotherapist, but also as qualities defining what it means to become a person in the fullest sense of the word.

[5] An expression often used by Dallas Willard.

[6] Rogers was one of the founders of humanistic or person-centered psychotherapy; Plato (or Socrates), along with Aristotle, the founders of Western philosophy; Freud, the founder of classical psychoanalysis; Frankl, the founder of logotherapy; and Sorokin, the founder of modern sociology.

[7] Although I generally use "moral" and "spiritual" interchangeably, I define spiritual as disembodied personal power, which is not opposed to it being tangibly embodied in the lives of both individuals and groups. I have in mind primarily the spirit of a person as the life of a person which is more than one's body. It is that which most defines what it means to be a person in the fullest, most evolved, or actualized sense. It refers to the essence or nature of being human, which includes above all a capacity for moral freedom, i.e., to know and embrace (as well as willingly reject) truth and true goodness. I am defining *morality* as the fruit or manifestation of this spirit in and through human intentions and actions in relation to a subjectively and objectively perceived reality of moral values. Given this freedom and these values, an actualized spiritual and moral life manifests itself in terms of

8   *moral character*, i.e., a *will* sufficiently guided or conscientiously governed by its fidelity to truth and what is truly good that it permeates all one thinks, feels, and does as it extends beyond one's self to influence all reality.

9   In way of example, consider the position of "The Four Horsemen" (Hitchens et al. 2019).

10 Parents commonly acknowledge some difference between what they call the world of children and the "real" world. In the former, they generally have in mind a world in which goodness reigns and anything seems possible—a world of fantasy conveyed in the story books we read to them and the movies we watch with them. By the latter, they generally have in mind a world permeated by selfish cold indifference, i.e., a ruthless, unscrupulous world, akin to a prison, in which we must sacrifice conscience to survive if not thrive.

11 My aim in using this case is to direct the reader's attention less to the characteristics that define his subjective experience than to those attributes of his experience actually or potentially shared with others—especially value qualities such as authenticity, empathy, and unconditional love. My aim is to bring these latter qualities to the foreground of our investigation to enable the reader to see for themselves whether and to what extent those features are, or potentially may be, embedded in their own "lived experience". These "empirically", i.e., experientially, verified value data provide, I claim, the necessary ground for any sound theory of addiction.

12 A period that began shortly before the COVID-19 pandemic.

13 Although when asked about the days, weeks, and months of such experiences of hope, he *intellectually* acknowledges those times, but says they generally seem so experientially distant it is as if they were little more than dreams.

14 He is currently smoking at least 10 cigarettes per day.

15 He managed to throw the rest away.

16 I remember putting my son on a block wall in our backyard and standing a foot or so away asking him to jump into my arms. And he did. I stood a step further away and asked him to jump again. And he did. But there was a point at which he could not jump, despite the fact that I knew I could catch him. It was beyond his present ability to trust that I could. An ability that could only be realized as he increasingly discovered he could trust me to that extent. Such examples, as we shall see, reveal an experiential process of moving from "faith to faith" by a rational form of experiential insight. That is, from lower forms of faith to higher forms by means of a fuller, more comprehensive awareness of reality or truth.

17 As we shall also see, moral power is distinctly different in kind from, e.g., physical, psychological, and social or political forms of power.

18 As we shall also see, such a "spiritual" appeal is not necessarily reducible to a "religious" appeal. See, for example, the atheist, Sam Harris' reference to such self-transcending experiences (Hitchens et al. 2019, pp. 48–49; Dennett, p. 51).

19 By this I mean that AA, or any other moral, religious, or spiritual approach, may itself be subject to its own forms of prejudice. It is true that the founders of AA, despite writing for a primarily Christian audience, were aware of the difficulty bound up with their appeal to a "higher power". It is also true that AA has evolved to include atheist, agnostic and non-Christian groups, allowing for broader interpretations of such a higher power. But such groups may still fall far short of providing sufficient access to that spirit of truth that alone provides the requisite power to overcome our suffering.

20 To avoid misinterpretation, I am not denying forms of pathological altruism. I am pointing to the sense in which the pervasive lack of healthy altruism or unconditional love, may tempt us to doubt its accessibility and realizability as the primary value of human life. Aristotle's, *Nicomachean Ethics*, for example, was an attempt to relativize an ethical life for most of us in view of the fact that even Socrates fell short of such a Good. It was not an attempt to deny its value insofar as it could be achieved. The same holds true for the history of Christianity, in which the majority of Christian denominations reacted to precisely this striving after "perfect love" as heretical (see, for example, references to the early Friends or Quakers). In a nutshell, how many of us can say with any genuine authority that we are truly and primarily oriented toward realizing, much less governed in all we think, plan, and do, by our love for truth and goodness? Yet, is that not the foundation upon which all religions purport to stand?

21 For a more in-depth look at this, see Willard (2018) and Wyner (1988).

22 As we shall see, Dodes' calls into question such a disease model, whether presented on scientific grounds or AA, in favor of an alternative account amenable to psychological moderation.

23 The point here is not whether there are, or may be, forms of reciprocal causality, i.e., behavior causing neurochemical and neuroanatomical changes which then causally influence behavior. It is the problem of limiting, reducing, or even emphasizing biological causes over psychological and, as we shall see, moral and spiritual causes.

24 Studies demonstrating that even with rats addiction is far more complex than appeals to biological causes alone.

25 Alternatively, one might interpret this "response" as an equally extreme prejudicial reaction to religious forms of prejudice.

26 Although I am not claiming that understanding the role the brain plays in addiction is not "useful" for understanding how addiction works, is the claim above that the ordinary person cannot understand the cause of their addictions and a way to overcome them without them understanding how their brains work? Does that mean that only "someday" (given such adequate understanding) will we have sufficient knowledge to heal our addictions? Moreover, are the only relevant factors here physical and psychological? In psychotherapy, for example, we may observe how different orientations focus on different aspects of a

26 Experienced peripherally in the act and moving into the foreground afterwards.

27 I realize that looking at AA through the lens of Dodes' criticism of AA potentially carries with it any misinterpretations he has about AA's actual theories. However, although my intention is not to misinterpret AA or Dodes' position (or interpretations of AA), I am not primarily concerned with either position. Rather, my concern is with a far broader or more generic problem.

28 Prejudice is not limited to its more obvious forms. Just as "experts" may be tempted to conflate (and, thereby, misrepresent) current forms of cognitive-behavioral-therapy or contemporary relational psychonalysis with their original classical forms, so too may one do the same with AA. Dodes, for example, seems to limit his attention to a more popular and narrow religious/Christian form of interpretation of AA tenets without acknowledging even the possibility of other, more rational, interpretations. More significantly, however, is his seeming use of such myths to reject any form of religious and moral basis for addiction.

29 Although "addict" is an objectifying term in contrast to "one suffering from an addiction", for simplicity's sake I will often use the former.

30 See, for example, Alloy and Abramson (1979) on "depressed realism".

31 As pointed out in the introduction, I can appreciate the offense taken by atheists to any reference to "religious witnesses", just as I can appreciate the offense taken by theists to "atheist witnesses". However, I would ask those on both sides to recall my definition of a reliable witness in terms of sincerity and insight and recognize these are attributes both sides can lay claim to. What marks such witnesses is precisely their tendency to embrace the spirit of religion above blind faith in any dogma and ritualistic practices.

32 This reality includes the nature and knowledge of numbers and numerical relations; logical propositions and logical relations; aesthetic and moral values; the nature of persons including the self, mind, our ideas and their lawful relationships; and so on.

33 As inconsistent as "unconscious thoughts" or "unconscious forms of consciousness" are or appear, we generally distinguish forms of consciousness or awareness of objects in the forefront of our minds from our awareness of objects in the periphery or background of our minds. One can be aware that one is breathing without focusing on or being mindful of one's breath. For a more in-depth look at how complex this issue tends to be, see Ellenberger (1970). With respect to these various layers of awareness, see also Assagioli (1965).

34 This is what we take Husserl to mean by phenomenology as a "presuppositionless philosophy": not an idealized assumption of us being able to undertake a phenomenological investigation from a position without presuppositions, but an ethical attitude or orientation willing to subject any and all presuppositions to an intersubjective rigorous evaluation of their truth.

35 See Wyner (1988) for an in-depth look at this issue.

36 I am claiming that there is a distinction between judgments and a judgmental attitude. No one should, can, or does avoid judgments, since that is how we distinguish one thing from another, but a judgmental or fault-seeking attitude should and can be avoided.

37 I should point out that every culture appeals to some doctrine of "original sin". My approach differs in its appeal to, or emphasis on, our own experience as the basis for any sound doctrine of this origin, rather than taking for granted, or exercising blind faith in, any particular religious theory and its traditionally accepted assumptions. This includes assumptions about a "phenomenological" approach. As I see it, the value of Husserl's "realist" vs. the generally accepted "idealist" approach is precisely its appeal to the use of experiential knowledge in its evaluation of the nature of knowledge itself.

38 Both specific and generic in the sense that the specific tangible character of the parent is experienced along with the generic character of that unconditional love that may tangibly manifested by others as well.

39 If it is not already clear, my general use of the male gender pronoun is not intended to reflect a male bias. It merely seemed to me more consistent or less confusing given the primacy placed on Brandon's case. In this regard, I do not attribute to a "God" male gender and in such contexts often use the female gender despite the conviction that "God" would include and transcend such gender limitations.

40 As per my previous claim, by "reason" here I have in view the kind of abstract reason Hume refers to when he claims "reason is the slave of the passions" (Wyner 1988).

41 See Maslow and Frankl's correspondence leading to the former's realization that without a self-transcendent good there can be no self-actualization.

42 As a psychologist patient once put it, "If my mother didn't hold me, kiss me, and tell me that she loved me, who is now going to do that in my life?".

43 I suggest that if one looks closely enough at the actual descriptions of *reality*—not just *humanity* in its present contingent state—by many "existentialist" philosophers one may observe no mere reference to any value-neutral "meaninglessness" but precisely a *cold* indifference, i.e., an *opposition* to true goodness. Note, for example, Sartre's description of reality in his *Nausea* (Sartre 1964). "Had I dreamed of this enormous presence?... all soft, sticky, soiling everything ... I hated this ignoble mess ... spilling over, filling everything with its gelatinous slither ... I knew it was the World, the naked World suddenly revealing itself, and I choked with rage at this gross, absurd being ... I shouted "filth! what rotten filth!" and shook myself to get rid of this sticky filth ... I had already detected everywhere a sort of conspiratioral air ... it was there, waiting, looking at one ... I had learned all I could know about existence" (pp. 134–35).

44 As previously mentioned, Brandchaft et al. (2010) uses the expression "pathological accommodation" to refer to instances such as this in which a child feels forced to subordinate his own *emerging* experiential sense of what is true, right, and good (i.e., his own voice or true sense of self) for the sake of retaining needed relational ties. See also Winnicott's (1965) appeal to a false vs. true self. New Testament authors refer to the contrast between the "carnal mind" and the "mind of the spirit".

45 This is evident in the way an adopted child, over time, tends to take on characterological qualities of his non-biological parents in the same way as the biological children. As previously described, how the child initially sees and values reality and himself primarily depends upon this parent–child relationship, regardless of any inherited biological characteristics.

46 With respect to this original relational inheritance, I am not claiming that we can erase or in that sense "cure" any form of trauma, much less severe relational trauma. I am, however, claiming we have the capacity to transcend this relational trauma. There is a form and degree of moral goodness that has sufficient power to enable us to transcend not only physical and psychological but even moral trauma. Insofar as one's capacity for moral growth is not entirely lost, one has some form and measure of access to this primary value underlying real and substantial moral and spiritual transformation.

47 To be clear, I am not at all suggesting that substantial personality change is limited to the young. I merely have in mind the way the young are initially more open to such change whereas insofar as we are increasingly subjected to prejudicial conformity with the world, we may be tempted to doubt this possibility.

48 Gandhi contrasts this predominant empty form of Christian *profession* with a "truly" spiritual Christianity incarnated in the life of his dear friend C. F. Andrews (Gandhi 1993; Gandhi and Andrews 1989) and other friends such as Jones (1976, p. 44): "The decision of the Mahatma not to be a Christian was arrived at in South Africa ... How could he really see Christ through all this racism? He did see Christ in C.F. Andrews ... this racism was often very deeply religious and held to in the name of religion ... his (Christ's) followers made him the sponsor of white rule and white ascendancy. How could Gandhi see Christ through that?" In Gandhi's words, "The church did not make a favorable impression on me ... They were not an assembly of devout souls ... going to church for recreation and in conformity to custom ... I soon gave up attending the service" (ibid., p. 45). From a Sikh perspective, see (Andrews 1934, p. 35): "Neither would he (Sadhu) separate either Hinduism or the Sikh religion by hard and fast lines from the Christian Faith. They were woven out of one texture by the Divine Spirit, and they needed to be interwoven again into one perfect fabric".

49 As in the case of the atheist Four Horsemen.

50 For a more in-depth look at the difference between *moral* and mere *social* power, see Wyner (2012).

51 For we wrestle not against flesh and blood, but against principalities, against powers, against the rulers of the darkness of this world, against spiritual wickedness in high places (Ephesians 6:12).

52 We must acknowledge that for more than 100 years we have focused on the wrong factors in psychotherapy ... we must teach students how to create a caring therapeutic environment that emphasizes the personal and interpersonal dimensions of therapy ... The aim would be to cultivate the trainee's capacity to connect with clients at a profound level so that clients feel deeply accepted, supported, and understood (Elkins 2015, p. 414).

References

Alloy, Lauren B., and Lyn Y. Abramson. 1979. Judgment of contingency in depressed and nondepressed students: Sadder but wiser? *Journal of Experimental Psychology: General* 108: 441–85. [CrossRef]

Amery, Jean. 1980. *At the Mind's Limits: Contemplations by a Survivor on Auschwitz and Its Realities*. Translated by Sidney Rosenfeld, and Stella P. Rosenfeld. Bloomington: Indiana University Press.

Andrews, Charles F. 1934. *Sadhu Sundar Singh: A Personal Memoir*. New York: Harper & Brothers Publishers.

Aristotle. 1962. *Nicomachean Ethics*. Translated by Martin Ostwald. New York: The Bobbs-Merrill Company, Inc.

Assagioli, Roberto. 1965. *Psychosynthesis: A Manual of Principles and Techniques*. New York: Hobbs.

Brandchaft, Bernard, Shelley Doctor, and Dorienne Sorter. 2010. *Toward an Emancipatory Psychoanalysis: Brandchaft's Intersubjective Vision*. New York: Routledge.

Buber, Martin. 1958. *Hasidism and Modern Man*. Translated and Edited by Maurice S. Friedman. New York: Horizon Press.

Buber, Martin. 1970. *I and Thou*. Translated by Walter Kaufmann. New York: Charles Scribner's Sons.

Dodes, Lance. M. 2002. *The Heart of Addiction*. New York: Harper Collins.

Elkins, David. 2015. Toward a common focus in psychotherapy research. In *The Handbook of Humanistic Psychology: Theory, Research, and Practice*, 2nd ed. Edited by Kirk Schneider, J. Fraser Pierson and James Bugental. Thousand Oaks: Sage Publications.

Ellenberger, Henri F. 1970. *The Discovery of the Unconscious: The History and Evolution of Dynamic Psychiatry*. New York: Basic Books, Inc.

Gandhi, Mohandes, and Charles F. Andrews. 1989. *Gandhi and Charlie: The Story of a Friendship. As Told through the Letters and Writings of Mohandes K. Gandhi and the Rev'd Charles Freer Andrews*. Edited by David McI Gracie. Cambridge: Cowley Publications.

Gandhi, Mohandes. 1993. *Gandhi on Christianity*. Edited by Robert Ellsberg. Maryknoll: Orbis Books.

Heilig, Markus, James MacKillop, Diana Martinez, Jürgen Rehm, Lorenzo Leggio, and Louk J. M. J. Vanderschuren. 2021. Addiction as a brain disease revised: Why it still matters, and the need for consilience. *Neuropsychopharmacology* 46: 1715–23. [CrossRef] [PubMed]

Hitchens, Christopher, Richard Dawkins, Sam Harris, and Daniel Dennett. 2019. *The Four Horsemaen: The Conversation that Sparked an Atheist Revolution*. New York: Random House.

Jones, E. Stanley. 1976. *Gandhi: Portrait of a Friend*. Nashville: Abingdon Press.
Levi, Primo. 1986. *The Drowned and the Saved*. Translated by Raymond Rosenthal. New York: Summit Books.
Merton, Thomas. 1966. Letter to an innocent bystander. In *Raids on the Unspeakable*. New York: New Directions.
Nhat Hanh, Thich. 1999. *Going Home: Jesus and Buddha as Brothers*. New York: Riverhead Books.
Oakley, Barbara, Ariel Knafo, Guruprasad Madhavan, and David S. Wilson, eds. 2012. *Pathological Altruism*. Oxford: Oxford University Press.
Peele, Stanton, and Bruce Alexander. 1998. Theories of addiction. In *The Meaning of Addiction: An Unconventional View*. Edited by Stanton Peele. San Francisco: Jossey-Bass.
Rogers, Carl. 1961. *On Becoming a Person: A Therapist's View of Psychotherapy*. Boston: Houghton Mifflin Company.
Sartre, Jean Paul. 1964. *Nausea*. Translated by Lloyd Alexander. New York: New Directions Publishing Corporation.
Sorokin, Pitirim A. 1954. *The Ways and Power of Love: Types, Factors, and Techniques of Moral Transformation*. Boston: Beacon Press.
Stolorow, Robert D. 2011. *World, Affectivity, Trauma: Heidegger and Post-Cartesian Psychoanalysis*. New York: Routledge.
Willard, Dallas. 2018. *The Disappearance of Moral Knowledge*. Edited by Steven Porter, Aaron Preston and Gregg A. Ten Elshof. New York: Routledge.
Winnicott, Donald W. 1965. *The Maturational Processes and the Facilitating Environment: Studies in the Theory of Emotional Development*. London: Karnac Books.
Wyner, Gary. 1988. Toward a Phenomenology of Conscientious Action and a Theory of the Practicality of Reason. Ph.D. thesis, University of Southern California, Los Angeles, CA, USA.
Wyner, Garret. 2012. *The Wounded Healer: Finding Meaning in Suffering*. Santa Barbara: Antioch University.

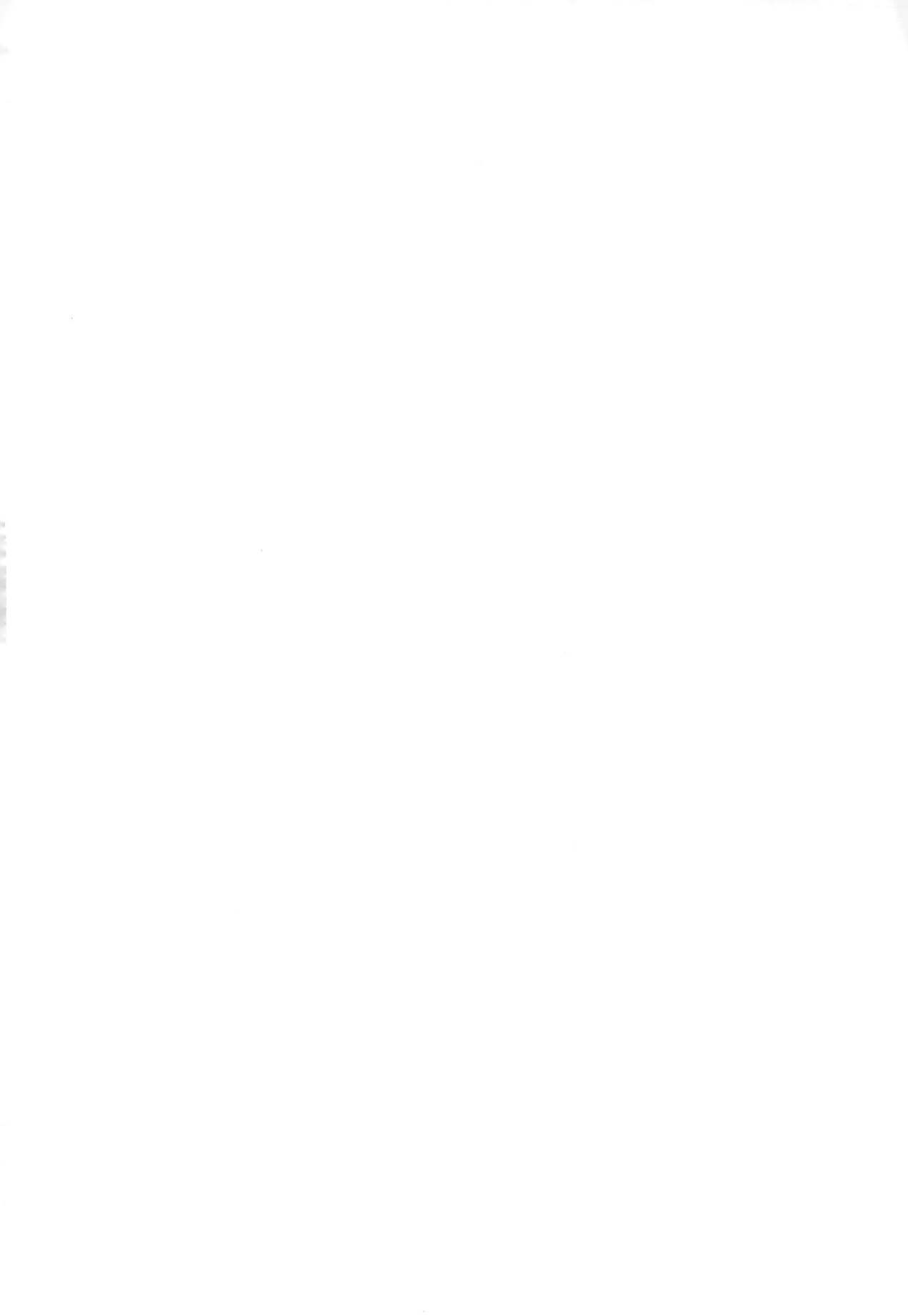

MDPI
St. Alban-Anlage 66
4052 Basel
Switzerland
Tel. +41 61 683 77 34
Fax +41 61 302 89 18
www.mdpi.com

Religions Editorial Office
E-mail: religions@mdpi.com
www.mdpi.com/journal/religions

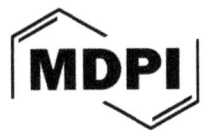

www.ingramcontent.com/pod-product-compliance
Lightning Source LLC
LaVergne TN
LVHW070657100526
838202LV00013B/985